T0205656

SPECIFIC GENE EXPRESSION AND EPIGENETICS
AND EPIGENETICS
THE INTERPLAY BETWEEN THE GENOME AND ITS ENVIRONMENT

SPECIFIC GENE EXPRESSION AND EPIGENETICS
THE INTERPLAY BETWEEN THE GENOME AND ITS ENVIRONMENT

Edited by
Kasirajan Ayyanathan, PhD

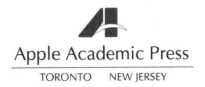

Apple Academic Press

TORONTO   NEW JERSEY

Apple Academic Press Inc. | Apple Academic Press Inc.
3333 Mistwell Crescent | 9 Spinnaker Way
Oakville, ON L6L 0A2 | Waretown, NJ 08758
Canada | USA

©2014 by Apple Academic Press, Inc.

First issued in paperback 2021

Exclusive worldwide distribution by CRC Press, a member of Taylor & Francis Group
No claim to original U.S. Government works

ISBN 13: 978-1-77463-352-6 (pbk)
ISBN 13: 978-1-77188-036-7 (hbk)

Library of Congress Control Number: 2014932131

Library and Archives Canada Cataloguing in Publication

Specific gene expression and epigenetics: the interplay between the genome and its environment/edited by Kasirajan Ayyanathan, PhD.

Includes bibliographical references and index.
ISBN 978-1-77188-036-7 (bound)
1. Gene expression. 2. Epigenetics. 3. Genomes. 4. DNA--Methylation.
5. Eukaryotic cells. 6. Genomics. 7. Mental illness--Genetic aspects.
I. Ayyanathan, Kasirajan, editor of compilation

QH450.S64 2014   572.8'65   C2014-900801-5

Apple Academic Press also publishes its books in a variety of electronic formats. Some content that appears in print may not be available in electronic format. For information about Apple Academic Press products, visit our website at **www.appleacademicpress.com** and the CRC Press website at **www.crcpress.com**

ABOUT THE EDITOR

KASIRAJAN AYYANATHAN, PhD

Kasirajan Ayyanathan, PhD, received his PhD degree from the Department of Biochemistry, Indian Institute of Science, one of the premier research institutions in India. Subsequently, at Temple University School of Medicine, Philadelphia, Pennsylvania, USA, he conducted post-doctoral research on the signal transduction by purinergic receptors, a class of G-Protein Coupled Receptors (GPCR), in erythroleukemia cancer cells. Next, he was trained as a staff scientist at the Wistar Institute, Philadelphia, for almost ten years and studied transcription regulation, chromatin, and epigenetic regulatory mechanisms in cancer before becoming an Associate Professor at Florida Atlantic University (FAU). Currently, he is at the Center for Molecular Biology and Biotechnology as a Research Associate Professor at FAU.

He is the recipient of Chern Memorial Award, presented by the Wistar Institute, and Howard Temin Career Research Award, presented by the National Cancer Institute, USA. Dr. Ayyanathan is well trained in molecular biology, cell biology, and biochemistry with main focus on studying transcription factors and gene regulation. He has contributed to several projects such as on the generation of conditional transcriptional repressors that are directed against the endogenous oncogenes to inhibit malignant growth, on the establishment of stable cell lines that express chromatin integrated transcriptional repressors and reporter genes in order to study the epigenetic mechanisms of KRAB repression, and on identification of novel SNAG repression domain interacting proteins in order to understand their roles in transcriptional repression and oncogenesis. Dr. Ayyanathan has published several research articles in peer-reviewed articles in these subject areas.

CONTENTS

Part II: Integrating Genomic Medicine into the Clinical Practice

ACKNOWLEDGMENT AND HOW TO CITE

The editor and publisher thank each of the authors who contributed to this book, whether by granting their permission individually or by releasing their research as open source articles. The chapters in this book were previously published in various places in various formats. To cite the work contained in this book and to view the individual permissions, please refer to the citation at the beginning of each chapter. Each chapter was read individually and carefully selected by the editors. The result is a book that provides a nuanced study of the recent advances in epigenetics.

LIST OF CONTRIBUTORS

David Anderson
Ignyta, Inc., San Diego, CA, USA

Marianne Andersson
Department of Surgery, Institute of Clinical Sciences, Sahlgrenska Academy, Sahlgrenska University Hospital, Gothenburg, Sweden

Annika Gustafsson Asting
Department of Surgery, Institute of Clinical Sciences, Sahlgrenska Academy, Sahlgrenska University Hospital, Gothenburg, Sweden

Gianmaria Barresi
University Hospital Tuebingen, Department of Obstetrics and Gynecology, Tuebingen, Germany

Nilima Biswas
Departments of Medicine and Pharmacology, and Institute for Genomic Medicine, University of California at San Diego, CA, USA

Michael Bonin
University Hospital Tuebingen, Department of Medical Genetics, Microarray Facility, Tuebingen, Germany

Josee Bouchard
Service de Néphrologie, Département de médecine, Hôpital du Sacré-Coeur de Montréal, Université de Montréal, Montreal, Quebec, Canada

David L. Boyle
Division of Rheumatology, Allergy and Immunology, UCSD School of Medicine, La Jolla, CA, USA

Sara Brucker
University Hospital Tuebingen, Department of Obstetrics and Gynecology, Tuebingen, Germany

Ralf Bundschuh
Departments of Physics and Biochemistry, The Ohio State University, Columbus, Ohio, USA

Helena Carén
Department of Clinical Genetics, Institute of Biomedicine, University of Gothenburg, Sweden

Shuang Chang
USDA, ARS, Avian Disease and Oncology Laboratory, East Lansing, MI 48823, USA

Hans H. Cheng
USDA, ARS, Avian Disease and Oncology Laboratory, East Lansing, MI 48823, USA

Jen-hwa Chu
Channing Laboratory, Brigham and Women's Hospital, Harvard Medical School, Boston, MA, USA

Jesús Delgado-Calle
Department of Internal Medicine, H.U. Marqués de Valdecilla-IFIMAV-University of Cantabria, Santander 39008, Spain

Asok K. Dasmahapatra
National Center for Natural Products Research, Research Institute of Pharmaceutical Sciences, School of Pharmacy, University of Mississippi, University, MS 38677, USA and Department of Pharmacology, University of Mississippi, MS 38677, USA

John Curfman
Comprehensive Cancer Center, The Ohio State University, Columbus, Ohio, USA

Amy Damask
Novartis, Cambridge, MA, USA

Xin-Sheng Deng
Department of Pathology, University of Colorado Anschutz Medical Campus School of Medicine, Aurora, CO, USA

Gary S. Firestein
Division of Rheumatology, Allergy and Immunology, UCSD School of Medicine, La Jolla, CA, USA

David Frankhouser
Comprehensive Cancer Center, The Ohio State University, Columbus, Ohio, USA

Valentina Gallo
Department of Epidemiology and Public Health, Imperial College, London, UK and Department of Social and Environmental Research, London School of Hygiene and Tropical Medicine, UK

Sara Geneletti
Department of Statistics, London School of Economics, Houghton Street, London, UK

Karina Haebig
University Hospital Tuebingen, Department of Medical Genetics, Microarray Facility, Tuebingen, Germany

Josh Hillman
Division of Rheumatology, Allergy and Immunology, UCSD School of Medicine, La Jolla, CA, USA

Blanca E. Himes
Channing Laboratory, Brigham and Women's Hospital, Harvard Medical School, Boston, MA, USA

Takae Hirasawa
Department of Epigenetics Medicine, Interdisciplinary Graduate School of Medicine and Engineering, University of Yamanashi, Yamanashi, 1110 Shimokato, Chuo, Yamanashi 409-3898, Japan

Sun Woo Kang
Department of Nephrology, Inje University, Busan, South Korea

Ikhlas A. Khan
National Center for Natural Products Research, Research Institute of Pharmaceutical Sciences, School of Pharmacy, University of Mississippi, University, MS 38677, USA and Department of Pharmacognosy, University of Mississippi, University, MS 38677, USA

Shabana I. Khan
National Center for Natural Products Research, Research Institute of Pharmaceutical Sciences, School of Pharmacy, University of Mississippi, University, MS 38677, USA and Department of Pharmacognosy, University of Mississippi, University, MS 38677, USA

Srikrishna Khandrika
Division of Nephrology and Hypertension, Department of Medicine, University of California San Diego Medical Center, San Diego, CA, USA

Muin J. Khoury
National Office of Public Health Genomics, Centers for Disease Control and Prevention, Atlanta, USA

Takeo Kubota
Department of Epigenetics Medicine, Interdisciplinary Graduate School of Medicine and Engineering, University of Yamanashi, Yamanashi, 1110 Shimokato, Chuo, Yamanashi 409-3898, Japan

Kristina Lagerstedt
Department of Surgery, Institute of Clinical Sciences, Sahlgrenska Academy, Sahlgrenska University Hospital, Gothenburg, Sweden

Choon-Kee Lee
The Myeloma and Amyloidosis Program, Department of Medicine, University of Colorado Anschutz Medical Campus School of Medicine, Aurora, CO, USA

Augusto A. Litonjua
Channing Laboratory, Brigham and Women's Hospital, Harvard Medical School, Boston, MA, USA and Division of Pulmonary and Critical Care Medicine, Brigham and Women's Hospital, Harvard Medical School, Boston, MA, USA

Bolin Liu
Department of Pathology, University of Colorado Anschutz Medical Campus School of Medicine, Aurora, CO, USA

Christina Lönnroth
Department of Surgery, Institute of Clinical Sciences, Sahlgrenska Academy, Sahlgrenska University Hospital, Gothenburg, Sweden

Kent Lundholm
Department of Surgery, Institute of Clinical Sciences, Sahlgrenska Academy, Sahlgrenska University Hospital, Gothenburg, Sweden

Juan Luo
Animal & Avian Sciences Department, University of Maryland, College Park, Maryland, 20740, USA

Jian Ma
International Medical Centre of PLA General Hospital, Beijing, PR China

Manjula Mahata
Departments of Medicine and Pharmacology, and Institute for Genomic Medicine, University of California at San Diego, CA, USA

Rakesh Malhotra
Division of Nephrology and Hypertension, Department of Medicine, University of California San Diego Medical Center, San Diego, CA, USA

Guido Marcucci
Comprehensive Cancer Center, The Ohio State University, Columbus, Ohio, USA

Roy O. Mathew
Veterans Affairs Medical Center, Albany, NY, USA

Ravindra L. Mehta
Division of Nephrology and Hypertension, Department of Medicine, University of California San Diego Medical Center, San Diego, CA, USA

Kunio Miyake
Department of Epigenetics Medicine, Interdisciplinary Graduate School of Medicine and Engineering, University of Yamanashi, Yamanashi, 1110 Shimokato, Chuo, Yamanashi 409-3898, Japan

Mark Murphy
Comprehensive Cancer Center, The Ohio State University, Columbus, Ohio, USA

Daniel T. O'Connor
Departments of Medicine and Pharmacology, and Institute for Genomic Medicine, University of California at San Diego, CA, USA and Division of Nephrology and Hypertension, Department of Medicine, University of California San Diego Medical Center, San Diego, CA, USA

Miquel Porta
Institut Municipal d'Investigació Mèdica, and School of Medicine, Universitat Autònoma de Barcelona, Catalonia, Spain

Sven Poths
University Hospital Tuebingen, Department of Medical Genetics, Microarray Facility, Tuebingen, Germany

Katharina Rall
University Hospital Tuebingen, Department of Obstetrics and Gynecology, Tuebingen, Germany

Fangwen Rao
Departments of Medicine and Pharmacology, and Institute for Genomic Medicine, University of California at San Diego, CA, USA

José A. Riancho
Department of Internal Medicine, H.U. Marqués de Valdecilla-IFIMAV-University of Cantabria, Santander 39008, Spain

Olaf Riess
University Hospital Tuebingen, Department of Medical Genetics, Microarray Facility, Tuebingen, Germany

Benjamin A.T. Rodriguez
Comprehensive Cancer Center, The Ohio State University, Columbus, Ohio, USA

Karin Schaeferhoff
University Hospital Tuebingen, Department of Medical Genetics, Microarray Facility, Tuebingen, Germany

Birgitt Schoenfisch
University Hospital Tuebingen, Department of Obstetrics and Gynecology, Tuebingen, Germany

Pei-an Betty Shih
Department of Nephrology, Inje University, Busan, South Korea

Robert Shoemaker
Ignyta, Inc., San Diego, CA, USA

Jiuzhou Song
Animal & Avian Sciences Department, University of Maryland, College Park, Maryland, 20740, USA

Kelan G. Tantisira
Channing Laboratory, Brigham and Women's Hospital, Harvard Medical School, Boston, MA, USA and Division of Pulmonary and Critical Care Medicine, Brigham and Women's Hospital, Harvard Medical School, Boston, MA, USA

Fei Tian
Animal & Avian Sciences Department, University of Maryland, College Park, Maryland, 20740, USA

Ashita Tolwani
Division of Nephrology, University of Alabama at Birmingham, AL, USA

Michael P. Trimarchi
Comprehensive Cancer Center, The Ohio State University, Columbus, Ohio, USA

Paolo Vineis
Department of Epidemiology and Public Health, Imperial College, London, UK and HuGeF, Via Nizza 52, 10126 Torino, Italy

Diethelm Wallwiener
University Hospital Tuebingen, Department of Obstetrics and Gynecology, Tuebingen, Germany

Larry A. Walker
National Center for Natural Products Research, Research Institute of Pharmaceutical Sciences, School of Pharmacy, University of Mississippi, University, MS 38677, USA, Department of Pharmacology, University of Mississippi, MS 38677, USA, and University of Mississippi Cancer Institute, University of Mississippi, University, MS 38677, US

Michael Walter
University Hospital Tuebingen, Department of Medical Genetics, Microarray Facility, Tuebingen, Germany

Shuiliang Wang
Department of Pathology, University of Colorado Anschutz Medical Campus School of Medicine, Aurora, CO, USA

Wei Wang
Department of Chemistry and Biochemistry, University of California San Diego, La Jolla, CA, USA

Scott T. Weiss
Channing Laboratory, Brigham and Women's Hospital, Harvard Medical School, Boston, MA, USA

John W. Whitaker
Department of Chemistry and Biochemistry, University of California San Diego, La Jolla, CA, USA

Ann Wu
Channing Laboratory, Brigham and Women's Hospital, Harvard Medical School, Boston, MA, USA

Mousheng Xu
Channing Laboratory, Brigham and Women's Hospital, Harvard Medical School, Boston, MA, USA
and Bioinformatics Program, Boston University, Boston, MA, USA

Liying Yan
EpigenDx, Worcester, MA, USA

Pearlly Yan
Comprehensive Cancer Center, The Ohio State University, Columbus, Ohio, USA

Xiao-Dan Yu
Department of Stress Medicine, Institute of Basic Medical Sciences, Beijing, PR China

Ying Yu
Animal & Avian Sciences Department, University of Maryland, College Park, Maryland, 20740, USA
and College of Animal Sciences, China Agricultural University, Haidian, Beijing, 100193, P.R. China

Huanmin Zhang
USDA, ARS, Avian Disease and Oncology Laboratory, East Lansing, MI 48823, USA

Jianping Zhao
National Center for Natural Products Research, Research Institute of Pharmaceutical Sciences, School
of Pharmacy, University of Mississippi, University, MS 38677, USA

Ming Zhao
Department of Stress Medicine, Institute of Basic Medical Sciences, Beijing, PR China

INTRODUCTION

This new volume on gene expression and epigenetics discusses how environment affects specific gene expression. The book also shows methods for bioinformatic analysis of the epigenome. The book is broken into two sections: the first looks at eukaryotic DNA methylation and the second at how to integrate genomic medicine into clinical practice.

Renal kallikrein (KLK1) synthesis and urinary excretion are reportedly diminished during AKI (acute kidney injury) in animal models and provision of kallikrein abrogates renal injury in this setting, but data in human AKI is limited. In Chapter 1, therefore, Kang and colleagues first examined KLK1 renal excretion in human AKI, and then probed potential endocrine and epigenetic mechanisms for its alterations. KLK1 enzymatic activity excretion was evaluated in urine from patients with established or incipient AKI, versus healthy/non-hospital as well as ICU controls. Endocrine control of KLK1 excretion was then probed by catecholamine and aldosterone measurements in established AKI versus healthy controls. To examine epigenetic control of KLK1 synthesis, the authors tested blood and urine DNA for changes in promoter CpG methylation of the KLK1 gene, as well as LINE-1 elements, by bisulfite sequencing. Patients with early/incipient AKI displayed a modest reduction of KLK1 excretion, but unexpectedly,established AKI displayed substantially elevated urine KLK1 excretion, ~11-fold higher than healthy controls, and ~3-fold greater than ICU controls. The authors then probed potential mechanisms of the change. Established AKI patients had lower SBP, higher heart rate, and higher epinephrine excretion than healthy controls, though aldosterone excretion was not different. Promoter KLK1 CpG methylation was higher in blood than urine DNA, while KLK1 methylation in blood DNA was significantly higher in established AKI than healthy controls, though KLK1 methylation in urine tended to be higher in AKI, directionally consistent with earlier/incipient but not later/established changes in KLK1 excretion in AKI. On multivariate ANOVA, AKI displayed coordinate changes in

KLK1 excretion and promoter methylation, though directionally opposite to expectation. Control (LINE-1 repetitive element) methylation in blood and urine DNA was similar between AKI and controls. Unexpectedly, increased KLK1 excretion in AKI patients was found; this increase is likely to be due in part to increments in adrenergic tone during BP depression. Epigenetic changes at KLK1 may also play a role in early changes of KLK1 expression and thus AKI susceptibility or recovery.

Increased cyclooxygenase activity promotes progression of colorectal cancer, but the mechanisms behind COX-2 induction remain elusive. Chapter 2, by Asting and colleagues, was therefore aimed to define external cell signaling and transcription factors relating to high COX-2 expression in colon cancer tissue. Tumor and normal colon tissue were collected at primary curative operation in 48 unselected patients. COX-2 expression in tumor and normal colon tissue was quantified including microarray analyses on tumor mRNA accounting for high and low tumor COX-2 expression. Cross hybridization was performed between tumor and normal colon tissue. Methylation status of up-stream COX-2 promoter region was evaluated. Tumors with high COX-2 expression displayed large differences in gene expression compared to normal colon. Numerous genes with altered expression appeared in tumors of high COX-2 expression compared to tumors of low COX-2. COX-2 expression in normal colon was increased in patients with tumors of high COX-2 compared to normal colon from patients with tumors of low COX-2. IL1β, IL6 and iNOS transcripts were up-regulated among external cell signaling factors; nine transcription factors (ATF3, C/EBP, c-Fos, Fos-B, JDP2, JunB, c-Maf, NF-κB, TCF4) showed increased expression and 5 (AP-2, CBP, Elk-1, p53, PEA3) were decreased in tumors with high COX-2. The promoter region of COX-2 gene did not show consistent methylation in tumor or normal colon tissue. Transcription and external cell signaling factors are altered as covariates to COX-2 expression in colon cancer tissue, but DNA methylation of the COX-2 promoter region was not a significant factor behind COX-2 expression in tumor and normal colon tissue.

Marek's disease virus (MDV) is an oncovirus that induces lymphoid tumors in susceptible chickens, and may affect the epigenetic stability of the CD4 gene. The purpose of Chapter 3, by Luo and colleagues, was to find the effect of MDV infection on DNA methylation status of the CD4 gene differed between MD-resistant (L63) and –susceptible (L72) chicken lines. Chickens from each line were divided into two groups with one group infected by MDV and the other group as uninfected controls. Then, promoter DNA methylation levels of the CD4 gene were measured by Pyrosequencing; and gene expression analysis was performed by quantitative PCR. Promoter methylation of the CD4 gene was found to be down-regulated in L72 chickens only after MDV infection. The methylation down-regulation of the CD4 promoter is negatively correlated with up-regulation of CD4 gene expression in the L72 spleen at 21 dpi. The methylation fluctuation and mRNA expression change of CD4 gene induced by MDV infection suggested a unique epigenetic mechanism existed in MD-susceptible chickens.

The Mayer-Rokitansky-Küster-Hauser (MRKH) syndrome is present in at least 1 out of 4,500 female live births and is the second most common cause for primary amenorrhea. It is characterized by vaginal and uterine aplasia in an XX individual with normal secondary characteristics. It has long been considered a sporadic anomaly, but familial clustering occurs. Several candidate genes have been studied although no single factor has yet been identified. Cases of discordant monozygotic twins suggest that the involvement of epigenetic factors is more likely. In Chapter 4, Rall and colleagues identified differences in gene expression and methylation patterns of uterine tissue between eight MRKH patients and eight controls using whole-genome microarray analyses. Results obtained by expression and methylation arrays were confirmed by qRT-PCR and pyrosequencing. The authors delineated 293 differentially expressed and 194 differentially methylated genes of which nine overlap in both groups. These nine genes are mainly embryologically relevant for the development of the female genital tract. This study used, for the first time, a combined whole-genome expression and methylation approach to reveal the etiology of the MRKH syndrome. The findings suggest that either deficient estrogen receptors or the ectopic expression of certain HOXA genes might lead to abnormal development of the female reproductive tract. In utero exposure to endocrine disruptors or abnormally high maternal hormone levels might cause ectopic expression or anterior transformation of HOXA genes. It is, however, also possible that different factors influence the anti-Mullerian hormone promoter activity during embryological development causing regression of the Müllerian ducts. Thus, our data stimulate new research directions to decipher the pathogenic basis of MRKH syndrome.

Bone is a complex connective tissue characterized by a calcified extracellular matrix. This mineralized matrix is constantly being formed and resorbed throughout life, allowing the bone to adapt to daily mechanical loads and maintain skeletal properties and composition. The imbalance between bone formation and bone resorption leads to changes in bone mass. This is the case of osteoporosis and osteoarthritis, two common skeletal disorders. While osteoporosis is characterized by a decreased bone mass and, consequently, higher susceptibility to fractures, bone mass tends to be higher in patients with osteoarthritis, especially in the subchondral bone region. It is known that these diseases are influenced by heritable factors. However, the DNA polymorphisms identified so far in GWAS explain less than 10% of the genetic risk, suggesting that other factors, and specifically epigenetic mechanisms, are involved in the pathogenesis of these disorders. Chapter 5, by Delgado-Callee and Riancho, summarizes current knowledge about the influence of epigenetic marks on bone homeostasis, paying special attention to the role of DNA methylation in the onset and progression of osteoporosis and osteoarthritis.

DNA methylation is an important epigenetic mark and dysregulation of DNA methylation is associated with many diseases including cancer. Advances in next-generation sequencing now allow unbiased methylome profiling of entire patient cohorts, greatly facilitating biomarker discovery and presenting new opportunities to understand the biological mechanisms by which changes in methylation contribute to disease. Enrichment-based sequencing assays such as MethylCap-seq are a cost effective solution for genome-wide determination of methylation status, but the technical reliability of methylation reconstruction from raw sequencing data has not been well characterized. In Chapter 6, Trimarchi and colleagues analyze three MethylCap-seq data sets and perform two different analyses to assess data quality. First, they investigate how data quality is affected by excluding samples that do not meet quality control cutoff requirements. Second, they consider the effect of additional reads on enrichment score, saturation, and coverage. Lastly, the authors verify a method for the determination of the global amount of methylation from MethylCap-seq data by comparing to a spiked-in control DNA of known methylation status. They show that rejection of samples based on our quality control parameters leads to a significant improvement of methylation calling. Additional reads beyond ~13 million unique aligned reads improved coverage, modestly improved saturation, and did not impact enrichment score. Lastly, the authors find that a global methylation indicator calculated from MethylCap-seq data correlates well with the global methylation level of a sample as obtained from a spike-in DNA of known methylation level. This paper shows that with appropriate quality control MethylCap-seq is a reliable tool, suitable for cohorts of hundreds of patients, that provides reproducible methylation information on a feature by feature basis as well as information about the global level of methylation.

Observational studies of human health and disease (basic, clinical and epidemiological) are vulnerable to methodological problems—such as selection bias and confounding—that make causal inferences problematic. Gene-disease associations are no exception, as they are commonly investigated using observational designs. A rich body of knowledge exists in medicine and epidemiology on the assessment of causal relationships involving personal and environmental causes of disease; it includes seminal causal criteria developed by Austin Bradford Hill and more recently applied directed acyclic graphs (DAGs). However, such knowledge has seldom been applied to assess causal relationships in clinical genetics and genomics, even in studies aimed at making inferences relevant for human health. Conversely, incorporating genetic causal knowledge into clinical and epidemiological causal reasoning is still a largely unexplored area. As the contribution of genetics to the understanding of disease aetiology becomes more important, causal assessment of genetic and genomic evidence becomes fundamental. The method Geneletti and colleagues develop in Chapter 7 provides a simple and rigorous first step towards this goal. The present paper is an example of integrative research, i.e., research that integrates knowledge, data, methods, techniques, and reasoning from multiple disciplines, approaches and levels of analysis to generate knowledge that no discipline alone may achieve.

Personalized health-care promises tailored health-care solutions to individual patients based on their genetic background and/or environmental exposure history. To date, disease prediction has been based on a few environmental factors and/or single nucleotide polymorphisms (SNPs), while complex diseases are usually affected by many genetic and environmental factors with each factor contributing a small portion to the outcome. Xu and colleagues hypothesized that the use of random forests classifiers to select SNPs would result in an improved predictive model of asthma exacerbations. Chapter 8 tests this hypothesis in a population of childhood asthmatics. In this study, using emergency room visits or hospitalizations as the definition of a severe asthma exacerbation, the authors first identified a list of top Genome Wide Association Study (GWAS) SNPs ranked by Random Forests (RF) importance score for the CAMP (Childhood Asthma Management Program) population of 127 exacerbation cases and 290 non-exacerbation controls. They predict severe asthma exacerbations using the top 10 to 320 SNPs together with age, sex, pre-bronchodilator FEV1 percentage predicted, and treatment group. Testing in an independent set of the CAMP population shows that severe asthma exacerbations can be predicted with an Area Under the Curve (AUC) = 0.66 with 160-320 SNPs in comparison to an AUC score of 0.57 with 10 SNPs. Using the clinical traits alone yielded AUC score of 0.54, suggesting the phenotype is affected by genetic as well as environmental factors. This study shows that a random forests algorithm can effectively extract and use the information contained in a small number of samples. Random forests, and other machine learning tools, can be used with GWAS studies to integrate large numbers of predictors simultaneously.

Aromatase, the key enzyme in estrogen biosynthesis, converts androstenedione to estrone and testosterone to estradiol. The enzyme is expressed in various tissues such as ovary, placenta, bone, brain, skin, and adipose tissue. Aromatase enzyme is encoded by a single gene CYP 19A1and its expression is controlled by tissue-specific promoters. Aromatase mRNA is primarily transcribed from promoter I.4 in normal breast tissue and physiological levels of aromatase are found in breast adipose stromal fibroblasts. Under the conditions of breast cancer, as a result of the activation of a distinct set of aromatase promoters (I.3, II, and I.7) aromatase expression is enhanced leading to local overproduction of estrogen that promotes breast cancer. Aromatase is considered as a potential target for endocrine treatment of breast cancer but due to nonspecific reduction of aromatase activity in other tissues, aromatase inhibitors (AIs) are associated with undesirable side effects such as bone loss, and abnormal lipid metabolism. Inhibition of aromatase expression by inactivating breast tumor-specific aromatase promoters can selectively block estrogen production at the tumor site. Although several synthetic chemical compounds and nuclear receptor ligands are known to inhibit the activity of the tumor-specific aromatase promoters, further development of more specific and efficacious drugs without adverse effects is still warranted. Plants are rich in chemopreventive agents that have a great potential to be used in chemotherapy for hormone dependent breast cancer which could serve as a source for natural AIs. In Chapter 9, Khan and colleagues provide a brief review of the studies on phytochemicals such as biochanin A, genistein, quercetin, isoliquiritigenin, resveratrol, and grape seed extracts related to their effect on the activation of breast cancer-associated aromatase promoters and discuss their aromatase inhibitory potential to be used as safer chemotherapeutic agents for specific hormone-dependent breast cancer.

Cladribine or 2-chlorodeoxyadenosine (2-CDA) is a well-known purine nucleoside analog with particular activity against lymphoproliferative disorders, such as hairy cell leukemia (HCL). Its benefits in multiple myeloma (MM) remain unclear. In Chapter 10, Ma and colleagues report the inhibitory effects of cladribine on MM cell lines (U266, RPMI8226, MM1.S), and its therapeutic potential in combination with a specific inhibitor of the signal transducer and activator of transcription 3 (STAT3). MTS-based proliferation assays were used to determine cell viability in response to cladribine. Cell cycle progression was examined by flow cytometry analysis. Cells undergoing apoptosis were evaluated with Annexin V staining and a specific ELISA to quantitatively measure cytoplasmic histone-associated DNA fragments. Western blot analyses were performed to determine the protein expression levels and activation. Cladribine inhibited cell proliferation of MM cells in a dose-dependent manner, although the three MM cell lines exhibited a remarkably different responsiveness to cladribine. The IC50 of cladribine for U266, RPMI8226, or MM1.S cells was approximately 2.43, 0.75, or 0.18 μmol/L, respectively. Treatment with cladribine resulted in a significant G1 arrest in U266 and RPMI8226 cells, but only a minor increase in the G1 phase for MM1.S cells. Apoptosis assays with Annexin V-FITC/PI double staining indicated that cladribine induced apoptosis of U266 cells in a dose-dependent manner. Similar results were obtained with an apoptotic-ELISA showing that cladribine

dramatically promoted MM1.S and RPMA8226 cells undergoing apoptosis. On the molecular level, cladribine induced PARP cleavage and activation of caspase-8 and caspase-3. Meanwhile, treatment with cladribine led
to a remarkable reduction of the phosphorylated STAT3 (P-STAT3), but
had little effect on STAT3 protein levels. The combinations of cladribine
and a specific STAT3 inhibitor as compared to either agent alone significantly induced apoptosis in all three MM cell lines. Cladribine exhibited inhibitory effects on MM cells in vitro. MM1.S is the only cell line
showing significant response to the clinically achievable concentrations
of cladribine-induced apoptosis and inactivation of STAT3. The data suggest that MM patients with the features of MM1.S cells may particularly
benefit from cladribine monotherapy, whereas cladribine in combination
with STAT3 inhibitor exerts a broader therapeutic potential against MM.

Epigenetics is a mechanism that regulates gene expression independently of the underlying DNA sequence, relying instead on the chemical modification of DNA and histone proteins. Although environmental
and genetic factors were thought to be independently associated with disorders, several recent lines of evidence suggest that epigenetics bridges
these two factors. Epigenetic gene regulation is essential for normal development, thus defects in epigenetics cause various rare congenital diseases.
Because epigenetics is a reversible system that can be affected by various
environmental factors, such as drugs, nutrition, and mental stress, the epigenetic disorders also include common diseases induced by environmental
factors. In Chapter 11, Kubota and colleagues discuss the nature of epigenetic disorders, particularly psychiatric disorders, on the basis of recent
findings: 1) susceptibility of the conditions to environmental factors, 2)
treatment by taking advantage of their reversible nature, and 3) transgenerational inheritance of epigenetic changes, that is, acquired adaptive epigenetic changes that are passed on to offspring. These recently discovered
aspects of epigenetics provide a new concept of clinical genetics.

A DNA methylation signature has been characterized that distinguishes rheumatoid arthritis (RA) fibroblast like synoviocytes (FLS) from osteoarthritis (OA) FLS. The presence of epigenetic changes in long-term
cultured cells suggest that rheumatoid FLS imprinting might contribute to
pathogenic behavior. To understand how differentially methylated genes
(DMGs) might participate in the pathogenesis of RA, Whitaker and

colleagues evaluated the stability of the RA signature and whether DMGs are enriched in specific pathways and ontology categories in Chapter 12. To assess the RA methylation signatures the Illumina HumanMethylation450 chip was used to compare methylation levels in RA, OA, and normal (NL) FLS at passage 3, 5, and 7. Then methylation frequencies at CpGs within the signature were compared between passages. To assess the enrichment of DMGs in specific pathways, DMGs were identified as genes that possess significantly differential methylated loci within their promoter regions. These sets of DMGs were then compared to pathway and ontology databases to establish enrichment in specific categories. Initial studies compared passage 3, 5, and 7 FLS from RA, OA, and NL. The patterns of differential methylation of each individual FLS line were very similar regardless of passage number. Using the most robust analysis, 20 out of 272 KEGG pathways and 43 out of 34,400 GO pathways were significantly altered for RA compared with OA and NL FLS. Most interestingly, the authors found that the KEGG 'Rheumatoid Arthritis' pathway was consistently the most significantly enriched with differentially methylated loci. Additional pathways involved with innate immunity (Complement and Coagulation, Toll-like Receptors, NOD-like Receptors, and Cytosolic DNA-sensing), cell adhesion (Focal Adhesion, Cell Adhesion Molecule), and cytokines (Cytokine-cytokine Receptor). Taken together, KEGG and GO pathway analysis demonstrates non-random epigenetic imprinting of RA FLS. The DNA methylation patterns include anomalies in key genes implicated in the pathogenesis of RA and are stable for multiple cell passages. Persistent epigenetic alterations could contribute to the aggressive phenotype of RA synoviocytes and identify potential therapeutic targets that could modulate the pathogenic behavior.

PART I

EUKARYOTIC DNA METHYLATION

CHAPTER 1

RENAL KALLIKREIN EXCRETION AND EPIGENETICS IN HUMAN ACUTE KIDNEY INJURY: EXPRESSION, MECHANISMS AND CONSEQUENCES

SUN WOO KANG, PEI-AN BETTY SHIH, ROY O. MATHEW, MANJULA MAHATA, NILIMA BISWAS, FANGWEN RAO, LIYING YAN, JOSEE BOUCHARD, RAKESH MALHOTRA, ASHITA TOLWANI, SRIKRISHNA KHANDRIKA, RAVINDRA L. MEHTA, AND DANIEL T. O'CONNOR

1.1 BACKGROUND

The incidence of acute kidney injury (AKI) in hospitalized patients is estimated to be 5-10%, and is much higher in the critically ill [1,2]. Despite the potential for recovery of kidney function, acute kidney injury is associated with substantial morbidity and even mortality. AKI, due to ischemia or nephrotoxic agent exposure, may lead to death or sublethal injury of proximal tubular cells, after which surviving cells may repolarize and/or de-differentiate, proliferate, migrate to denuded areas, re-differentiate, and

This chapter was originally published under the Creative Commons Attribution License. Kang SW, Shih PA, Mathew RO, Mahata M, Biswas N, Rao F, Yan L, Bouchard J, Malhotra R, Tolwani A, Khandrika S, Mehta RL, and O'Connor DT. Renal Kallikrein Excretion and Epigenetics in Human Acute Kidney Injury: Expression, Mechanisms and Consequences. BMC Nephrology *12,27 (2011). doi:10.1186/1471-2369-12-27*

restore nephron structure (including the tubular epithelium) and function [3,4].

The serine protease kallikrein (KLK1; E.C.-3.4.21.35; OMIM 147910), excreted from kidney into urine, catalyzes the cleavage of low molecular weight kininogen to lysyl-bradykinin (kallidin), which exhibits both vasodilator and natriuretic pharmacological properties in the kidney; if these properties occur in vivo, the potential of the system for regulating blood pressure is clear [5].

Renal kallikrein levels were markedly reduced in an aminoglycoside-induced AKI animal model [6], and KLK1 gene transfer protected against aminoglycoside-induced nephropathy by diminishing apoptosis and inflammation [7]. In addition, KLK1 infusion during aminoglycoside treatment attenuated drug-induced renal dysfunction, cortical damage, and apoptosis in the rat [8]. Previously, we have reported that urinary KLK1 excretion was diminished in renal allograft recipients with a clinical diagnosis of acute tubular necrosis (ATN) [9]; since urinary KLK1 originates in the kidney, reduced urinary kallikrein levels may reflect impaired renal function. However, this finding has not been pursued in humans.

In mammals, cytosine methylation occurs almost exclusively at CpG dinucleotides, which are enriched at CpG islands, often are located at 5'-/ promoter regions of functional genes [10]. Cytosine methylation may result in transcriptional repression either by interfering with transcription factor binding or by inducing a repressive chromatin structure [11]. Apoptotic pathways are targets for such "epigenetic" silencing, and several apoptosis-linked genes that are regulated directly or indirectly by methylation have been described [12].

In this study, we first probed whether KLK1 excretion is altered in human AKI, and if so what mechanisms (endocrine or epigenetic) might be driving the change. Since kidney repair after injury may recapitulate normal morphogenesis, we hypothesized that urinary kallikrein levels would be associated with severity of AKI and with epigenetic changes in the renal kallikrein-1 (KLK1) promoter. We considered that changes in kallikrein excretion or the KLK1 promoter might predict renal functional recovery and thus serve as biomarkers of recovery from AKI, thereby facilitating timely diagnosis and treatment. We therefore examined patients with AKI for urinary expression of KLK1 enzymatic activity, as well as genomic DNA from blood and urine for CpG methylation pattern at the KLK1 gene promoter.

1.2 METHODS

1.2.1 ESTABLISHED AKI CASES

Cases were ascertained from a single center prospective non-concurrent observational cohort of inpatients who were identified as having suffered acute kidney injury (AKI) during a hospital admission. The institutional review board of the University of California, San Diego (UCSD) reviewed and approved the study as well as the consent document. Primary providers referred potentially eligible patients to investigators and study coordinators. Patients were eligible for enrollment if they were greater than 18 years of age and met the serum creatinine criteria for acute kidney injury as set out by the Acute Kidney Injury Network (AKIN) [13]: an abrupt rise by ≥ 0.3 mg/dl within a 48-hour period. Patients were excluded if they received chronic renal replacement therapy (hemodialysis or peritoneal dialysis) within the 6 months prior to admission; had ever been in receipt of a kidney transplant; pregnant or breast feeding; currently incarcerated or otherwise institutionalized (nursing home, rehabilitation); were placed under hospice/comfort care; or did not have reasonable expectation of survival past the present hospitalization. If eligible, the patient or authorized representative was presented the study and consent for participation was obtained. All relevant patient data were derived from the electronic and paper medical records, as well as direct interview of the patient or surrogate. Basic demographic information and co-morbid conditions were recorded on enrollment. Etiology of AKI was determined by chart review of provider diagnosis, and verification by study personnel; diagnosis followed the categories set by the Project to Improve Care of Acute Renal Disease (PICARD) study investigators [1]. Daily assessment included medication review, physical exam (as recorded in medical record or assessed by study personnel when missing), vital signs, intake and output, and labs. Clinical data elements were collected daily and the need for and utilization pattern of renal replacement therapy was also monitored and recorded. Blood and urine samples were collected at time of entry, daily for 7 days maximum, and at hospital discharge. Twenty-four hour urine collections were performed at study entry and hospital discharge for creatinine/urea clearance (in approximation of glomerular filtration rate—GFR) as well as urinary kallikrein activity. One sample of whole blood was collected for genomic DNA preparation (and genetic analysis of the *KLK1* locus) at the time of study entry. At the time of discharge, follow-up appointments with either the primary care physician or a nephrologist (not all patients were seen by a nephrologist during the hospitalization), extent of renal recovery, and dialysis dependence (if needed during hospitalization) were ascertained. Recovery: pre-defined study endpoints were 12 months of follow-up, start of maintenance hemodialysis or peritoneal dialysis, receipt of a kidney transplant, or death; recovery of renal function was the primary outcome, defined as a return to within 10% of baseline eGFR or lowest eGFR prior to AKI event. Recovery was assessed at 6 months of follow-up.

1.2.2 HEALTHY (NON-HOSPITAL) CONTROLS

In addition, we obtained data for a control group of 38 healthy adult subjects. Each healthy control was selected from only one member from each of 38 twin pair sets. Twin pairs were recruited by a population-based twin registry in southern California [14], and by newspaper advertisement. These twins are of European, African-American, and Asian biogeographic ancestry. Ethnicity was established by self-identification. Self-reported zygosity was confirmed by extensive SNP genotyping. There was no clinical evidence for kidney disease or any other cardiovascular disorder in any of the controls. Untimed (spot) urine collections were performed, and one sample of EDTA-anticoagulated whole blood was collected for genetic analysis of the *KLK1* locus at the time of study entry.

1.2.3 REPLICATION: INCIPIENT (EARLY) AKI CASES IN AN INTENSIVE CARE UNIT (ICU), WITH ICU CONTROL SUBJECTS

An additional sample of controls was ascertained for replication of findings, in an ICU setting. In brief, the replication sample consisted of n = 44 subjects ("ICU controls") who did not develop AKI during a 7-day observation period after hospital ICU admission, as well as n = 11 subjects (ICU cases) who did develop AKI, as defined above. Patients were screened at ICU admission for potential study participation at three academic medical centers (University of California San Diego, University of Alabama, and Université de Montréal) between July 2006 and December 2008. Patients were eligible for enrollment if they were age 18 or older and had a life expectancy of at least 48 hours. Controls were excluded if they had AKI according to the AKIN criteria [13], were admitted to the ICU > 48 hours prior to screening, transferred from another ICU, had a serum creatinine > 2 mg/dl ≤ 3 days before ICU admission, were prisoners, received dialysis within the 12 months prior to admission, had a functioning kidney transplant, were on anticoagulants or warfarin within the last 7 days, suffered from decompensated cirrhosis, had CKD stage 5, were anemic (hemoglobin < 9.0 mg/dl or hematocrit < 27%), or were already enrolled in another research project.

The study was approved by the Institutional Review Boards at each institution, and written informed consent was obtained from all participants or their health care surrogates. Following informed consent, data on past medical history were collected once, and clinical, laboratory and process-of-care elements were collected daily. Each institution's local laboratory measured serum creatinine values. AKI was defined as an increase in serum creatinine level of more than 0.3 mg/dL or more than 50% from a reference creatinine within 48 hours (AKIN criteria) [13]. Patients without AKI within the first 4 days had continued blood and urine samples twice daily, for a total study observation period of 7 days.

1.2.4 BIOCHEMICAL ASSAYS

Urine was assayed for kallikrein by an alkaline amidolytic activity assay as previously described (4), using the chromogenic substrate S-2266:

[D] Val-Leu-Arg-paranitroanilide (Kabi Pharmacia; Franklin, OH, USA) [5,15]. The activity of kallikrein per liter of urine (units per liter, U/L) is calculated from the formula: $U/L = (9.55 \cdot A)$, where A = absorbance, after a 30-min assay incubation of the paranitroanilide product in a spectrophotometer at 405 nm [5,15]. Inclusion or exclusion of the kallikrein inhibitor aprotinin (Trasylol, Miles Inc., West Haven, CT, USA) indicated that a fraction of human urinary S-2266 amidolytic activity in the absence of aprotinin was non-kallikrein (likely urokinase) [15]; thus, aprotinin (20 kallikrein inhibitory U/mL) was systematically included in the assay blank, to assure specificity for kallikrein measurement. The inter-assay coefficient of variation was 18.1%, and activities from n = 20 samples measured on two separate occasions correlated highly (Spearman R = 0.92, P< 0.01). In n = 87 subjects, activity correlated (Spearman R = 0.82, P< 0.0001) when results were compared for kallikrein excretion normalized to time versus creatinine excretion. Specificity of the S-2266 amidolytic assay for glandular (KLK1, including renal, pancreas, and salivary) kallikrein activity in urine arises from two features: first, the substrate S-2266 is cleaved only by a particular subset of serine proteases, including KLK1; and second, the inclusion of aprotinin in the assay blank, which specifically inhibits serine proteases including KLK1; nonetheless, only an immunoassay specific for lysyl-bradykinin (the kinin product of KLK1) generation could provide absolute assurance of specificity for KLK1.

Clinical chemistries (serum or urine, electrolytes or creatinine) were measured by spectrophotometric autoanalyzer. Urine aldosterone concentration was determined by enzyme immunoassay (Alpco Diagnostics, Salem, NH, USA). Urine catecholamine concentration was determined by commercial ELISA kit (Labor Diagnostika Nord GmBH & Co. KG, Nordhorn, Germany). Urine values were normalized to creatinine concentration in the same sample.

1.2.5 DNA EXTRACTION AND BISULFITE TREATMENT OF CPG SITES

A sample of EDTA-anticoagulated whole blood was obtained from participants and stored at -70°C prior to DNA extraction. Timed and spot urine

AGGTATATGGGGCTTTGTACCAGGGGTCACTGATTCCTCCGTCTTCCTGTTTCTGCTTCCCCTCAGTC
CCCCCTTGCCTCACTGGCTGCTCCCCAGAGCAAAGCCCCAGAGCCACAGGCCCTGCCCCACCTGGCTT
CAACCCCAGGAATGCG(POS#1)TCCAGCG(POS#2)TGATCCAGGGCCTGCAGAACAGGTGCTGGTTCTCC
CTCCCCG(POS#3)TCTACAGCTCTGGGGATCG(POS#4)GRGGGGGGGSGGCAATTGTCCAGCCCCCAGG
CAACAGGGGAAGGGCCTTGGCCAACATCTGGGTGCCAGCAGGGCAGGGGTGGGGCTCTGAGGGGATAA
GGGCTTTTAAAAGGCTCCCCAGGGAGGTTCCCCAGTTCCTCCACCTGCTGGCCCCTGGACACCTCTGT

FIGURE 1: Map of CpG sites studied in the human KLK1 proximal promoter. Letters highlighted in gray are the target regions complementary to amplified PCR primers. The CpGs analyzed are numbered as Pos#1 - Pos#4 and colored yellow. Green underlined sequences are target regions complementary to sequencing primers. Green highlighted A is the transcriptional initiation ("cap") site. Sequences following the transcription initiation site are colored pink.

samples were obtained and frozen at -70°C before assay. Blood DNA was prepared from blood leukocytes with a commercial kit (QIAamp® DNA Mini Kit; Qiagen, USA). Urine DNA was prepared from the urine pellet with spun columns (urine DNA isolation kit; Norgen, Canada). Both DNAs were subjected to sodium metabisulfite ($Na_2S_2O_5$) treatment (Imprint™ DNA Modification Kit; Sigma, USA), and then eluted in 20 µL elution buffer. Bisulfite converts cytosine residues to uracil, but leaves 5-methylcytosine residues unaffected.

1.2.6 KLK1 *PROMOTER CPG METHYLATION ANALYSIS*

Pyrosequencing for allele discrimination (Pyrosequencing; Qiagen, USA) provides real-time extension-based DNA analysis that can evaluate multiple CpG sites [16]. CpG methylation analysis at the 5'/upstream/proximal promoter region of human kallikrein serine protease 1 (*KLK1*) gene was performed. The *KLK1* gene was analyzed by a single PCR amplicon spanning 4 CpGs in a 263 bp region, with two biotinylated sequencing (extension) primers (Figure 1). The consecutive 4 CpGs were located -203 to -135 bp from the transcription initiation site: sequentially at -203, -196, -154, and -135 bp (Figure 1).

As a control, global CpG methylation analysis was completed using PyroMark LINE-1 reagents (Pyrosequencing; Qiagen, USA). We thus determined the methylation status of three CpG sites in LINE-1 repetitive (LTR-like) elements, wherein methylation levels of CpG sites represent global methylation status across the genome, because of the repetitive nature of LINE-1 elements [17,18].

PCR amplification was performed using 10X PCR buffer, 3.0 mM $MgCl_2$, 200 µM of each dNTP, 0.2 µM each of forward and reverse primers, HotStar DNA polymerase (Qiagen, USA) 1.25 U, and ~10 ng of bisulfite-converted DNA per 50 µl reaction. PCR cycling conditions were: 94°C 15 min; 45 cycles of 94°C 30 s, 56°C 30 s, 72°C 30 s; 72°C 5 min; and then products were held at 4°C. The PCR was performed with one of the PCR primers biotinylated to convert the PCR product to single-stranded DNA template. PCR products (each 10 µl) were sequenced by Pyrosequencing PSQ96 HS System (Pyrosequencing, Qiagen, USA). The methylation status of each locus was analyzed individually as a T/C SNP using Pyro-QCpG™ software (Pyrosequencing).

AKI case samples were evaluated at study entry (baseline, time of diagnosis). After bisulfite modification and PCR amplification, *KLK1* blood DNA promoter methylation data from 13 AKI patients and 30 controls were obtained. *KLK1* urine DNA promoter methylation data from 9 AKI and 22 controls were available. LINE-1 blood DNA methylation data from 14 AKI patients and 32 controls were available for evaluation. LINE-1 urine DNA methylation data from 15 AKI patients and 32 controls were obtained.

1.2.7 STATISTICAL ANALYSES

Results are expressed as the mean value ± one standard error of the mean (SEM) for continuous variables. For comparisons of two groups, unpaired two-sided t-tests or one-way ANOVA (enabling adjustment for covariates of age, sex, and ethnicity) were performed. Non-parametric Wilcoxon Rank Sum test was used to confirm parametric tests in the face of relatively small sample sizes. Proportions were evaluated by Fisher's exact test (2×2 tables) or chi-square test (3×2 tables). Statistical analyses were performed in R2.10.1 <http://www.r-project.org/> or SPSS-17 (Statistical Package for the Social Sciences; Chicago, IL, USA). A P value of < 0.05 was considered significant. Multiple linear regression was performed with default criteria of entry ($p < 0.05$) and exit ($p > 0.10$) from the multivariate regression model, using stepwise or forward options. Recovery from AKI was pre-defined as return (within 6 months follow-up) to within 10% of baseline eGFR, or lowest eGFR prior to AKI event.

1.3 RESULTS

1.3.1 RENAL KLK1 EXCRETION AND EGFR IN THE 4 SUBJECT GROUPS: AKI CASES AND CONTROLS

Demographic and anthropometric description of the study samples is presented in Table 1. Baseline demographic characteristics (age, sex) were similar across groups.

TABLE 1: Clinical characteristics of cases and controls: Established versus incipient AKI cases, and ICU versus healthy controls

Characteristics	P < 0.05 (*)	AKI		Controls	
		Established	Incipient (early, ICU)	ICU	Healthy (non-hospital)
		n = 20	n = 11	n = 44	n = 38
Age, years	*	48.8 ± 3.5	68.1 ± 3.8	52.9 ± 2.3	46.3 ± 1.5
Sex (male/female)		15/5	5/6	26/18	28/10
Ethnicity, n	*				
White		11	5	28	20
Black		3	4	8	6
Hispanic		5	0	7	6
Other		1	2	1	6
Lab findings at enrollment					
sCr, mg/dl	*	2.67 ± 0.43	1.29 ± 0.12	0.81 ± 0.05	0.9 ± 0.04
eGFR, ml/min	*	44.4 ± 7.3	60.9 ± 5.7	98.2 ± 4.9	97.5 ± 3.5
uCr/sCr, ratio	*	42.4 ± 7.2	83.3 ± 18.1	106.6 ± 18.3	119.6 ± 5.2
Urine kallikrein (U/gm creatinine)	*	6.74 ± 1.92	1.17 ± 0.16	2.04 ± 0.47	0.63 ± 0.08
Vital signs at enrollment					
Systolic BP, mmHg	0.08	119.8 ± 4.4	126.9 ± 8.7	124.3 ± 3.4	131.4 ± 1.7
Diastolic BP, mmHg	*	70.7 ± 3.4	61.8 ± 5.1	68.6 ± 2.3	74.7 ± 1.5
Heart rate, beats/min	*	89.3 ± 3.6	86.5 ± 7.4	81.3 ± 2.4	68.0 ± 1.6
Co-morbid conditions (Y/N)					
Diabetes mellitus		6/14	6/5	12/32	0/38
Hypertension	*	10/10	8/3	20/22	8/30
Coronary artery disease		1/19	4/7	10/34	0/38
Congestive heart failure	*	0/20	3/8	4/40	0/38
Chronic liver disease	*	6/14	0/11	4/40	0/38
Chronic lung disease	*	4/16	3/8	7/37	0/38
Chronic kidney disease	*	8/12	3/8	1/43	0/38
HIV positive		2/18	0/11	3/41	0/38
Malignancy		3/17	1/10	12/32	0/38
Smoker	*	8/12	3/8	16/28	4/34

TABLE 1: *Cont.*

	P < 0.05 (*)	AKI		Controls	
		Established	Incipient (early, ICU)	ICU	Healthy (non-hospital)
Characteristics		n = 20	n = 11	n = 44	n = 38
Primary treating service, n					
Medical/Surgical		14/6	11/0	34/10	-
Other characteristics while hospitalized (Y/N)					
ICU admission	*	13/7	11/0	44/0	-
Ventilator at enrollment		5/15	3/8	13/31	-
Pressor infusions	*	3/17	9/2	12/32	-
Norepinephrine	*	2/18	8/3	11/33	-
Epinephrine + dopamine	*	1/19	9/2	12/32	-
Diuretics at enrollment	*	3/17	5/6	2/42	-
AKI outcomes					
Required dialysis for AKI		3/17	1/10	-	-
Recovery from AKI	*	17/3	11/0	-	-
Remained dialysis-dependent at follow-up		1/19	0/11	-	-
Final eGFR at follow-up		66.5 ± 8.0	76.6 ± 5.5	-	-
eGFR Δ at follow-up		+16.5 ± 2.2	+22.2 ± 5.4	-	-
sCr Δ at follow-up	0.08	-1.0 ± 0.3	-0.25 ± 0.05	-	-

ICU = intensive care unit, AKI = acute kidney injury, n = number of study subjects, BMI = body mass index, s = serum, u = urine, Cr = creatinine, FeNa+ = fractional excretion of sodium, SBP = systolic blood pressure, DBP = diastolic blood pressure, HR = heart rate, bpm = beats per minute. Δ = change at discharge (from initial value). *P values calculated with Fisher's exact test for categorical variables and ANOVA (log-transformed and covariates adjusted: age, sex) for continuous variables. *: Symbol indicates $P \leq 0.05$ comparing across all available groups. Recovery of renal function was the primary outcome, defined as a return to within 10% of baseline eGFR or lowest eGFR prior to AKI event. Plus-minus values are mean ± SEM.

As compared to healthy/outpatient controls (Table 1, Figure 2), ICU/ inpatient controls displayed unaltered eGFR, though a modest ~3.2-fold increase in urinary KLK1 excretion. ICU subjects with incipient AKI had a modest fall in eGFR (down ~38% compared to ICU controls), coupled

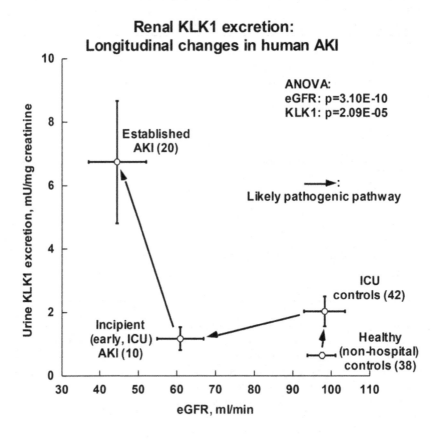

FIGURE 2: Urinary kallikrein activity in AKI: Cases versus controls. Results are shown for both KLK1 excretion and eGFR in 4 groups: established AKI, incipient (early, ICU) AKI, ICU controls, and healthy (non-hospital) controls. Results (shown as mean ± 1 SEM) were analyzed by ANOVA, factoring for age, sex and race.

with a ~43% fall in KLK1 excretion. However, subjects with established (more severe) AKI exhibited a ~6.9-fold increase in KLK1 excretion (p = 2.09E-05), coupled with a further ~27% fall in eGFR (p = 3.10E-10).

1.3.2 ESTABLISHED AKI: CLINICAL CHARACTERISTICS

We then turned our attention to clinical features (Table 2) of the AKI subjects that might account for the KLK1 elevation. In clinical laboratory findings at study enrollment (entry), patients with AKI had significantly higher serum creatinine (2.67 ± 0.43 vs. 0.9 ± 0.04 mg/dl; p < 0.001), and fractional excretion of sodium (FeNa+; 1.7 ± 0.4 vs. 0.8 ± 0.06%; p = 0.05), than healthy controls, with lower eGFR (44.4 ± 7.5 vs. 97.5 ± 3.6 ml/min; p = 0.0001).

At study enrollment, AKI patients had lower SBP (119.8 ± 4.4 vs. 131.4 ± 1.7 mmHg; p = 0.02) and higher heart rate (89.3 ± 3.6 vs. 68.0 ± 1.6 beats/min; p = 1.73E-05) than healthy controls. Within the AKI group (n = 20), acute kidney injury was attributed to ischemia in 7 patients, nephrotoxins in 4, sepsis in 1, and multifactorial causes in 8 (Table 2); KLK1 excretion did not vary by AKI causal group (ANOVA p = 0.83). Six patients had diabetes mellitus, 10 had hypertension, 1 had coronary artery disease, 6 had chronic liver disease, 4 had chronic lung disease, 8 had chronic kidney disease (previous eGFR < 60 ml/min), 13 required admission to an ICU during hospitalization, 5 required mechanical ventilation at enrollment, and 5 had oliguria at enrollment. At study entry, 3 patients required infusion of vasopressors (2 norepinephrine, 1 dopamine and epinephrine combination), and 3 took diuretics (2 furosemide, 1 thiazide). In the evaluation of primary outcome, 17 patients attained recovery of renal function (see Methods) at 6 months of follow-up (Table 1).

1.3.3 ESTABLISHED AKI: KALLIKREIN, CATECHOLAMINES, AND ALDOSTERONE

Here we probed potential hormonal mechanisms whereby KLK1 excretion was elevated in established AKI, focusing on such known KLK1 stimulators as catecholamines [19] and aldosterone.

TABLE 2: Mechanistic studies: Characteristics of the AKI study subjects versus healthy controls

Characteristics	Established AKI patients (n = 20)	Healthy controls (n = 38)	P value*
Age, years	48.8 ± 3.5	46.3 ± 1.5	0.52
Sex (male/female), n	15/5	30/8	1
Ethnicity, n			0.6
White	11	20	
Black	3	6	
Hispanic	5	6	
Other	1	6	
Weight, kg	91.2 ± 6.2	93.9 ± 3.7	0.293
BMI, kg/m^2	31.1 ± 2.2	27.8 ± 1	0.177
Laboratory findings at enrollment			
sCr, mg/dl	2.7 ± 0.47	0.9 ± 0.04	0.0007
eGFR, ml/min	44.4 ± 7.5	97.5 ± 3.6	< 0.0001
uNa+/uCr, mEq/gm	127.6 ± 22.5	125.4 ± 9.4	0.347
uCr/sCr, ratio	42.4 ± 7.2	119.6 ± 11.4	< 0.0001
FeNa+, %	1.7 ± 0.4	0.8 ± 0.1	0.05
Vital signs at enrollment			
Systolic BP, mmHg	119.8 ± 4.4	131.4 ± 1.7	0.02
Diastolic BP, mmHg	70.7 ± 3.4	74.7 ± 1.5	0.3
Heart rate, beats/min	89.3 ± 3.6	68.0 ± 1.6	< 0.0001
Contributing causes to AKI, n (with urine KLK1 activity excretion, U/gm creatinine, mean ± SEM)		0.83	
Ischemia	7 (6.0 ± 3.7)	-	-
Nephrotoxins	4 (7.2 ± 3.9)	-	-
Septic	1 (4.6)	-	-
Multifactorial causes/other	8 (7.6 ± 2.9)	-	-

AKI = acute kidney injury, n = number of study subjects, BMI = body mass index, s = serum, u = urine, Cr = creatinine, FeNa+ = fractional excretion of sodium, SBP = systolic blood pressure, DBP = diastolic blood pressure, HR = heart rate, bpm = beats per minute, ICU = intensive care unit. *P values were calculated with Fisher's exact test for categorical variables, and ANOVA (log-transformed, adjusted for covariates: age, sex) for continuous variables. Plus-minus values are mean ± one SEM. Bold: $p \leq 0.05$.

TABLE 3: Mechanistic studies: Urinary biochemistries in established AKI cases versus healthy controls

	AKI patients	n available	Healthy controls	n available	T-test P	ANOVA P†	Wilcoxon rank P
Urine kallikrein (U/gm creatinine)	6.74 ± 1.92	18	0.63 ± 0.08	37	0.0058	0.00029	0.0012
Urine aldosterone (pg/mg creatinine)	9269.9 ± 2652.31	16	12982.4 ± 2619.78	38	0.325	0.65	0.1282
Urine epinephrine (ng/mg creatinine)	20.1 ± 2.4	14	7.48 ± 1.07	32	1.11E-06	0.00016	1.79E-05
Urine norepinephrine, (ng/mg creatinine)	37.15 ± 8.14	14	26.85 ± 3.2	32	0.344	0.16	0.4424
Urine kallikrein/ urine aldosterone ratio (mU/μg)	872.0 ± 277.5	15	160.5 ± 76.7	38	0.00027	8.45E-05	3.62E-05
Urine kallikrein/ urine epinephrine ratio (mU/ng)	0.32 ± 0.13	13	0.18 ± 0.04	31	0.8465	0.8	0.899

Plus-minus values are covariate-adjusted mean ± one SEM. N is the number of study subjects available to conduct each experiment. †Results are analyzed by one-way ANOVA, factoring for age, sex and race. Bold: $p ≤ 0.05$.

1.3.4 URINARY KALLIKREIN ENZYMATIC ACTIVITY

From the 20 established AKI patients and 38 healthy controls, urine was available for kallikrein measurement (Table 3) in 18 patients and 37 controls. Unexpectedly, established AKI subjects displayed substantially elevated kallikrein excretion (Figure 2, Table 1), about ~10 times higher than that of controls (activity: 6132.9 ± 2302 vs. 623.0 ± 88.2 mU/L, $p < 0.001$; urine kallikrein activity/creatinine ratio: 6.74 ± 1.92 vs. 0.63 ± 0.08 U/gm, $p < 0.001$). To exclude the possibility that diuretic treatment at study entry increased urinary kallikrein excretion [20], we conducted statistical analysis again by exclusion of the 3 diuretic cases (Tables 1); urinary kallikrein excretion remained significantly different between AKI and controls (urine kallikrein/urine creatinine ratio: 7.14 ± 2.18 vs. 0.63 ± 0.08 mU/mg; p = 0.001). We measured the urinary non-kallikrein amidolytic activity (likely urokinase) by inclusion or exclusion of the kallikrein inhibitor aprotinin. The percentage of kallikrein activity within total S-2266 amidolytic activity was not different between AKI patients and controls (78.0 ± 4.8% vs. 69.0 ± 2.4%; p = 0.072).

Since black and white subjects differ in reported KLK1 excretion [5,15], we evaluated the role of ethnicity in our samples (Table 1). Although cases and controls each included several biogeographic ancestries, KLK1 excretion did not differ significantly in black versus white cases (p = 0.26) or black versus white controls (p = 0.69), perhaps reflecting the relatively small sample sizes. Disease analyses were adjusted for biogeographic ancestry as a covariate.

1.3.5 URINARY ALDOSTERONE AND CATECHOLAMINE EXCRETIONS

We measured urinary aldosterone, epinephrine and norepinephrine excretions (Table 3), since these hormones are known to increase urinary kallikrein. Established AKI subjects exhibited substantially elevated epinephrine excretion, ~2.7 times higher than that of healthy controls (Table 3, Figure 3; 20.1 ± 2.4 vs. 7.48 ± 1.07 ng/mg creatinine; ANOVA p = 0.00016). Urinary kallikrein/epinephrine ratio did not differ between groups (Table 3); parallel elevations of KLK1 and epinephrine suggest that the epinephrine excess in AKI may be sufficient to account for the increased KLK1. To exclude the possibility that epinephrine infusion (in one case, Tables 1) increased urinary excretion, in a subsequent analysis we excluded that case, but urinary epinephrine remained different between AKI and controls (19.99 ± 2.62 vs. 7.48 ± 1.07 ng/mg creatinine; ANOVA p = 0.001). Indeed, Figure 3 illustrates parallel elevations of renal kallikrein and epinephrine excretion in the AKI group.

Urinary aldosterone excretion did not differ between established AKI and healthy controls (Table 3) (9269.9 ± 2652.31 vs. 12982.4 ± 2619.78 pg/mg creatinine; ANOVA p = 0.65). Since urinary kallikrein/aldosterone

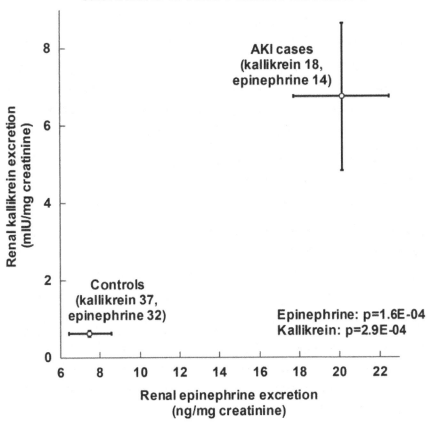

FIGURE 3: Coordinate effects of AKI on kallikrein and epinephrine excretion. Results (shown as mean ± 1 SEM) were analyzed by one-way ANOVA, factoring for age, sex and race. The numbers studied for kallikrein are 18 established AKI patients and 37 healthy controls. The numbers studied for epinephrine are 14 established AKI patients and 32 healthy controls.

ratio was also elevated in AKI (Table 3), increments in aldosterone could not explain the rise in KLK1 excretion in AKI. Urinary norepinephrine excretion did not differ in AKI (Table 3) (37.15 ± 8.14 vs. 26.85 ± 3.20 ng/ mg creatinine; ANOVA $p = 0.16$); nor did urine kallikrein/norepinephrine excretion ratios.

1.3.6 URINE ALBUMIN EXCRETION

Quantitative urine albumin excretion was evaluated in established AKI cases and healthy controls. Albumin values in cases ranged from 2.0-4490 mg/gm creatinine (mean, 1090 mg/gm), but kallikrein and albumin excretions did not correlate (Pearson $r = 0.006$, $p = 0.54$), rendering it unlikely that elevated kallikrein activity in AKI arose simply from pathological excretion of plasma proteases. In healthy controls, albumin excretion was 6.27 ± 0.39 mg/gm creatinine.

1.3.7 ICU CONTROLS: URINARY KALLIKREIN ACTIVITY AND CLINICAL FINDINGS

44 "ICU controls" were available to evaluate the specificity of urinary kallikrein elevation in AKI. Table 1 shows demographic, laboratory and clinical findings of these ICU controls. The kallikrein increment in AKI persisted when studied with ICU controls (6.74 ± 1.92 vs. 2.04 ± 0.47 U/ gm creatinine; $p = 0.028$), though kallikrein excretion was modestly elevated in ICU- compared to healthy controls (2.04 ± 0.47 vs. 0.63 ± 0.08 U/gm creatinine; $p = 0.005$).

Compared with established AKI, ICU controls had significantly lower serum creatinine (0.81 ± 0.05 vs. 2.67 ± 0.43 mg/dl; $p = 0.0005$). Compared with healthy controls, ICU controls were older (54.2 ± 2.2 vs. 46.3 ± 1.5 years; $p = 0.005$), with higher heart rate (81.3 ± 2.4 vs. 68.0 ± 1.6 bpm; $p < 0.0001$), but lower DBP (68.6 ± 2.3 vs. 74.7 ± 1.5 mmHg; $p = 0.029$). Even though not significantly different, SBPs of ICU controls tended to be lower than those in healthy controls (124.3 ± 3.4 vs. 131.4 ± 1.7 mmHg; $p = 0.066$). The ICU controls had variable primary diseases (Table 1). 13

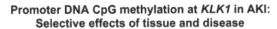

Promoter DNA CpG methylation at *KLK1* in AKI:
Selective effects of tissue and disease

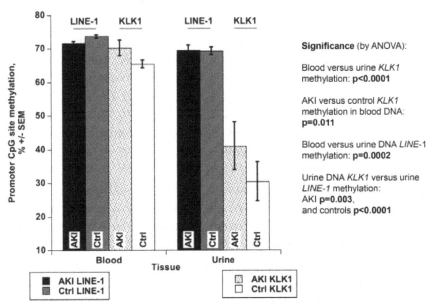

Significance (by ANOVA):

Blood versus urine *KLK1*
methylation: **p<0.0001**

AKI versus control *KLK1*
methylation in blood DNA:
p=0.011

Blood versus urine DNA *LINE*-1
methylation: **p=0.0002**

Urine DNA *KLK1* versus urine
LINE-1 methylation:
AKI **p=0.003**,
and controls **p<0.0001**

FIGURE 4: CpG methylation analyzed by bisulfite sequencing: Results at the KLK1 promoter, as well as a global control (LINE-1 repetitive elements), in genomic DNA from urine or blood (mononuclear cells). Results (shown as mean ± one SEM), from established AKI cases or healthy controls, were analyzed by ANOVA, factoring for age, sex and race. LINE-1 reagents (Pyromark, Biotage) were used to analyze the 3 CpG sites in LINE-1 repetitive elements, while the KLK1 gene was analyzed by a separate PCR covering 4 promoter CpGs. Promoter KLK1 specific methylation was substantially higher in blood than urine DNA (blood 66.38 ± 1.00 vs. urine $33.43 \pm 4.67\%$; ANOVA p < 0.0001). Promoter KLK1 methylation in blood DNA was higher in AKI than controls (AKI, 70.32 ± 2.27 vs. controls, $65.36 \pm 1.05\%$; ANOVA p = 0.011). Promoter KLK1 methylation in urine DNA did not differ in AKI versus controls (AKI, 40.95 ± 7.06 vs. controls, $30.35 \pm 5.88\%$; ANOVA p = 0.22). Global LINE-1 methylation was greater in both blood than urine DNA (blood 73.11 ± 0.38 vs. urine $69.37 \pm 0.86\%$, p = 0.0002). LINE-1 methylation in blood DNA did not differ in AKI and controls (AKI, 71.71 ± 0.44 vs. controls, $73.67 \pm 0.41\%$; ANOVA p = 0.08). LINE-1 methylation in urine DNA did not differ in cases/controls (AKI, 69.53 ± 1.54 vs. controls, $69.29 \pm 1.05\%$; ANOVA p = 0.79).

among them required mechanical ventilation, while 12 required vasopressor infusion during ICU admission (Table 1).

1.3.8 KLK1 *PROMOTER DNA CPG METHYLATION PATTERNS*

KLK1 promoter CpG methylation (positions in Figure 1) was studied in established AKI and healthy controls. Promoter KLK1 CpG methylation (Figure 4) was higher in blood than urine DNA (blood 66.38 ± 1.00 vs. urine $33.43 \pm 4.67\%$; ANOVA p < 0.0001). Promoter KLK1 methylation in blood DNA was also higher in AKI than controls (70.32 ± 2.27 vs. $65.36 \pm 1.05\%$; ANOVA p = 0.011), while promoter *KLK1* methylation in urine DNA trended to be higher in AKI than controls (40.95 ± 7.06 vs. $30.35 \pm 5.88\%$; ANOVA p = 0.22; Figure 4).

Global CpG methylation, examined by LINE-1, was high in both blood and urine, though even higher in blood (blood 73.11 ± 0.38 vs. urine $69.37 \pm 0.86\%$, p = 0.0002). LINE-1 CpG methylation in blood DNA was similar between AKI and controls (71.71 ± 0.44 vs. $73.67 \pm 0.41\%$; ANOVA p = 0.08), as was LINE-1 methylation in urine DNA (AKI 69.53 ± 1.54 vs. control $69.29 \pm 1.05\%$; ANOVA p = 0.79) (Figure 4). In AKI blood DNA, *KLK1*-specific methylation was similar to global LINE-1 methylation (70.32 ± 2.27 vs. $71.71 \pm 0.44\%$; p = 0.56). In controls, however, *KLK1* CpG methylation in blood DNA was significantly lower than global LINE-1 methylation in blood DNA (65.36 ± 1.05 vs. $73.67 \pm 0.41\%$; p < 0.0001) (Figure 4). In both AKI and controls, *KLK1* specific methylation in urine DNA was significantly lower than global LINE-1 methylation in urine DNA (AKI 40.95 ± 7.06 vs. $69.53 \pm 1.54\%$; p = 0.003; controls 30.35 ± 5.88 vs. $69.29 \pm 1.05\%$; p < 0.0001) (Figure 4).

Urine *KLK1* promoter CpG methylation did not predict KLK1 activity excretion. However, in a multivariate analysis, disease status jointly predicted both *KLK1* promoter methylation and enzyme activity excretion, with higher values for each in cases (multivariate p = 0.004; Figure 5. Since increased *KLK1* promoter methylation would be predicted to decrease gene expression, this joint effect cannot explain (and indeed runs counter to) the elevated KLK1 excretion observed in our AKI cases (Figure 5).

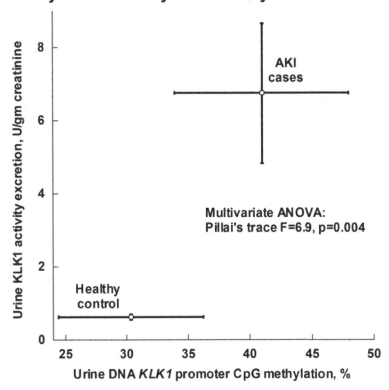

FIGURE 5: AKI: Coordinate effects of disease on KLK1 promoter CpG methylation and KLK1 enzymatic activity excretion in urine. The multivariate analysis compared established AKI cases with healthy controls.

1.4 DISCUSSION

1.4.1 OVERVIEW

Several previous lines of investigation link alterations in KLK1 expression to AKI, in both experimental animals and humans. A decrease in urinary kallikrein excretion occurs in rodents with AKI after methemoglobin [21]; rats treated with aminoglycosides have dramatically reduced levels of urinary kallikrein [6], and a transient decrease in urinary kallikrein excretion occurs during chromate-induced AKI in the rat [22]. Renal kallikrein mRNA expression was specifically reduced in the post-ischemic rodent kidney, with persistently altered expression even after functional recovery from ischemic acute renal failure [23]. In humans, we reported previously that urinary kallikrein excretion was diminished in acute tubular necrosis (ATN) after renal transplantation [9].

Studies in rodents suggest beneficial effects of exogenous KLK1 replacement in the setting of experimental AKI. *KLK1* gene transfer protected against aminoglycoside-induced nephropathy, with inhibition of apoptosis and inflammation [7]. *KLK1* replacement after gentamicin attenuated drug-induced renal dysfunction, cortical damage, and apoptosis in the rat [8]. Furthermore, KLK1 reduced gentamicin-induced renal dysfunction and fibrosis, with decreased myofibroblast and collagen accumulation [8]. These findings indicate that the renal kallikrein/kinin system prevents and promotes recovery of aminoglycoside-induced renal injury by inhibiting apoptosis, inflammatory cell recruitment, and fibrotic lesions.

Thus, we expected that AKI patients would have diminished urinary kallikrein excretion, since urinary kallikrein originates in the kidney; further, we anticipated that kallikrein increments might be associated with superior outcomes in AKI. Unexpectedly our established AKI subjects displayed substantially elevated (by as much as ~11-fold; ANOVA p = 0.00029; Figure 2; Tables 1,3) kallikrein excretion.

1.4.2 ORIGIN OF INCREASED KLK1 EXCRETION IN ESTABLISHED AKI

Although previous reports of KLK1 excretion in AKI indicated diminished excretion in both rodent models [6,21,22] and AKI/ATN in the setting of human renal transplantation [9], we noted a ~11-fold elevation of KLK1 excretion in our established AKI subjects (Tables 1-3; Figure 2). Why might KLK1 excretion be elevated in human AKI? Here we examined hormonal factors known to increase KLK1 excretion: catecholamines and aldosterone [5,19,20,24-26]. We found that an elevation in epinephrine excretion paralleled that for kallikrein (Figure 3), while norepinephrine and aldosterone excretions were unchanged (Table 3). In experimental animals, kallikrein excretion is regulated by adrenergic receptors, with stimulation by β-receptors and inhibition by α-receptors [19]. While diuretics can also elevate kallikrein excretion [20,27], the KLK1 excretion increment in AKI persisted after exclusion of the 3 subjects on diuretics.

Why was epinephrine elevated in our AKI subjects? AKI patients had lower systolic BP than controls (119.8 ± 4.4 vs. 131.4 ± 1.7 mmHg; $p = 0.02$) and higher heart rate (89.3 ± 3.6 vs. 68.0 ± 1.6 bpm; $p = 1.73E\text{-}05$) (Table 2). While the mechanism cannot be readily probed in the setting of acute human illness, we suspect that that lower BP in AKI may stimulate baroreceptors, with resulting increase in endogenous production of epinephrine, and consequently increased heart rate and kallikrein excretion (Figure 6).

1.4.3 KLK1 EPIGENETICS

Promoter *KLK1* specific CpG methylation was higher in blood than urine DNA (blood 66.38 ± 1.00 vs. urine $33.43 \pm 4.67\%$; ANOVA $p < 0.0001$; Figure 4), consistent with kidney-specific expression of the *KLK1* gene, in that renal kallikrein is synthesized in the distal tubule and released into urine and peritubular interstitium [20], and cytosine methylation results in transcriptional repression either by interfering with transcription factor binding or by inducing a repressive chromatin structure [11].

**Human AKI: Hypothetical schema for steps
eventuating in increased renal kallikrein (KLK1) excretion**

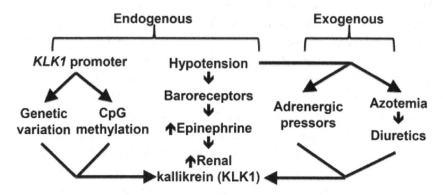

FIGURE 6: Hypothetical schema integrating experimental findings in this study of KLK1 in AKI. This diagram is presented not as established fact, but rather to generate hypotheses for further investigation. Endogenous factors may influence KLK1 synthesis and renal excretion: lower BP in AKI may activate baroreceptors, thus increasing endogenous secretion of epinephrine, thereby increasing both heart rate and urinary kallikrein excretion. KLK1 promoter genetic variants or CpG methylation can influence renal kallikrein production. Finally, exogenous factors such as adrenergic pressor infusions or diuretic treatment can also increase renal kallikrein production; indeed, since a subset of our AKI cases received such treatments (Table 1), we cannot exclude this possibility.

KLK1 promoter methylation in blood DNA was higher in AKI than controls (70.32 ± 2.27 vs. 65.36 ± 1.05%; p = 0.011), and there was also a trend towards higher urine *KLK1* methylation in AKI than controls, but the difference was not significant (40.95 ± 7.06 vs. 30.35 ± 5.88%; p = 0.22). While a multivariate analysis indicated a joint effect of AKI on both KLK1 excretion and urine *KLK1* CpG methylation (Figure 5), elevated *KLK1* methylation would be predicted to decrease KLK1 excretion in AKI, as occurs in early/incipient AKI (Figure 2). Increased KLK1 excretion in later/established AKI (Figure 2) thus highlights the influence of epinephrine (Figure 3) to elevate KLK1, even in the face of opposing epigenetic influence.

LINE-1 methylation results enabled comparisons of *KLK1* to global genomic patterns of CpG methylation [18]. In AKI blood DNA, *KLK1*-specific methylation was similar to global LINE-1 methylation (70.32 ± 2.27 vs. 71.71 ± 0.44%; p = 0.56). In control blood DNA, however, *KLK1*-specific methylation was lower than global LINE-1 methylation (65.36 ± 1.05 vs. 73.67 ± 0.41%; p < 0.0001) (Figure 4).

We investigated the 4 most proximal consecutive CpG sites in *KLK1* promoter (Figure 1). This proximal promoter region is unusually polymorphic, containing a poly-guanine length polymorphism coupled with multiple base-substitution variants that constitute at least ten different alleles or haplotypes [28]. Functional/transfection analysis of several alleles in this region suggests that different variants lead to alterations in expression of the *KLK1* gene [29]. Since genetic variation may contribute to AKI susceptibility [30], this hypothesis warrants future studies of *KLK1* promoter variants in larger cohorts, assessing the effects of such variants on both susceptibility and recovery in AKI, since exogenous KLK1 does exert protective effects against aminoglycoside-induced AKI [7,8].

It should be noted that the sources of DNA for these epigenetic studies in blood and urine are likely to be heterogeneous—blood DNA could emerge from any leukocyte subpopulation, while DNA in urine can emerge from cell types other than renal. Nor have we established whether the promoter CpG methylation events we observed have functional consequences for transcription.

1.4.4 ADVANTAGES AND LIMITATIONS OF THIS STUDY

Our conclusions are derived from analysis of four subject groups (Figure 2): two degrees of AKI (established versus incipient/early), and two kinds of controls (ICU versus healthy/non-hospital). Furthermore, we were able to probe clinical and biochemical characteristics of cases and controls to identify elevated epinephrine as a likely driver of increased KLK1 excretion (Figure 3, Table 3). While we were able to evaluate epigenetic factors in control of KLK1 excretion in the form of promoter CpG methylation (Figures 1, 4), we did not study other epigenetic mechanisms, such as histone modifications, nor could we probe gene expression more directly by evaluating transcript abundance in tissue, since biopsies would have been hazardous. Furthermore, the established AKI cases were ascertained at a later time point than either AKI cases or controls in the ICU cohorts. Finally, the results would benefit from replication, given the numbers of subjects studied (Figure 2, Table 1), as well as evaluation of additional mediators of AKI risk and repair.

1.5 CONCLUSIONS

In conclusion, human patients with established AKI display an unexpected increase in urinary KLK1 enzymatic activity excretion (Figure 2); the effect is reproducible across control groups, and seems to be driven by epinephrine excess in the setting of hemodynamic instability (Figures 3, 6). AKI and controls differed in *KLK1* promoter CpG methylation in blood DNA (AKI > controls), and *KLK1* CpG methylation differed systematically from global control (LINE-1 element) methylation, suggesting a potential role of epigenetic factors in AKI susceptibility (Figure 4).

REFERENCES

1.   Mehta RL, Pascual MT, Soroko S, Savage BR, Himmelfarb J, Ikizler TA, Paganini EP, Chertow GM: Spectrum of acute renal failure in the intensive care unit: the PICARD experience. Kidney Int 2004, 66(4):1613-1621.
2.   Nash K, Hafeez A, Hou S: Hospital-acquired renal insufficiency. Am J Kidney Dis 2002, 39(5):930-936.
3.   Nony PA, Schnellmann RG: Mechanisms of renal cell repair and regeneration after acute renal failure. J Pharmacol Exp Ther 2003, 304(3):905-912.
4.   Liu KD, Brakeman PR: Renal repair and recovery. Crit Care Med 2008, 36(4 Suppl):S187-192.
5.   Song CK, Martinez JA, Kailasam MT, Dao TT, Wong CM, Parmer RJ, O'Connor DT: Renal kallikrein excretion: role of ethnicity, gender, environment, and genetic risk of hypertension. J Hum Hypertens 2000, 14(7):461-468.
6.   Higa EM, Schor N, Boim MA, Ajzen H, Ramos OL: Role of the prostaglandin and kallikrein-kinin systems in aminoglycoside-induced acute renal failure. Braz J Med Biol Res 1985, 18(3):355-365.
7.   Bledsoe G, Crickman S, Mao J, Xia CF, Murakami H, Chao L, Chao J: Kallikrein/ kinin protects against gentamicin-induced nephrotoxicity by inhibition of inflammation and apoptosis. Nephrol Dial Transplant 2006, 21(3):624-633.

8. Bledsoe G, Shen B, Yao YY, Hagiwara M, Mizell B, Teuton M, Grass D, Chao L, Chao J: Role of tissue kallikrein in prevention and recovery of gentamicin-induced renal injury. Toxicol Sci 2008, 102(2):433-443.

9. O'Connor DT, Barg AP, Amend W, Vincenti F: Urinary kallikrein excretion after renal transplantation: relationship to hypertension, graft source, and renal function. Am J Med 1982, 73(4):475-481.

10. Weber M, Davies JJ, Wittig D, Oakeley EJ, Haase M, Lam WL, Schubeler D: Chromosome-wide and promoter-specific analyses identify sites of differential DNA methylation in normal and transformed human cells. Nat Genet 2005, 37(8):853-862.

11. Jaenisch R, Bird A: Epigenetic regulation of gene expression: how the genome integrates intrinsic and environmental signals. Nat Genet 2003, 33(Suppl):245-254.

12. Jones PA: Cancer. Death and methylation. Nature 2001, 409(6817):143-144.

13. Mehta RL, Kellum JA, Shah SV, Molitoris BA, Ronco C, Warnock DG, Levin A: Acute Kidney Injury Network: report of an initiative to improve outcomes in acute kidney injury. Crit Care 2007, 11(2):R31.

14. Cockburn M, Hamilton A, Zadnick J, Cozen W, Mack TM: The occurrence of chronic disease and other conditions in a large population-based cohort of native Californian twins. Twin Res 2002, 5(5):460-467.

15. Wong CM, O'Connor DT, Martinez JA, Kailasam MT, Parmer RJ: Diminished renal kallikrein responses to mineralocorticoid stimulation in African Americans: determinants of an intermediate phenotype for hypertension. Am J Hypertens 2003, 16(4):281-289.

16. Brakensiek K, Wingen LU, Langer F, Kreipe H, Lehmann U: Quantitative high-resolution CpG island mapping with Pyrosequencing reveals disease-specific methylation patterns of the CDKN2B gene in myelodysplastic syndrome and myeloid leukemia. Clin Chem 2007, 53(1):17-23.

17. Gonzalgo ML, Liang G: Methylation-sensitive single-nucleotide primer extension (Ms-SNuPE) for quantitative measurement of DNA methylation. Nat Protoc 2007, 2(8):1931-1936.

18. Yang AS, Estecio MR, Doshi K, Kondo Y, Tajara EH, Issa JP: A simple method for estimating global DNA methylation using bisulfite PCR of repetitive DNA elements. Nucleic Acids Res 2004, 32(3):e38.

19. Olsen UB: Changes of Urinary Kallikrein and Kinin Excretions Induced by Adrenaline Infusion in Conscious Dogs. Scand J Clin Lab Inv 1980, 40(2):173-178.

20. O'Connor DT: Response of the renal kallikrein-kinin system, intravascular volume, and renal hemodynamics to sodium restriction and diuretic treatment in essential hypertension. Hypertension 1982, 4(5 Pt 2):III72-78.

21. Martin R, Nesse A, de Muchnik EE: Urinary kallikrein and pathophysiology of acute renal failure in the rat. Medicina (B Aires) 1976, 36(3):223-228.

22. Girolami JP, Orfila C, Pecher C, Cabos-Boutot G, Bascands JL, Moatti JP, Adam A, Colle A: Inverse relationship between renal and urinary kallikrein during chromate-induced acute renal failure in rat: urinary kallikrein excretion as a possible recovery index. Biol Chem Hoppe Seyler 1989, 370(12):1305-1313.

23. Basile DP, Fredrich K, Alausa M, Vio CP, Liang M, Rieder MR, Greene AS, Cowley AW Jr: Identification of persistently altered gene expression in the kidney after

functional recovery from ischemic acute renal failure. Am J Physiol Renal Physiol 2005, 288(5):F953-963.

24. Ohman KP: Circulating kallikreins in normotensive and hypertensive humans: effects of mineralocorticoid administration. Blood Press 1997, 6(4):214-222.

25. O'Connor DT, Preston RA: Urinary kallikrein activity, renal hemodynamics, and electrolyte handling during chronic beta blockade with propranolol in hypertension. Hypertension 1982, 4(5):742-749.

26. Yasujima M, Abe K, Tanno M, Sato K, Kasai Y, Seino M, Chiba S, Goto T, Omata K, Tajima J, et al.: Chronic Effects of Norepinephrine and Vasopressin on Urinary Prostaglandin-E and Kallikrein Excretions in Conscious Rats. Clin Exp Hypertens A 1984, 6(7):1297-1310.

27. Olshan AR, O'Connor DT, Preston RA, Frigon RP, Stone RA: Involvement of kallikrein in the antihypertensive response to furosemide in essential hypertension. J Cardiovasc Pharmacol 1981, 3(1):161-167.

28. Hua H, Zhou S, Liu Y, Wang Z, Wan C, Li H, Chen C, Li G, Zeng C, Chen L, et al.: Relationship between the regulatory region polymorphism of human tissue kallikrein gene and essential hypertension. J Hum Hypertens 2005, 19(9):715-721.

29. Song Q, Chao J, Chao L: DNA polymorphisms in the 5'-flanking region of the human tissue kallikrein gene. Hum Genet 1997, 99(6):727-734.

30. Alam A, O'Connor DT, Perianayagam MC, Kolyada AY, Chen Y, Rao F, Mahata M, Mahata S, Liangos O, Jaber BL: Phenylethanolamine N-methyltransferase gene polymorphisms and adverse outcomes in acute kidney injury. Nephron Clin Pract 2010, 114(4):c253-259.

CHAPTER 2

COX-2 GENE EXPRESSION IN COLON CANCER TISSUE RELATED TO REGULATING FACTORS AND PROMOTER METHYLATION STATUS

ANNIKA GUSTAFSSON ASTING, HELENA CARÉN,
MARIANNE ANDERSSON, CHRISTINA LLINNROTH,
KRISTINA LAGERSTEDT, AND KENT LUNDHOLM

2.1 BACKGROUND

Colorectal cancer is common in Western countries with unanimous findings that prostaglandins are important for both carcinogenesis and progression [1-3]. It has been repeatedly observed that Cyclooxygenase-1/-2 inhibition attenuates appearance of epithelial cancer in experimental models and in part also in patients. Both primary and secondary prevention with cyclooxygenase (COX) inhibitors demonstrate and confirm decreased incidence of colorectal carcinoma in both retrospective and randomized patient cohorts [4-7]. Thus, a large number of observations emphasize that induced prostaglandin production, particularly PGE_2, is involved in cell signaling through prostanoid receptors, where our own observations suggested subtype EP_2 receptor expression in colon cancer tissue to predict reduced survival [2]. An important issue behind the appearance and progression of colorectal cancer seems to be increased production of PGE_2 secondary to COX-2 induction in both transformed epithelial cells and host stroma [2,4,8-11]. Mechanisms behind COX-2 gene induction in colorectal cancer disease remain elusive, although a lot of information is available on the regulation of COX-2 gene expression [12,13]. Most such information has, however, been obtained in isolated cell culture experiments with obvious limitations compared to the in vivo situation based on uninterrupted host and tumor cell signaling. Therefore, the aim of the present study was to relate well-recognized external cell- and transcription factor expression to elevated tumor COX-2 expression in colorectal cancer tissue at primary operations aimed at cure.

2.2 METHODS

2.2.1 PATIENTS

Tumor and colon tissue samples were collected from 48 unselected patients at primary operation for colorectal carcinoma between 2001 to 2004 in Uddevalla county of Sweden. All patients underwent surgery as the only curative treatment and none received neoadjuvant radio-chemotherapy, according to individual decisions and institutional indications. Normal colon tissue was collected as a minimum of 10 cm away from the macroscopically seen tumor tissue. The group of patients consisted of 54% males and 46% females with a mean age of 72.5 years (range 40 to 91 years) at surgery. Mean survival time was 27.3 ± 4.2 months (range 0 to 73 months) following surgery according to a recent update of survival (Dec 2008), where 21 patients were still alive. Tumors were histologically classified as Dukes A (8), Dukes B (19), Dukes C (11) and Dukes D (10). PCR analysis was performed to quantify COX-2 mRNA expression [2]. Mean COX-2 expression in tumor tissue for the entire group was 6.27 ± 0.60 mol/mol GAPDH (range 0.11 to 24.67) (n = 48) and 14.6 ± 1.7 (range 1.7 to 38.08) (n = 29) in normal colon tissue. Patients used in subsequent experiments were selected according to COX-2 expression in tumors; one group of 10

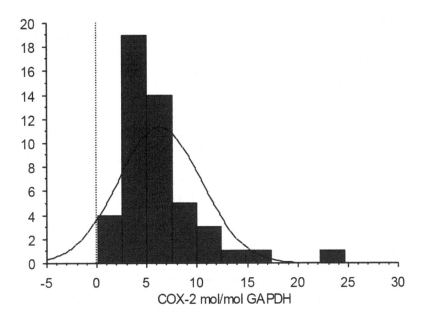

FIGURE 1: Distribution of COX-2 among patients (n = 48). COX-2 expressions of tumors used in this study were distributed at the top and bottom quartile.

patients with highest and one group of 10 patients with lowest COX-2 expression (Figure 1, Table 1).

2.2.2 RNA AND DNA EXTRACTION

Tumor and normal colon tissue samples were collected down to the serosa layer during surgery and kept fresh frozen in liquid nitrogen and stored in -80°C until analysis. Certified pathologists staged all tumors. Tumor samples were secured by the surgeon in charge and contained around 55-75% tumor cells according to random visual inspection. RNA extraction and cDNA synthesis were performed as described [2]. A quality check of RNA in all samples was done in Bioanalyzer 2100 with limit RIN 6.0 for further analysis (Agilent). DNA was extracted with QIAamp® DNA Mini Kit (Qiagen) according to instructions. RNase A solution (Promega) was used as extra step in DNA purification. Concentration of RNA and DNA was determined in NanoDrop® ND-1000 Spectrophotometer (NanoDrop Technologies).

TABLE 1: Classification of patients with high or low COX-2 expression in tumor tissue

	COX-2 expression in tumor tissue	
	High (10)	Low (10)
COX-2 T	12.5 ± 1.5	2.6 ± 0.4
(mol/mol GAPDH) NM	5.06 ± 3.0	12.3 ± 4.0
Dukes[1]	3 A, 6 B, 1 D	3 B, 5 C, 2 D
Age at surgery	71 ± 2.5	73 ± 3.4
Gender	6 M, 4 F	4 M, 6 F
Postoperative survival (months)	23 ± 5.8	29 ± 8.0
Right/left colon	4/6	4/6

Mean ± SEM
T = tumor tissue
NM = Normal colon tissue
[1]Approx. TNM; A = T1, N0, M0; B = T2/T3, N0, M0; C = T2/T3/T4, N1/N2, M0; D = T2/T3/T4, N1/N2, M1

2.2.3 GENE EXPRESSION ANALYSIS

Microarray analysis was performed on pooled tumor mRNA from 9 out of 10 patients with high COX-2 mRNA expression versus 9 out of 10 patients with low COX-2 mRNA expression. The two patients were excluded due to low RIN indicating poor RNA quality. 500 ng of mRNA from tumors with high COX-2 patients was labeled with Cy-3-dCTP (Amersham Bio-Sciences) in a cDNA synthesis reaction with Agilent Flourescent Direct Label. Tumor samples with low COX-2 expression (500 ng) were labeled with Cy-5-dCTP. Pooled tumor cDNA from patients with high COX-2 versus pooled DNA from patients with low COX-2 expression were then hybridized on whole human oligo genome microarrays (4 × 44K expression arrays, Agilent) during 18 hrs followed by post-hybridization washes according to in situ instructions (Hybridization Kit Plus, Agilent).

Microarrays were quantified on Agilent G2565 AA microarray scanner and data were pre-processed in Feature Extraction 9.1 software program (Agilent). The same procedures were performed with normal colon mucosa tissue from all patients with only 4 patients per pool due to poor RNA quality. One hybridization with high COX-2 tumor expression versus corresponding normal colon mucosa tissue was also performed. Four technical replicates of all tumor tissue analyses and two technical replicates of normal colon tissue and tumor versus normal colon tissue analyses were performed. Dye-normalized, outlier- and background subtracted values were analyzed in GeneSpring GX 10 software program (Agilent) according to standard procedures. A quality control was performed with QC metrics. Analysis used were filter on flags (present or marginal) were 27194 probes (out of 41078) passed in 2 out of 4 technical replicates with tumor tissue. In normal tissue 25735 probes passed and in tumor vs normal tissue 27919 probes passed filter on flags for further analysis with t-test ($p < 0.05$). Fold change 1.5 of log2 transformed ratios was considered a statistically significant change in gene expression. Significant pathway analysis with entity list FC 1.5 was used to define significantly altered pathways. PCR analyses were performed at Tataa Biocenter (Gothenburg, Sweden) in a LightCycler 480 Probe Master (Roche). PCR assays (AKT1 HS00178289_m1, IL1B HS01555410_m1, IL6 HS00985639_m1, TRA@ HS 00612292_m1, CARD11 HS01060626_m1, Applied Biosystems) were tested and validated for efficiency and specificity. All samples were run in duplicate and negative controls were negative. Results were related to assay efficiency and GAPDH (GAPDH assay from Tataa Biocenter's Reference Gene Panel Human) and calculated according to comparative Ct method.

2.2.4 DNA METHYLATION ANALYSIS WITH BISULFITE SEQUENCING

Methylation analysis was performed with tag-modified bisulfite genomic sequencing [14]. EpiTect® Bisulfite kit (Qiagen) was used for bisulphite modification of 1 µg tumor and normal colon tissue DNA from each patient (n = 20) according to instructions. Modified DNA samples were amplified with two different sets of primers (Table 2) directed towards two areas of the COX-2 promoter region using touchdown PCR (1 × Reaction Buffer, 0.5 mM dNTPs, 2.0 mM $MgCl_2$, 0.4 µM forward and reverse primers resp., and 1 unit HotStart Taq (Qiagen). Primer pair 1 was taken from Hur et al. and primer pair 2 was designed with BiSearch [15,16]. PCR reactions were denatured at 95°C for 10 min, then 20 cycles of 95°C 45 s, 60°C/65°C annealing temperature with a decrease of half a degree per cycle for 45 s, 68°C 60 s followed by 15-20 cycles of 95°C 45 s, 50°C/55°C 45 s and 68°C 60 s ended with a 7 min extension at 68°C. EpiTect® PCR Controls (Qiagen) was used to ensure that the reaction worked properly; one methylated control sample, one unmethylated control and a 50/50 mixture of methylated and unmethylated controls were included in each PCR to ensure that methylated and unmethylated template were both equally amplified. The specificity of PCR products was inspected by use of 2100 Bioanalyzer according to protocol for DNA 1000 (Agilent). PCR products were then purified using Agencourt AMPure magnetic beads (Agencourt Bioscience Corporation) using the Biomek NX pipetting robot (Beckman Coulter) and eluted in distilled water. Sequence PCR was performed using forward or reverse primer with the ABI Prism BigDye™ cycle sequencing Ready Reaction Kit v1.1 (Applied Biosystems). Sequence PCR was run in 10 µl reactions under following conditions: 96°C 1 min, followed by 25 cycles of 96°C 10 s and 50°C 4 min. Sequencing products were purified using CleanSeq magnetic beads (Agencourt) using the Biomek NX and re-suspended in 10 µl of High Dye formamide (Applied Biosystems). The sequencing products were separated with gel electrophoresis on a 3730 DNA analyser (Applied Biosystems) and the output data were viewed and analysed using Sequence Analysis v5.2 (Applied Biosystems) and BiqAnalyzer [17].

2.2.5 STATISTICS

Results are presented as mean ± SEM. Statistical analyses were performed by ANOVA and $p < 0.05$ was regarded significant in two-tailed tests. This study was approved by the board of Ethics at University of Gothenburg

(NCT00473980). Accordingly, all patients participated with informed consent.

TABLE 2: Primers used for methylation analysis

	Tag	Primer Sequence (5'-3')	Bp
1	FP1692	CCACTCACTCACCCACCCGAAGAAGAAAAGATATTTGG	448
1	RP2104	GGGTGGGAGGTGGGAGGGATAAACTTTACTATCTAAAA	
2	B1(1595)	CCACTCACTCACCCACCCTTGGAGAGGAAGTTAAGTGTTT	223
2	b1(1782)	GGGTGGGAGGTGGGAGGGATCCCCACTCTCCTATCTAAT	

2.3 RESULTS

2.3.1 COX-2 EXPRESSION

Large difference in gene expression was observed when comparing tumor tissue with high COX-2 expression to normal colon mucosa tissue from the same patients (2557↑, 3182↓) (Table 3). A large number of genes with altered expression appeared also in colon cancer tissue of tumors with high COX-2 expression when compared to tumors with low COX-2 expression (3086↑, 3031↓) (Table 4). Expression of COX-2 in normal colon mucosa tissue was significantly increased in patients with tumors of high COX-2 expression compared with mucosa from patients with low COX-2 expression in tumors (776↑, 804↓). Highly expressed genes in tumor tissue with high COX-2 expression were associated to cell motility, cell structure, muscle proteins, and energy homeostasis while down-regulated genes in such tumors seemed to be related to tumor antigens as Melanoma antigen and Chondrosarcoma ass. Gene, etc (Table 4). Several factors of immune response as serpin peptidase inhibitor and inducible metric oxide synthase 2 with antitumoral activities were either up- or down-regulated in normal colon tissue from patients with tumors of high COX-2 expression (Table 5). Patients with tumors with high COX-2 expression did not in the present material display significantly reduced survival compared to patients with tumors with low COX-2 expression (Table 1). However, COX-2 expression predicted survival at borderline significance in a larger patient material [2].

TABLE 3: Genes listed according to the magnitude of most altered expression between tumor tissue and normal mucosa from the same patients with tumors of high intrinsic COX-2 expression

Gene	↑/↓	FC	Function	Gene Symbol (GeneID)
Matrix metallopeptidase 7	↑	110	Breakdown of extracellular matrix, metastasis	MMP7 (4316)
Keratin 23	↑	77	Structural integrity of epithelial cells	KRT23 (25984)
Myosin	↑	63	Muscle, heavy polypeptide 2	MYH2 (4620)
Claudin 1	↑	38	Integral membrane protein, component of tight junction strands	CLDN1 (9076)
Actin α1, skeletal	↑	36	Cell motility, structure and integrity	ACTA1 (58)
Forkhead box Q1	↑	34	Transcription factor (i.e. TGF-beta2)	FOXQ1 (94234)
Proprotein convertase subtilisin/kexin type 1	↑	22	Regulating insulin biosynthesis, obesity, activate precursor protein, associated with carcinoid tumors	PCSK1 (5122)
Sarcolipin	↑	25	Regulates several sarcoplasmic reticulum Ca(2+)-ATPases	SLN (6588)
Matrix metallopeptidase 1	↑	14	Breakdown of extracellular matrix, metastasis	MMP1 (4312)
Myosin, cardiac, beta	↑	25	Heavy chain, also expressed in skeletal muscle tissues rich in slow-twitch type I muscle fibers	MYH7 (4625)
Hydroxy-δ-5-steroid dehydrogenase	↓	79	Biosynthesis of steroid hormones, polymorphisms related to prostate cancer	HSD3B2 (3284)
Hydroxy-δ-5-steroid dehydrogenase	↓	30	Biosynthesis of steroid hormones, diagnostic trophoblastic marker	HSD3B1 (3283)
similar to 3 β-hydroxysteroid dehydrogenase	↓	28	Pseudogene	LOC391081 (391081)
-	↓	24	unknown	CR627415
Butyrylcholinesterase	↓	21	Homozygoutics sustain prolonged apnea after administration of the muscle relaxant suxamethonium	BCHE (590)

TABLE 3: *Cont.*

Gene	↑/↓	FC	Function	Gene Symbol (GeneID)
Neuronal pentraxin	↓	19	Excitatory synapse remodelling, mediate neuronal death induced by reduction in neuronal activity in mature neurons	NPTX1 (4884)
Dipeptidyl-peptidase 6	↓	18	Binds and alters specific voltage-gated potassium channels expression and biophysical properties	DPP6 (1804)
ATP-binding cassette, sub-family G	↓	17	Breast cancer resistance protein, xenobiotic transporter may play a major role in multidrug resistance	ABCG2 (9429)
Insulin like-5	↓	17	Relaxin/Insulin family, ligand for GPCR142	INSL5 (10022)
Regenerating islet-derived 1 β	↓	16	Highly similar to REG1A protein (islet cell regeneration and diabetogenesis)	REG1B (5968)

↑ *increased expression*
↓ *decreased expression*

TABLE 4: Genes listed according to the magnitude of most altered expression in tumor tissue of high intrinsic COX-2 expression

Gene	↑/↓	FC	Function	Gene Symbol (GeneID)
Unknown	↑	156	unknown	W60781
Myosin	↑	107	Muscle, heavy polypeptide 2	MYH2 (4620)
Desmin	↑	49	Muscle filament	DES (1674)
Creatine kinase	↑	46	Muscle, energy homeostasis, serum marker for myocardial infarction	CKM (1158)
Troponin T type 3	↑	41	Skeletal	TNNT3 (7140)
Actin α, cardiac	↑	37	Muscle, contractile, cell motility	ACTC1 (70)
Actin α1, skeletal	↑	35	Cell motility, structure and integrity	ACTA1 (58)
Synaptopodin 2	↑	28	Cell-shape regulation, homolog with Myopodin (a tumor suppressor; inhibits growth and metastasis)	SYNPO2 (171024)
Nebulin	↑	25	Cytoskeletal matrix	NEB (4703)
Calponin	↑	23	Differentiation marker, reduced in tumor vessels associated with tumor progression	CNN1 (1264)
Growth diff. factor 10	↓	28	Regulation of cell growth and differentiation	GDF10 (2662)

TABLE 4: *Cont.*

Gene	↑/↓	FC	Function	Gene Symbol (GeneID)
Unc-13 homolog A	↓	19	diacylglycerol and phorbol ester receptors, essential role in synaptic vesicle priming	UNC13A (23025)
LOC553137	↓	16	miscRNA, unknown function	LOC553137 (553137)
Melanoma antigen family B, 2	↓	14	Tumor-associated antigen, expressed only in testis and tumors, regulated by demethylation	MAGEB2 (4113)
Chondrosarcoma associated gene 1	↓	13	Tumor antigen, expressed in testis and in chondrosarcomas	CSAG1 (158511)
Folate receptor 1	↓	13	Involvement in cancer prognosis	FOLR1 (2348)
Renin	↓	13	Blood pressure and electrolyte balance	REN (5972)
Small proline-rich protein 3	↓	12	Epithelial homeostatis, aberrant expression contribute to tumorigenesis of esophageal squamous cell carcinoma	SPRR3 (6707)
Heat shock 27kDa protein 3	↓	12	Muscle	HSPB3 (8988)
Chromogranin B	↓	11	Precursor for biological active peptides, involved early in breast cancer	CHGB (1114)

↑ *increased expression*
↓ *decreased expression*

TABLE 5: Genes listed according to the magnitude of most altered expression in normal mucosa from patients with tumors of high intrinsic COX-2 expression

Gene	↑/↓	FC	Function	Gene Symbol (GeneID)
Pancreatic derived factor (PANDER)	↑	79	Cytokine, induces apoptosis of alpha and beta cells, implicated in diabetes	FAM3B (54097)
Regenerating islet-derived 1 α	↑	40	Secreted by the exocrine pancreas, associated with islet cell regeneration and diabetogenesis	REG1A (5967)
Ribosomal protein S4, Y-linked 2	↑	40	Translation	RPS4Y2 (140032)
Serpin peptidase inhibitor, ovalbumin	↑	35	Cytoprotective, cell survival factor, monocyte regulation, potential cancer marker (elevated in plasma)	SERPINB2 (5055)

TABLE 5: *Cont,*

Gene	↑/↓	FC	Function	Gene Symbol (GeneID)
Nitric oxide synthase 2, inducible	↑	19	reactive free radical, biologic mediator in several processes, incl. neurotransmission, antimicrobial and antitumoral activities	NOS2A (4843)
Pentraxin-related gene	↑	16	Immune response, inflammation, rapidly induced by IL-1β	PTX3 (5806)
Regenerating islet-derived 1 β	↑	16	highly similar to REG1A protein	REG1B (5968)
Hydroxy-delta-5-steroid dehydrogenase	↑	10	Biosynthesis of steroid hormones, polymorphisms related to prostate cancer	HSD3B2 (3284)
Hydroxy-delta-5-steroid dehydrogenase	↑	10	Biosynthesis of steroid hormones, diagnostic trophoblastic marker	HSD3B1 (3283)
ADAM metallopeptidase	↑	10	cleavage of proteoglycans, control of organ shape during development, and inhibition of angiogenesis	ADAMTS9 (56999)
Unknown	↓	15	unknown	ENST00000343
6-phosphofructo-2-kinase	↓	13	Produce fructose 2,6-P(2), involved in Warburg effect	PFKFB3 (5209)
hemoglobin, γ A	↓	8	Normally expressed in the fetal liver, spleen and bone marrow	HBG1 (3047)
matrix metallopeptidase 7	↓	8	Breakdown of extracellular matrix, metastasis	MMP7 (4316)
Fc receptor-like 4	↓	7	Immune regulation	FCRL4 (83417)
Chemokine receptor 5	↓	6	B cell migration and localization	BLR1 (643)
Fibroblast growth factor 5	↓	6	Mitogenic and cell survival activities, involved in a variety of biological processes, incl. cell growth, morphogenesis, tissue repair, tumor growth and invasion, oncogene	FGF5 (2250)
Family with sequence similarity 129, member C	↓	6	B-cell novel protein, BCNP1 completely unknown protein with 3 predicted transmembrane domains	FAM129C (199786)
selectin L	↓	6	Leukocyte-endothelial cell interactions	SELL (6402)
Zinc finger protein	↓	5	DNA binding	ZNF683 (257101)

↑ *increased expression*
↓ *decreased expression*

2.3.2 *TRANSCRIPTION FACTORS*

A large number of transcription factors with reported importance for regulation of the COX-2 gene in human cells were evaluated and are listed in Table 6. Eight of these transcription factors showed increased expression, while 5 transcription factors were down-regulated in tumors with high COX-2 expression.

TABLE 6: Significant alterations in expression of previously reported important transcription factors in tumors of high intrinsic COX-2 expression

Gene	Product	FC 1.5	FC 2.0	FC 3.0	Reference[a]
TFAP2C	AP-2γ	↓	-	-	[12]
TFAP2E	AP-2ε	-	-	-	[12]
ATF1	ATF1	-	-	-	[13]
ATF2	ATF2/CREB2	-	-	-	[13]
ATF3	ATF3/AP1	↑	-	-	[13]
BATF	B-ATF	-	-	-	[13]
CREBBP	CBP/p300 co-activator	-	-	-	[12]
CDX2	CDX2	↓	-	-	[29]
CEBPA	C/EBP-α	-	-	-	[13]
CEBPB	C/EBP-β	-	-	-	[13]
CEBPD	C/EBP-δ	↑	↑	-	[13]
CREB5	CRE-BPA	-	-	-	[13]
CREB1	CREB	-	-	-	[13]
ELK1	Elk-1	↓	-	-	[13]
FOS	c-Fos/AP1	↑	-	-	[12]
FOSB	Fos-B/AP1	↑	↑	↑	[12]
FOSL1	Fra-1/AP1	-	-	-	[12]
FOSL2	Fra-2/AP1	-	-	-	[12]
DNAJC12	JDP1	-	-	-	[12]
JDP2	JDP2	↑	-	-	[12]
JUN	Jun/AP1	-	-	-	[12]
JUNB	JunB/AP1	-	-	-	[12]
JUND	JunD/AP1	↑	-	-	[12]
MAF	c-Maf/AP1	↑	↑	-	[12]
NFATC1	NFATc1/NFAT2	-	-	-	[12]
NFATC4	NFAT3	-	-	-	[12]

TABLE 6: *Cont.*

Gene	Product	FC 1.5	FC 2.0	FC 3.0	Reference[a]
NFATC3	NFAT4	-	-	-	[12]
NFAT5	NFAT5	-	-	-	[12]
NFKB1	NF-κB, p105/p50	-	-	-	[12,13]
NFKB2	NF-κB, p100	-	-	-	[12,13]
RELA	NF-κB, RelA (p65)	-	-	-	[12,13]
RELB	NF-κB, RelB	-	-	-	[12,13]
REL	NF-κB, c-Rel	-	-	-	[12,13]
NFKBIA	NF-κB, IκBα	↑	↑	-	[12,13]
NFKBIB	NF-κB, IκBβ	-	-	-	[12,13]
NFKBIE	NF-κB, IκBε	-	-	-	[12,13]
CHUK	NF-κB, IKK-α	-	-	-	[12,13]
IKBKB	NF-κB, IKK-β	-	-	-	[12,13]
IKBKG	NF-κB, IKK-γ	-	-	-	[12,13]
TP53	p53	↓	↓	-	[30]
ETV4	PEA3	↓	-	-	[13]
PPARA	PPARα	-	-	-	[12]
PPARD	PPARβ/δ	-	-	-	[12]
PPARG	PPARγ	-	-	-	[12]
SP1	SP-1	-	-	-	[12]
TBP	TATA-binding protein	-	-	-	[12]
TCF4	TCF4	↑	↑	-	[13]

AP-2α, AP-2β, AP-2δ, NFAT1 and Retinoic acid receptor were also tested, but no expression were found. ↑ increased expression; ↓ decreased expression; FC is log2 fold changes
[a] *published report with emphasis on transcription factor in regulation of COX-2 gene.*

2.3.3 EXTERNAL FACTORS

Genes with reported functions in external cell signaling indicated 6 genes with increased expression, while no gene indicated down-regulation related to high COX-2 expression in tumor tissue (Table 7). Table 8 describes genes with significantly altered expression of transcription factors and external cell signaling factors in normal mucosa from patients with tumors of increased COX-2 expression. IL1-β, IL6, and iNOS were up-regulated, probably inducing a variety of transcription factors.

TABLE 7: Significant alterations in expression of previously reported important external cell signaling factors and enzymes in tumors of high intrinsic COX-2 expression

Gene	Product	FC 1.5	FC 2.0	FC 3.0	Reference[a]
DNMT1	DNA MTase 1	-	-	-	[26]
DNMT3A	DNA MTase 3A	↑	↑	-	[26]
DNMT3B	DNA MTase 3B	-	-	-	[26]
MDM2	hdm2	-	-	-	[30]
HPGD	HPGD	-	-	-	[1]
HNRPD	HuR	-	-	-	[31]
IL1B	IL1b	↑	↑	-	[32,33]
IL6	IL6	↑	↑	↑	[34]
IL6R	IL6 receptor	↑	-	-	[34]
NOS2A	iNOS	-	-	-	[13]
MAPK14	p38 MAPK	-	-	-	[35]
PTGES	mPGES-1	-	-	-	[1]
PRKCB1	Protein kinas Cβ1	↑	↑	↑	[12]
RALA	Ras family (oncogene)	-	-	-	[12]
RASA4	Ras p21 protein activator	-	-	-	[12]
RASSF1	Ras ass. (tumor supr.)	-	-	-	[12]
RIN2	Ras and Rab interact. 2	-	-	-	[12]
TINP1	TGF-β	-	-	-	[13]
TNF	TNF-α	↑	-	-	[13]

↑ *increased expression*
↓ *decreased expression*
FC is log2 fold change
[a] published report with emphasis on the current factors

2.3.4 PATHWAY ANALYSIS

Significantly altered metabolic and signaling pathways (FC 1.5) in tumors with high COX-2 expression were mainly related to immunity according to algorithm analyses (GeneSpring GX 10, Agilent). Five genes that were significantly changed in arrays (AKT1, CARD11, IL1B, IL6, and TRA@) and involved in significantly changed pathways according to the algorithm analyses (TCR, BCR, IL1, and IL6) were tested individually (Table 9). All results from individual PCR analyses agreed with array results with one exception; in tumor tissue with high compared to low COX-2 expression AKT1 expression was significantly higher in PCR analyses, with opposite direction in array analysis.

TABLE 8: Significant alterations in expression of transcription factors and cell signaling factors in normal colon mucosa from patients with tumors of high intrinsic COX-2 expression

Gene	Product	FC 1.5	FC 2.0	FC 3.0
PTGS2	COX-2	↑	↑	↑
Transcription				
ATF3	ATF3/AP1	↑	-	-
CEBPD	C/EBP-δ	↑	↑	-
CREB1	CREB	↑	-	-
FOSB	Fos-B/AP1	↑	↑	-
DNAJC12	JDP1	↑	-	-
NFATC1	NFATc1/NFAT2	↓	-	-
PPARG	PPARγ	↓	-	-
BATF	B-ATF	↓	-	-
External cell factors				
IL1B	IL1b	↑	↑	↑
IL6	IL6	↑	↑	↑
NOS2A	iNOS	↑	↑	↑

All factors listed in Table 6 and 7 were evaluated.

2.3.5 DNA METHYLATION

A majority of tumor tissue specimens displayed no methylation of the promoter region of the COX-2 gene in tumor tissue; only 2 tumors showed methylation of the promoter region (low COX-2, Dukes B tumors with intermediate differentiation). Methylation of the promoter region of the COX-2 gene was not observed in any of the normal colon mucosa specimens.

TABLE 9: Gene expressions in tumor tissue with high COX-2 expression compared to tumor tissue with low COX-2 expression confirmed by q-PCR

	CARD 11		TRA@		IL6		IL1B		AKT1	
	High COX-2 (9)	Low COX-2 (9)	High COX-2 (9)	Low COX-2 (9)	High COX-2 (9)	Low COX-2 (9)	High COX-2 (9)	Low COX-2 (9)	High COX-2 (9)	Low COX-2 (9)
Mean	0.40 ± 0.08	0.42 ± 0.24	2.87 ± 0.63	0.55 ± 0.14	1.97 ± 0.79	0.09 ± 0.03	1.61 ± 0.49	0.27 ± 0.06	1.09 ± 0.13	0.62 ± 0.07
Median	0.39	0.07	3.12	0.44	0.87	0.05	1.01	0.21	0.96	0.59
Variance	0.06	0.50	3.57	0.18	5.65	0.008	2.16	0.04	0.14	0.04
P-value*	ns		0.002		0.03		0.02		0.005	

ANOVA analysis
CARD11 = caspase recruitment domain family, member 11
TRA@ = T cell receptor alpha locus
IL6 = Interleukin 6
IL1B = Interleukin 1β
AKT1 = v-akt murine thymoma viral oncogene homolog 1 or protein kinase B

2.4 DISCUSSION

Increased prostanoid activity is a well recognized characteristic of colorectal cancer [4,8,10,18-20]. Early, it was claimed that such tumors have increased COX-2 expression deduced from immunohistochemical evaluations of tumor tissue specimens. More recent investigations have however emphasized that increased COX-2 expression in colorectal cancer is preferentially a local phenomenon with uneven distribution among transformed cells without overall increased tissue content [11]. These findings imply heterogenous cell clones or that other factor are responsible for either up- or down-regulation of COX-2 in malignant cells. It is also important to underline that increased COX-2 expression in tumor tissue may well be confined to stroma and host cells. Such a complex condition supports cross-talk among cells with prostanoids as signals through specific receptors. Our previous investigations have demonstrated a statistically significant relationship between COX-2 expression and tumor tissue production of PGE_2, which is elevated in colon cancer tissue [11]. These kinds of findings agree with information that both primary and secondary intervention with cyclooxygenase inhibitors influenced on both local tumor growth and systemic effects in experimental and clinical cancer [4]. Of particular interest may be previous observations that subtype EP_2 receptor expression in colon cancer tissue predicted reduced survival [2]. Seen together, it seems that induction of COX-2 is a key-factor behind progression of epithelial cell transformation to invasive cancer in colon mucosa. This logic has been practically explored evaluating the role of COX-2 inhibition on epithelial dysplasia in esophageal mucosa, although without consistent results [21]. However, understanding in part complex cell to cell interactions and signaling in composed tissues it should not be expected to be isolated single factors behind local and systemic tumor progression. Therefore, we intended to evaluate relationships between high COX-2 expression in colon cancer tissue to other factors of known importance for tumor cell division, apoptosis, and metastasis. In this perspective microarray screening should be rewarding.

With this purpose we have quantified COX-2 expression in primary tumors from 48 unselected patients with R0 resected primary tumors. Then, tumor tissue with 10 highest and lowest COX-2 expressions was chosen for subsequent hybridization in various combinations. Such cross-combinations of tissues for microarray expression analyses revealed that tumors with high intrinsic COX-2 expression displayed pronounced up-regulation of genes related to muscle fibers and cytoskeleton matrix, perhaps reflecting matrix remodeling including angiogenesis. By contrast, down-regulated genes in such tumors were more related to functional proteins and eventual cellular antigens (Table 4). Similar findings were observed in comparisons between tumor tissue and normal mucosa from the corresponding patients (Table 3). Most interesting was however, findings that normal colon tissue from patients with high intrinsic COX-2 expression in tumor tissue revealed pronounced up- and down-regulation of several gene functions. Such observations led to the conclusion that colon tissue in patients with colon cancer is significantly altered in regards to functional aspects either primarily or secondary to the appearance of manifest tumor. Analysis of significantly altered pathways at high COX-2 displayed that most alterations were related to immune reactions in the present and previous analyses [22]. This confirms our previous results based on an alternative approach where preoperative COX inhibition by indomethacin mainly affected genes and pathways that involved the immunity [22,23].

It may be rewarding to understand the control of COX-2 gene expression behind complex in vivo interactions as emphasized. According to this line we evaluated a large number of proposed genes with importance for COX-2 expression as listed in Table 6. Fourteen out of 47 genes were found to have significantly altered expression defined at least as 1.5 fold change compared to normal mucosa or by chance variation in transcript expression. Fos-B/AP1 expression displayed the most pronounced alteration of up-regulated transcripts among transcription factors. A transcription complex known to regulate COX-2 gene expression via binding to CRE-sites in the promoter region is Activator protein 1 (AP-1), which consists of homo- or heterodimers of JUN- and FOS-families with roles in several different cancers. In colorectal cancer AP-1 may be activated by either K-RAS mutation or via Wnt signals. Different genes are transcribed controlling biological activities such as proliferation, apoptosis and differentiation depending on the sub-components of AP-1 [24,25]. Six of 19 factors with emphasized importance for external cell signaling were up-regulated in tumor tissue of high intrinsic COX-2 expression (Table 7). As expected, such experiments confirmed no significant transcript with decreased expression. IL6 and protein kinas Cβ1 appeared most up-regulated in such cross hybridizations, although transcription of NF-κB was not elevated. In this context it is important to emphasize that protein and gene activation may occur despite evidence of unchanged transcription levels, usually subsequent to phosphorylation changes. Again, it was observed that 9 transcription factors and IL1β, IL6 and iNOS were significantly altered in normal colon tissue from patients with tumors of high intrinsic COX-2 expression. Individual confirmation of array results by PCR determinations displayed also a significantly higher expression of IL1β and IL6 at high COX-2. This phenomenon demonstrates that overall COX-2 expression in primary colorectal carcinoma probably includes primary and secondary alterations in tumor un-involved colon tissue.

It is well recognized that methylation of CpG island located within promoter regions of genes may silence gene expression, described as a hallmark in human cancer. This represents findings early during carcinogenesis and is maintained by DNA methyltransferase (DNMTs) [26]. Such methylation of the COX-2 promoter region may be associated with loss of gene expression as reported for gastric cancer [15,27]. Similar evidence has been reported for COX-2 gene expression in colorectal cancer [27,28], although, statistical evaluations of reported observations do not give the impression that COX-2 expression in colon cancer tissue is related to COX-2 promoter methylation. Accordingly, we did not observe significant methylation in two well-defined parts of the COX-2 promoter region in tumor and normal colon tissues. However, DNA methyltransferase was expressed at increased levels in tumor tissue compared to the corresponding normal colon tissue. Therefore, it is unlikely that promoter methylation was a significant factor behind the lack of COX-2 expression in presently investigated areas of colon cancer tissue. It remains to be determined how COX-2 is either induced in tumor tissue with intrinsic high COX-2 expression or down-regulated in tumor cells with correspondingly low overall COX-2 expression to provide the well-recognised scattered pattern of expression observed in immunohistochemical cross tissue sections. Important is our observation that COX-2 expression in normal colon tissue was also significantly increased in patients with tumors of high COX-2 expression. This points to the possibility, that the mucosa or entire colon tissue may be altered as a general phenomenon in patients with certain kind of colon tumors. Perhaps, the inflammatory activation by some kind of bacterial flora(s) could be a speculative guess.

2.5 CONCLUSION

Our present study emphasized and confirmed our previous observations that increased COX-2 expression or tissue content is overall not a unanimous finding in colorectal cancer tissue. A scattered presence of COX-2 may rather represent different cell clones or different local conditions at the cellular level. Both transcription and external cell signaling factors were significantly altered as covariates to COX-2 expression in colon cancer tissue. DNA methylation of the COX-2 promoter region did not seem to be a significant factor behind COX-2 expression in either tumor tissue or normal colon tissue in the present material. Our results confirm that both local and systemic inflammation promote tumor growth and disease progression.

REFERENCES

1. Greenhough A, Smartt HJ, Moore AE, Roberts HR, Williams AC, Paraskeva C, Kaidi A: The COX-2/PGE2 pathway: key roles in the hallmarks of cancer and adaptation to the tumour microenvironment. Carcinogenesis 2009, 30(3):377-386.

2. Gustafsson A, Hansson E, Kressner U, Nordgren S, Andersson M, Wang W, Lonnroth C, Lundholm K: EP1-4 subtype, COX and PPAR gamma receptor expression in colorectal cancer in prediction of disease-specific mortality. Int J Cancer 2007, 121(2):232-240.

3. Gustafsson A, Hansson E, Kressner U, Nordgren S, Andersson M, Lonnroth C, Lundholm K: Prostanoid receptor expression in colorectal cancer related to tumor stage, differentiation and progression. Acta Oncol 2007, :1-6.

4. Cahlin C, Gelin J, Andersson M, Lonnroth C, Lundholm K: The effects of non-selective, preferential-selective and selective COX-inhibitors on the growth of experimental and human tumors in mice related to prostanoid receptors. Int J Oncol 2005, 27(4):913-923.

5. Thun MJ, Namboodiri MM, Calle EE, Flanders WD, Heath CW Jr: Aspirin use and risk of fatal cancer. Cancer Res 1993, 53(6):1322-1327.

6. Muscat JE, Stellman SD, Wynder EL: Nonsteroidal antiinflammatory drugs and colorectal cancer. Cancer 1994, 74(7):1847-1854.

7. Sandler RS, Halabi S, Baron JA, Budinger S, Paskett E, Keresztes R, Petrelli N, Pipas JM, Karp DD, Loprinzi CL, et al.: A randomized trial of aspirin to prevent colorectal adenomas in patients with previous colorectal cancer. N Engl J Med 2003, 348(10):883-890.

8. Gelin J, Andersson C, Lundholm K: Effects of indomethacin, cytokines, and cyclosporin A on tumor growth and the subsequent development of cancer cachexia. Cancer Res 1991, 51(3):880-885.

9. Lundholm K, Gelin J, Hyltander A, Lonnroth C, Sandstrom R, Svaninger G, Korner U, Gulich M, Karrefors I, Norli B, et al.: Anti-inflammatory treatment may prolong survival in undernourished patients with metastatic solid tumors. Cancer Res 1994, 54(21):5602-5606.

10. Hull MA, Ko SC, Hawcroft G: Prostaglandin EP receptors: targets for treatment and prevention of colorectal cancer? Mol Cancer Ther 2004, 3(8):1031-1039.

11. Cahlin C, Lonnroth C, Arvidsson A, Nordgren S, Lundholm K: Growth associated proteins in tumor cells and stroma related to disease progression of colon cancer accounting for tumor tissue PGE2 content. Int J Oncol 2008, 32(4):909-918.

12. Chun KS, Surh YJ: Signal transduction pathways regulating cyclooxygenase-2 expression: potential molecular targets for chemoprevention. Biochem Pharmacol 2004, 68(6):1089-1100.

13. Tsatsanis C, Androulidaki A, Venihaki M, Margioris AN: Signalling networks regulating cyclooxygenase-2. Int J Biochem Cell Biol 2006, 38(10):1654-1661.

14. Han W, Cauchi S, Herman JG, Spivack SD: DNA methylation mapping by tag-modified bisulfite genomic sequencing. Anal Biochem 2006, 355(1):50-61.

15. Hur K, Song SH, Lee HS, Ho Kim W, Bang YJ, Yang HK: Aberrant methylation of the specific CpG island portion regulates cyclooxygenase-2 gene expression in human gastric carcinomas. Biochem Biophys Res Commun 2003, 310(3):844-851.

16. Tusnady GE, Simon I, Varadi A, Aranyi T: BiSearch: primer-design and search tool for PCR on bisulfite-treated genomes. Nucleic Acids Res 2005, 33(1):e9.

17. Bock C, Reither S, Mikeska T, Paulsen M, Walter J, Lengauer T: BiQ Analyzer: visualization and quality control for DNA methylation data from bisulfite sequencing. Bioinformatics 2005, 21(21):4067-4068.

18. Cao Y, Prescott SM: Many actions of cyclooxygenase-2 in cellular dynamics and in cancer. J Cell Physiol 2002, 190(3):279-286.

19. Pradono P, Tazawa R, Maemondo M, Tanaka M, Usui K, Saijo Y, Hagiwara K, Nukiwa T: Gene transfer of thromboxane A(2) synthase and prostaglandin I(2) synthase antithetically altered tumor angiogenesis and tumor growth. Cancer Res 2002, 62(1):63-66.

20. Wang D, Dubois RN: Prostaglandins and cancer. Gut 2006, 55(1):115-122.

21. Zhi H, Wang L, Zhang J, Zhou C, Ding F, Luo A, Wu M, Zhan Q, Liu Z: Significance of COX-2 expression in human esophageal squamous cell carcinoma. Carcinogenesis 2006, 27(6):1214-1221.

22. Lonnroth C, Andersson M, Arvidsson A, Nordgren S, Brevinge H, Lagerstedt K, Lundholm K: Preoperative treatment with a non-steroidal anti-inflammatory drug (NSAID) increases tumor tissue infiltration of seemingly activated immune cells in colorectal cancer. Cancer Immun 2008, 8:5.

23. Gustafsson A, Andersson M, Lagerstedt K, Lonnroth C, Nordgren S, Lundholm K: Receptor and enzyme expression for prostanoid metabolism in colorectal cancer related to tumor tissue PGE2. Int J Oncol 2010, 36(2):469-478.

24. Ashida R, Tominaga K, Sasaki E, Watanabe T, Fujiwara Y, Oshitani N, Higuchi K, Mitsuyama S, Iwao H, Arakawa T: AP-1 and colorectal cancer. Inflammopharmacology 2005, 13(1-3):113-125.

25. Grau R, Iniguez MA, Fresno M: Inhibition of activator protein 1 activation, vascular endothelial growth factor, and cyclooxygenase-2 expression by 15-deoxy-Delta12,14-prostaglandin J2 in colon carcinoma cells: evidence for a redox-sensitive peroxisome proliferator-activated receptor-gamma-independent mechanism. Cancer Res 2004, 64(15):5162-5171.

26. Egger G, Liang G, Aparicio A, Jones PA: Epigenetics in human disease and prospects for epigenetic therapy. Nature 2004, 429(6990):457-463.

27. Castells A, Paya A, Alenda C, Rodriguez-Moranta F, Agrelo R, Andreu M, Pinol V, Castellvi-Bel S, Jover R, Llor X, et al.: Cyclooxygenase 2 expression in colorectal cancer with DNA mismatch repair deficiency. Clin Cancer Res 2006, 12(6):1686-1692.

28. Toyota M, Shen L, Ohe-Toyota M, Hamilton SR, Sinicrope FA, Issa JP: Aberrant methylation of the Cyclooxygenase 2 CpG island in colorectal tumors. Cancer Res 2000, 60(15):4044-4048.

29. Kim SP, Park JW, Lee SH, Lim JH, Jang BC, Jang IH, Freund JN, Suh SI, Mun KC, Song DK, et al.: Homeodomain protein CDX2 regulates COX-2 expression in colorectal cancer. Biochem Biophys Res Commun 2004, 315(1):93-99.

30. Cressey R, Pimpa S, Tontrong W, Watananupong O, Leartprasertsuke N: Expression of cyclooxygenase-2 in colorectal adenocarcinoma is associated with p53 accumulation and hdm2 overexpression. Cancer Lett 2006, 233(2):232-239.

31. Denkert C, Koch I, von Keyserlingk N, Noske A, Niesporek S, Dietel M, Weichert W: Expression of the ELAV-like protein HuR in human colon cancer: association with tumor stage and cyclooxygenase-2. Mod Pathol 2006, 19(9):1261-1269.

32. Lin DW, Nelson PS: The role of cyclooxygenase-2 inhibition for the prevention and treatment of prostate carcinoma. Clin Prostate Cancer 2003, 2(2):119-126.

33. Duque J, Diaz-Munoz MD, Fresno M, Iniguez MA: Up-regulation of cyclooxygenase-2 by interleukin-1 beta in colon carcinoma cells. Cell Signal 2006, 18(8):1262-1269.

34. Maihofner C, Charalambous MP, Bhambra U, Lightfoot T, Geisslinger G, Gooderham NJ: Expression of cyclooxygenase-2 parallels expression of interleukin-1 beta, interleukin-6 and NF-kappaB in human colorectal cancer. Carcinogenesis 2003, 24(4):665-671.

35. Gauthier ML, Pickering CR, Miller CJ, Fordyce CA, Chew KL, Berman HK, Tlsty TD: p38 regulates cyclooxygenase-2 in human mammary epithelial cells and is activated in premalignant tissue. Cancer Res 2005, 65(5):1792-1799.

DOWN-REGULATION OF PROMOTER METHYLATION LEVEL OF *CD4* GENE AFTER MDV INFECTION IN MD-SUSCEPTIBLE CHICKEN LINE

JUAN LUO, YING YU, HUANMIN ZHANG, FEI TIAN, SHUANG CHANG, HANS H. CHENG, AND JIUZHOU SONG

3.1 BACKGROUND

CD4 encodes a glycoprotein, located on the surface of T helper (Th) cells and regulatory T cells. Through interaction with MHC class II molecules, CD4 directs the linage development of Th cells in immune organs and activates the CD4[+] T cell maturation process [1]. Thus, the transcriptional level of *CD4* is directly related to T cell development [2]. In mice, *CD4* transcription is controlled by several cis-acting elements including enhancers, silencers and DNA methylation [3,4]. However, the epigenetic regulation of *CD4* gene in chicken and its relationship with any virus infection are still unclear.

Marek's disease (MD), a T cell lymphoma of chickens caused by the Marek's disease virus (MDV), is characterized by mononuclear cell-infiltration in various organs including peripheral nerves, skin, muscle, and

This chapter was originally published under the Creative Commons Attribution License. Luo J, Yu Y, Zhang H, Tian F, Chang S, Cheng HH, and Song J. Down-Regulation of Promoter Methylation Level of CD4 Gene After MDV Infection in MD-Susceptible Chicken Line. BMC Proceedings **5(Suppl 4)**,S7 *(2011). doi:10.1186/1753-6561-5-S4-S7.*

visceral organs [5], and is a worldwide problem for the poultry industry. A complex MDV life cycle was found in susceptible chickens during MD progression, which includes an early cytolytic phase (2-7 days post infection, dpi), latent phase (7-10 dpi), late cytolytic phase (from 18 dpi) and transformation phase (28 dpi and onwards) [6].

Epigenetics is the study of alterations that result in inherited changes in phenotypes despite the lack of DNA sequence polymorphisms and include DNA methylation, histone modification and chromatin remodeling [7]. It is described as the interaction between genes and environmental factors. Aberrant CpG methylation levels of the gene promoter region contribute to oncogenesis [8]. Viruses are one of the environmental agents that can cause alterations of DNA methylation level in host genes [9].

The focus of this study was to better understand the expression control of *CD4* by ascertaining the epigenetic status in the *CD4* promoter and the *CD4* expression in relation to MDV infection. Two inbred chicken lines, MD-resistant or –susceptible with the same MHC (major histocompatibility complex) haplotypes, from Avian Disease and Oncology laboratory (ADOL) were used [5]. We, therefore, measured the promoter methylation and transcription of the *CD4* gene before and after MDV infection of both lines. We found methylation alterations in the *CD4* promoter region after MDV infection differ between these two lines.

3.2 METHODS

3.2.1 ANIMALS, VIRUS INFECTION EXPERIMENTS AND SAMPLE COLLECTION

USDA, Avian Disease and Oncology Laboratory (ADOL) chicken lines 6 (L6$_3$) and lines 7 (L7$_2$) chickens, which are MD-resistant and MD-susceptible, respectively, were obtained. For each line, the chickens were divided into two groups with 30 chickens infected by MDV and 30 uninfected controls. A very virulent plus strain of MDV (648A passage 40, VV+) was injected intra-abdominally on the fifth day after hatching with 500 plaque-forming units (PFU). Spleen samples were collected at 5 dpi, 10 dpi and 21 dpi, put in RNAlater (Qiagen, USA) immediately, and then stored at -80°C. All procedures followed the standard animal ethics and user guidelines.

3.2.2 DNA EXTRACTION, BISULFITE TREATMENT AND PYROSEQUENCING

DNA was extracted from 20-30 mg spleen by NucleoSpin® Tissue Kits (Macherey-Nagel, Germany). 500 ng DNA was treated with sodium bisulfite and purified by EZ DNA Methylation-Gold Kit™ (ZYMO Research, USA). Primers for pyrosequencing were designed by PSQ Assay Design software (Biotage, Swedan) (Table 1). For cost reduction, a universal primer (5'-GGGACACCGCTGATCGTTTA-3') was used in the PCR assays [10]. DNA methylation level analysis was performed with Pyro Q-CpG system (PyroMark ID, Biotage, Sweden) as previously described [10,11].

TABLE 1: Primers used in Pyrosequencing and quantitative PCR

Genes	Primers	Sequence	Purpose
CD4	F	5'- TTGAGATTATAYGTATTTGGAAGA -3'	Pyrosequencing
	R	5'- GGGACACCGCTGATCGTTTA ACCTT-TATATCTCCTCCTCTCCA -3'	
	Sequencing	5'- AGTATTTATTGAGAGAAGTT -3'	
	Assay	5'- YGTAGATTGTAGTAGAGTTTGGATYG GTAGTAAGATYGTGTTGAYGTTTT -3'	
GAPDH	F	5'-GAGGGTAGTGAAGGCTGCTG-3'	quantitative PCR
	R	5'-ACCAGGAAACAAGCTTGACG-3'	
CD4	F	5'- TGTCAACGCCGGATGTATAA-3'	quantitative PCR
	R	5'- CTTGTCCATTGGCTCCTCTC-3'	

Y stands for C/T. Bold Y in the assay sequence is the CpG sites analyzed.

3.2.3 RNA EXTRACTION AND QUANTITATIVE REAL-TIME RT-PCR

RNA from 30-50mg spleen was extracted using the RNAeasy Mini Kit (Qiagen, USA). Reverse transcription was carried out in 20 μl with 1 μg of total RNA by using SuperScript™ III Reverse Transcriptase (Invitrogen, USA) and oligo (dT)$_{12-18}$ primers (Invitrogen, USA). Primers (Table 1) for quantitative real-time RT-PCR were designed by Primer3 online primer designer system (http://frodo.wi.mit.edu/). qPCR was performed on the iCycler iQ PCR system (Bio-Rad, USA) in a final volume of 20 μl using QuantiTect SYBR Green PCR Kit (Qiagen, USA) with the following procedure: denatured at 95°C for 15 min, followed by 40 cycles at 95 °C for 30 s, 60 °C for 30 s, 72 °C for 30 s, then extended at 72 °C for 10 min. Each reaction was replicated twice. The housekeeping gene *GAPDH* (glyceraldehyde-3-phosphate dehydrogenase) was used to normalize the assays.

3.2.4 STATISTICAL ANALYSIS

Promoter methylation levels and gene expression before and after MDV infection were compared by Student's t test. An exact F test was performed to distinguish different methylation patterns [10]. Correlation between *CD4* DNA methylation and expression was tested by Pearson's correlation coefficient.

3.3 RESULTS

3.3.1 CD4 PROMOTER METHYLATION ANALYSIS BEFORE AND AFTER MDV INFECTION

To determine the promoter methylation level of the *CD4* gene, a DNA sequence containing the CpG islands from the *CD4* gene promoter region (sequence shown in Table 1) was downloaded from UCSC (http://genome.ucsc.edu) and the methylation level was determined by pyrosequencing.

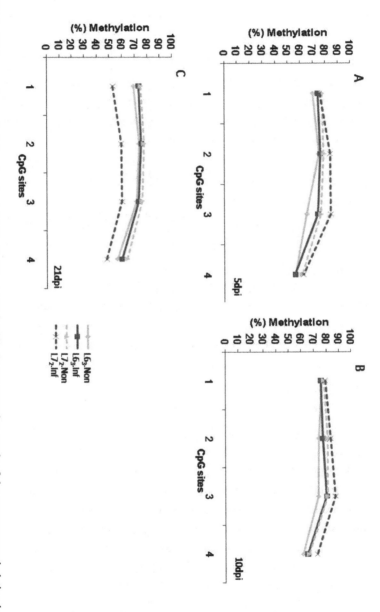

FIGURE 1: *CD4* promoter methylation levels at 5 (A), 10 (B) and 21dpi (C). Pyrosequencing result of the promoter methylation level of *CD4* gene before and after MDV infection at different time points. A decrease of promoter methylation level was observed only $L7_2$ chickens. 5dpi: 5 days post infection; 10dpi: 10 days post infection; 21dpi: 21 days post infection. $L6_3$.Non: noninfected control of $L6_3$ chicken; $L6_3$. Inf: infected $L6_3$ chicken; $L7_2$.Non: noninfected control of $L6_3$ chicken; $L6_3$.Inf: infected $L6_3$ chicken, n=4 for each line.

The CpGs in the promoter of *CD4* exhibits a high (>70%) methylation level in both L6$_3$ and L7$_2$ chickens before MDV infection. During MD progression, no significant methylation changes of *CD4* promoter were detected in L6$_3$ chickens at 5, 10 and 21 dpi or in L7$_2$ chickens at 5 and 10 dpi (P>0.05, Figure 1, and Figure 1A and 1B); however, the significant down-regulation of *CD4* promoter methylation level was observed at 21 dpi in L7$_2$ chickens (P< 0.05, Figure 1C). The result from the exact F test revealed that the *CD4* promoter methylation pattern in L7$_2$ infected samples at 21 dpi was significantly different from any other groups (Figure 2).

3.3.2 CD4 GENE EXPRESSION AT 21 DPI

To ascertain if the *CD4* gene transcription level is influenced by its promoter methylation changes at 21 dpi, we conducted quantitative PCR. We found a significantly higher expression of *CD4* gene in L7$_2$ infected samples compared with noninfected control samples (P<0.05) (Figure 3), whereas no significant up or down-regulation of *CD4* expression was detected in L6$_3$ chickens after MDV infection (P>0.05). Hereinafter, further correlation analysis showed that methylation level of all the detected CpG sites existed a negatively relationship with *CD4* gene expression in L7$_2$ chicken at 21dpi (Figure 4).

3.4 DISCUSSION

The *CD4* gene and its regulatory sequences are conserved [12]. In human and mouse, multiple protein or transcription factor binding sites, including the Myb binding site, Elf-1 binding site, and Ikaros binding site, were found in the promoter region of *CD4*, which is involved in the on/off switching of *CD4* gene expression [4]. These regulatory sites were also found in the chicken *CD4* promoter with potential functions in its expression [12]. It is well known that epigenetic factors such as DNA methylation and histone modifications play important roles in transcriptional regulation in mammals [7]. For example. the methylation change in at least one CpG site of *CD4* gene in mouse is related to CD4+ T cell differentiation [3]. In this study, we thus examined the methylation status in the promoter region of *CD4* gene in chickens related to MDV infection.

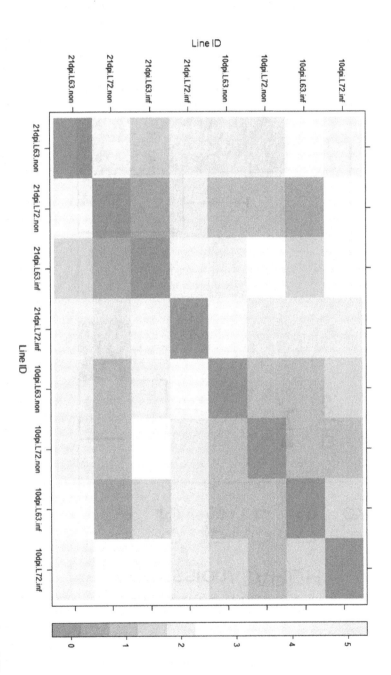

FIGURE 2: Exact F test for DNA methylation patterns of CD4. The methylation level of each of the CpG site in the promoter region of *CD4* gene was used to do an exact F test. P values matrix among L_6 and L_7 at 5, 10 and 21dpi. Color bar shows the significance level (P values with $-\log_{10}(P)$. e.g., $-\log_{10}(0.05) = 1.3$; $\log_{10}(0.01) = 2$).

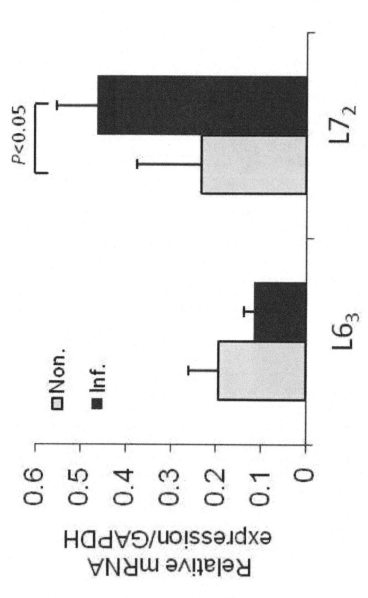

FIGURE 3: Relative mRNA expression of *CD4* gene at 21dpi. Real-time quantitative PCR was used to detect the mRNA expression level of *CD4* gene in different chicken lines with or without MDV infection at 21dpi. The relative expression level of *CD4* gene was normalized to a house keeping gene *GAPDH*. Non.: noninfected control samples; Inf.: infected samples. n=4 for each line and treatment.

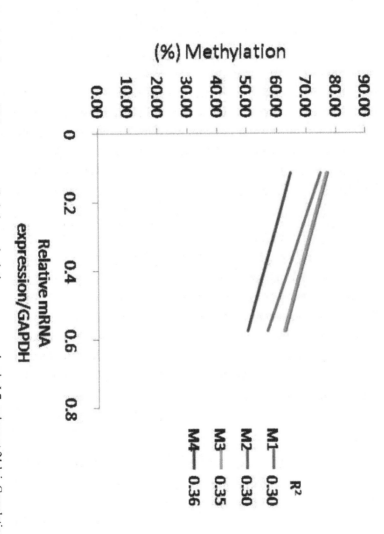

FIGURE 4: Correlation between CD4 promoter methylation and relative gene expression in $L7_2$ spleen at 21dpi. Correlation analysis of the relationship between methylation and CD4 gene mRNA expression level. R represents for the correlation coefficient. M1: CpG site 1; M2: CpG site 2; M3: CpG site3; M4: CpG site 4. n=4 for each line and treatment.

MDV is an oncovirus using CD4+ T cell as a target for latent infection and transformation, which may have interactions with the *CD4* gene at the epigenetic level [13]. In our previously study, two mutations (CG→TG) were identified in the *DNMT3b* gene between L63 and L72 chickens [10], which implied that the DNA methylation machinery may be different in the two lines in response to MDV infection. In this study, the methylation levels on the promoter region of the *CD4* gene were fluctuated over different time points of MDV infection in MD-susceptible chickens, especially during the late cytolytic phase. The quantitative PCR results confirmed that *CD4* expression in L72 chicken during the late stages of MDV infection was upregulated while the *CD4* promoter methylation was down-regulation. Since the expression of *CD4* is essential for CD4+ T cell development and activation, it may suggest that there are different epigenetic machineries of activation of CD4+ T cells by MDV infection through regulation of *CD4* methylation levels between MD-resistant and susceptible chicken lines. From previous studies, it was found that the number of infected CD4+ T cells were similar during the early phase (cytolytic phase) of MDV infection between MD-resistant and –susceptible chicken lines, but was increased during cytolytic phase in MD-susceptible chicken line and decreased in MD-resistant chicken line [14]. Additionally, in MD-resistant chicken line, CD4+ T cell is latently infected, but cannot be transformed, whereas in MD-susceptible chicken lines the infected CD4+ T cell can be transformed after the latent phase [5,15]. Taken together, the methylation change of *CD4* gene gives us an important clue that epigenetic alteration could associate with MD etiology. Therefore, future efforts will disclose the epigenetic landscapes, including genome-wide DNA methyltion and histone modifications, in immune organs and specific cell types, such as the CD4+ T cell, which will supply rich information to explore the epigenetic machinery related to chemical and physiological mechanisms of MD resistance or susceptibility.

3.5 CONCLUSIONS

In conclusion, the methylation fluctuation and mRNA expression of CD4 gene induced by MDV infection suggested a unique epigenetic mechanism existed in MD-susceptible chickens.

REFERENCES

1. Huang Z, Xie H, Ioannidis V, Held W, Clevers H, Sadim MS, Sun Z: Transcriptional regulation of CD4 gene expression by T cell factor-1/beta-catenin pathway. J Immunol 2006, 176(8):4880-4887.
2. Paillard F, Sterkers G, Vaquero C: Transcriptional and post-transcriptional regulation of TcR, CD4 and CD8 gene expression during activation of normal human T lymphocytes. Embo J 1990, 9(6):1867-1872.
3. Tutt Landolfi MM, Scollay R, Parnes JR: Specific demethylation of the CD4 gene during CD4 T lymphocyte differentiation. Mol Immunol 1997, 34(1):53-61.
4. Ellmeier W, Sawada S, Littman DR: The regulation of CD4 and CD8 coreceptor gene expression during T cell development. Annu Rev Immunol 1999, 17:523-524.
5. Davison F, Nair V: Marek's Disease: An Evolving Problem. Oxford: Elsevier Academic Press; 2004.
6. Calnek BW: Pathogenesis of Marek's disease virus infection. Curr Top Microbiol Immunol 2001, 255:25-55.
7. Allis CD, Jenuwein T, Reinberg D, Caparros M-L: Epigenetics. Cold Spring Harbor Laboratory Press; 2006.
8. Herman JG, Baylin SB: Gene silencing in cancer in association with promoter hypermethylation. N Engl J Med 2003, 349(21):2042-2054.
9. Amara K, Trimeche M, Ziadi S, Laatiri A, Hachana M, Sriha B, Mokni M, Korbi S: Presence of simian virus 40 DNA sequences in diffuse large B-cell lymphomas in Tunisia correlates with aberrant promoter hypermethylation of multiple tumor suppressor genes. Int J Cancer 2007, 121(12):2693-2702.
10. Yu Y, Zhang H, Tian F, Zhang W, Fang H, Song J: An integrated epigenetic and genetic analysis of DNA methyltransferase genes (DNMTs) in tumor resistant and susceptible chicken lines. PLoS ONE 2008, 3(7):e2672.
11. Colella S, Shen L, Baggerly KA, Issa JP, Krahe R: Sensitive and quantitative universal Pyrosequencing methylation analysis of CpG sites. Biotechniques 2003, 35(1):146-150.
12. Koskinen R, Salomonsen J, Tregaskes CA, Young JR, Goodchild M, Bumstead N, Vainio O: The chicken CD4 gene has remained conserved in evolution. Immunogenetics 2002, 54(7):520-525.

13. Rouse BT, Wells RJ, Warner NL: Proportion of T and B lymphocytes in lesions of Marek's disease: theoretical implications for pathogenesis. J Immunol 1973, 110(2):534-539.

14. Burgess SC, Basaran BH, Davison TF: Resistance to Marek's disease herpesvirus-induced lymphoma is multiphasic and dependent on host genotype. Vet Pathol 2001, 38(2):129-142.

15. Burgess SC, Davison TF: Identification of the neoplastically transformed cells in Marek's disease herpesvirus-induced lymphomas: recognition by the monoclonal antibody AV37. J Virol 2002, 76(14):7276-7292.

A COMBINATION OF TRANSCRIPTOME AND METHYLATION ANALYSES REVEALS EMBRYOLOGICALLY-RELEVANT CANDIDATE GENES IN MRKH PATIENTS

KATHARINA RALL, GIANMARIA BARRESI, MICHAEL WALTER, SVEN POTHS, KARINA HAEBIG, KARIN SCHAEFERHOFF, BIRGITT SCHOENFISCH, OLAF RIESS, DIETHELM WALLWIENER, MICHAEL BONIN, AND SARA BRUCKER

4.1 BACKGROUND

The Mayer-Rokitansky-Küster-Hauser (MRKH) syndrome (OMIM 277000) is the second most common cause of primary amenorrhea and affects at least 1 in 4,500 females. It is characterized by congenital absence of the uterus and the upper two thirds of the vagina in women with a normal female karyotype. As the ovaries are functional, women affected have physiological hormone levels and normal secondary sexual characteristics [1]. The MRKH syndrome may occur isolated (type I), or can be associated with renal or skeletal malformations, and, to a lesser extent, auditory and cardiac defects (type II) [2]. Although it is generally sporadic,

This chapter was originally published under the Creative Commons Attribution License. Rall K, Barresi G, Walter M, Poths S, Haebig K, Schaeferhoff K, Schoenfisch B, Riess O, Wallwiener D, Bonin M, and Brucker S. A Combination of Transcriptome and Methylation Analyses Reveals Embryologically-Relevant Candidate Genes in MRKH Patients. Orphanet Journal of Rare Diseases 6,32 (2011). doi:10.1186/1750-1172-6-32.

familial clustering has been described, indicating a genetic cause [3]. Familial cases have been explained by autosomal dominant inheritance with incomplete penetrance and variable expressivity or by small chromosomal aberrations undetectable in standard karyotypes [4]. However, the lack of families with informative genetic histories has not allowed the identification of any locus using standard genetic linkage analysis. Investigations have therefore used a candidate gene approach based on association with other genetic diseases or involvement during embryogenesis [4].

The association of abnormalities in Müllerian duct (MD) development with renal, skeletal, cardiac and auditory defects suggests that crucial genes of fetal development and sex differentiation such as *HOX, WNT* and those encoding anti-Müllerian hormone (AMH) and its receptor are potential candidates [5,6]. The WNT genes control the production of a large family of proteins involved in intercellular signaling during embryogenesis. Heterozygous mutations of WNT4 have been detected in a subgroup of patients, but these patients also show signs of hyperandrogenism [7-10]. *HOX* genes play key roles in body patterning and organogenesis, in particular during genital tract development and the differentiation of the kidneys and skeleton. Thus, expression or function defects in one or several *HOX* genes may account for this syndrome. Furthermore, several hormones regulate physiological processes in the adult female reproductive tract by regulating *HOX* gene expression. Alterations in *HOX* gene expression that persist in the adult are a molecular mechanism by which endocrine disruptors may affect reproductive tract development [11,12]. However, structural abnormalities in *HOX* genes or in hormones regulating *HOX* expression have not been identified in women with MRKH syndrome until today [13-17]. As a third group of genes, AMH and its receptor have been regarded as causative factors in MRKH syndrome as AMH initiates MD regression in the 6th gestational week [18-22]. Mutation analyses of the *AMH* gene, however, did not support a link between MRKH syndrome and AMH yet [18,23]. Finally, mutations in other genes with a broad spectrum of activity during early development such as *WT1, PAX2* and others have also been excluded in MRKH patients [4].

From the previous studies one can conclude that the targeted candidate gene approach has failed to decipher the causes of MRKH syndrome [2,5,24]. Recently, several recurrent copy number variants in patients with isolated and syndromic Müllerian aplasia have been described, but none of them was consistently found in a larger group of patients [25].

Cases of discordant monozygotic twins suggest that the involvement of epigenetic factors is more likely. Several studies have identified epigenetic differences, either for selected genes in monozygotic twins or in the overall epigenome [26,27].

We provide here the first study using a whole-genome approach to detect differences at the transcriptome and methylome level between MRKH patients and healthy controls. As integrated genomics becomes more and more important, the synergy between transcriptional and epigenetic gene regulation may be used to better understand the etiology of MRKH syndrome.

4.2 METHODS

4.2.1 PATIENTS

This study was approved by the ethics committee of the Eberhard-Karls-University of Tuebingen. Between July 2007 and December 2010, we had partly or completely excised 102 rudimentary uterine structures during laparoscopic-assisted neovagina in MRKH patients after informed consent was obtained [28]. As controls, we included 63 patients who underwent hysterectomy for benign disease in the same period.

Microarray analysis was performed in eight patients and eight controls to detect differentially expressed genes and seven patients and seven controls from the same group to detect differentially methylated CpG sites. Of these patients, four had MRKH type I and four had MRKH type II, including three patients with skeletal malformations, and amongst these, one with Fallot's tetralogy and one with ureter abnormalities. None of the patients had MURCS association or other complex malformations.

Analysis of serum samples at the time of surgery showed similar distribution between cycle phase one and two in the patients and control group.

Tissue samples were examined histologically before RNA and DNA were isolated. All tissue samples in both groups consisted of more than 80% myometrium.

4.2.2 RNA AND DNA ISOLATION

The total RNA from myometrial pieces of rudimentary uterine tissue or normal uterus was isolated using the RNeasy® Mini Kit (Qiagen, Hilden, Germany). RNA quality was checked by a Lab-on-a-Chip-System Bio-analyzer 2100 (Agilent, Boeblingen, Germany), and the concentration was determined using a BioPhotometer (Eppendorf, Hamburg, Germany). DNA was isolated using the DNeasy® purification Kit (Qiagen, Hilden, Germany) according to protocol and the concentration was determined using a BioPhotometer (Eppendorf).

4.2.3 AFFYMETRIX MICROARRAY ANALYSIS

Double-stranded cDNA was synthesized from 100 ng of total RNA and subsequently linearly amplified and biotinylated using the GeneChip® WT cDNA Synthesis and Amplification Kit (Affymetrix, Santa Clara, CA, USA) according to the manufacturer's instructions. 15 μg of labeled and fragmented cDNA was hybridized to GeneChip® Human Gene 1.0 ST arrays (Affymetrix). Arrays were scanned using the GCS3000 Gene Chip scanner (Affymetrix) and AGCC 3.0 software. Scanned images were inspected visually to check for hybridization artifacts and proper grid alignment and analyzed with Expression Console 1.0 (Affymetrix) to generate report files for quality control.

4.2.4 QUANTITATIVE REAL-TIME PCR

Relative expression of selected mRNA targets was determined by quantitative real-time PCR (qRT-PCR). 250-500 ng of total RNA was reverse transcribed using a QuantiTect Reverse Transcription Kit (Qiagen) according to the manufacturer. cDNA was diluted 1:10 before PCR amplification or preamplified using the TaqMan PreAmp Master Mix Kit (Applied Biosystems, Carlsbad, CA, USA) according to the manufacturer's protocol and diluted 1:20 for the subsequent PCR analysis. Primers were designed with Primer3 or PrimerBlast (http://biotools.umassmed.edu/bioapps/primer3_www.cgi, http://www.ncbi.nlm.nih.gov/tools/primer-blast/) and synthesized by Metabion (Metabion, Martinsried, Germany). Table 1 gives a list of PCR targets and primers.

TABLE 1: qRT-PCR targets with corresponding Affymetrix probeset ID and primer used for amplification

Target	Affymetrix cluster ID	Forward primer	Reverse primer
HOXA5	8138735	CGCCCAACCCCAGATCTA	GGCCGCCTATGTTGTCATG
HOXA9	8138749	GCTTGTGGTTCTCCTCCAGT	CCAGGGTCTGGTGTTTTGTA
PGR	7951165	TGGTGTTTGGTCTAGGATGGA	GGATCTGCCACATGGTAAGG
ESR1	8122840	GCAGGGAGAGGAGTTTGTGT	CAGGACTCGGTGGATATGG
OXTR	8085138	GCACGGTCAAGATGACTTTC	GCATGTAGATCCAGGGGTTG
PEG10	8134339	GACCCCATCCTTCCTGTCTT	GCTTCACTTCTGTGGGGATG
MFAP5	7960919	TGCTCTCGTCTTGTCTGTAAGG	ACAGGGAGGAAGTCGGAAGT
IRS1	8059470	GTTTCCAGAAGCAGCCAGAG	GGAAGATATGAGGTCCTAGTTGTGA
IRS2	7972745	CTTCTTGTCCCACCACTTGA	CAGTGCTGAGCGTCTTCTTTT
IGF2	7937772	ACACCCTCCAGTTCGTCTGT	CGGAAACAGCACTCCTCAA
WISP2	8062864	GCGACCAACTCCACGTCT	GTCTCCCCTTCCCGATACA
CDH5	7996264	ACAACGAGGGCATCATCAA	AATGACCTGGGCTCTGTTTC
SDHA	8104166	AGAAGCCCTTTGAGGAGCA	CGATTACGGGTCTATATTCCAGA
PDHB	8088384	GAGGCTGGCCACAGTTTG	GAAATTGAACGCAGGACCTT
PGRMC1	8169617	GGTGTTCGATGTGACCAAAG	TGAGGTCAGAAAGGTCATCGT
HISPPD1	8169617	TCCATCATCTGACGTTCCAC	TGGTGTTGGGAGGATCTTTG

Real-time detection of specific PCR products was performed on a LightCycler480 (Roche, Penzberg, Germany) with 5 μL of 2x QuantiTect SYBR Green PCR Kit (Qiagen). The PCR reaction was initiated by a 10 min hot start followed by 45 cycles of 95°C for 20 s, 58°C for 40 s, and 72°C for 20 s. Each PCR reaction was performed in three technical replicates. PCR efficiency was calculated from 4- or 5-fold serial dilutions of an equal mixture of all cDNAs using the following equation: $E = 10^{\wedge}[-1/slope]$ [29]. To calculate the relative expression of each target, the raw Cp values were imported into qBase [30]. Three suitable reference genes (*PDH, SDHA, PGRMC1* or *HISPPD1*) were selected according to their M-values and used for normalization of the qRT-PCR reactions [31,32].

4.2.5 ILLUMINA METHYLATION ARRAY ANALYSIS

200-500 ng DNA was bisulfite-converted using the EZ DNA Methylation Kit (Zymo Research, Orange, CA, USA) according to the manufacturer's protocol.

Seven patient and seven control probes were evaluated for genome-wide promoter methylation using the Illumina Infinium HumanMethylation27 BeadArray.

After bisulfite conversion, each sample was whole-genome amplified (WGA) and enzymatically fragmented. The bisulfite-converted WGA-DNA samples were purified and applied to the BeadChips. Allele-specific primer annealing is followed by single-base extension using DNP- and Biotin-labeled ddNTPs. DNA methylation values, described as beta values, are recorded for each locus in each sample via BeadStudio software [33].

Differential methylation was assessed by subtracting the mean methylation level (beta value) of the patient group from the mean beta value of the reference group using BeadStudio software.

4.2.6 PYROSEQUENCING METHYLATION ANALYSIS

PCR and sequencing primer were designed by Qiagen using the PyroMark Assay Design Software 2.0 and are shown in Table 2. For each gene, we selected the sequence of the CpG island region which had previously been identified as differentially methylated in the array experiments. One to five adjacent CpG sites were analyzed for each CpG island. Five patient and five control samples were included in the experiment. 200 ng of isolated DNA was bisulfite-converted using the EZ DNA Methylation Kit (Zymo). 24 ng of bisulfite-treated DNA were amplified in reaction mixture containing forward and reverse primer, 1 U of HotStarTaq DNA Polymerase (Qiagen), 200 µmol each of dNTP/l and nuclease-free water. The same cycling conditions were used for all assays: denaturing at 95°C for 15 min; 35 cycles at 95°C for 10 s, at 59, 3°C for 30 s, and at 72°C for 30 s; an additional elongation step was performed at 72°C for 3 min. Gel electrophoresis was carried out on all PCR products. All PCR reactions included a no-template control and four standardized methylation controls (0%, 30%, 70%, and 100% methylated DNA). Pyrosequencing was carried out using the Pyrosequencer PSQ 96 MA (Biotage AB, Uppsala, Sweden). Results were automatically analyzed using the PSQ 96MA 1.0 software (Allele Quantification mode).

TABLE 2: Pyrosequencing targets with corresponding Illumina probeset ID and primer used for amplification

Target	Illumina Target ID	Forward primer	Reverse primer	Sequencing primer
WISP2	cg03562120	GTGTGT-GTTTGGGAGT-GATTT	Bio-CT-CATATCCCCTA-CAAAACCAACTTTAA	GTTTGGGAGT-GATTTTATAGTT-GT
HOXA5	cg02248486	GGAATTAT-GATTTTTATAAT-TATGTAATTGG-TAGTT	Bio-AACCACAAAT-CAAACACACATATCA	AATTATGATTTT-TATAATTATGTA-ATTGGTAG
HOXA9	cg27009703	Bio-GTGGTGATG-GTGGTGGTATAT	ACTTCAACCCCTA-CAACTTCCAATCCA	TCAACCCCTA-CAACTTCCAATC-CAAAA
WT1	cg25094569	Bio-TGGATGT-GATTTTGGGATAG-GT	CCCATTTTTAAAAC-CAAACCATTTAACT	ATTTTTA-AAAAATAAA-CAACCTTCTC-TATC
GATA4	cg17795240	AAGGATTGGTT-TAGGGAGAGTTT-GTTTTG	Bio-TAAAATTTCAC-CATATTAAC-CAAAAACTCCTA-ACCTTA	GGTTTAGGGAGA-GTTTGTTTTG

4.2.7 PATHWAY ANALYSIS

Gene regulation networks were generated using Ingenuity Pathway analysis software (ingenuity® systems, http://www.ingenuity.com). The dataset with differentially regulated transcripts and their corresponding expression and methylation values were uploaded into the application. The genes were overlaid onto a global molecular network developed from information in the Ingenuity Pathways Knowledge Base. Networks of these focus genes were then algorithmically generated based on their connectivity. All edges are supported by at least one reference from the literature, from a textbook, or from canonical information stored in the Ingenuity Pathways Knowledge Base. Genes from the microarray dataset that met the fold change cutoff of 1.5 and that were associated with a relevant pathway in the Ingenuity Pathways Knowledge Base were included in the analysis.

4.2.8 STATISTICAL METHODS

With quantitative RT-PCR normalized values were obtained from qBase. The ratio of means of patients divided by means of controls was then calculated and the log2 of this ratio is shown. For the Affymetrix microarray analysis the means of patients were divided by the means of controls and the log2 was shown as log fold change. Measurement errors were calculated using Gaussian error propagation. As usual it is assumed that normalized values obtained from qBase are lognormal distributed and a t-test (i.e. the Welch test assuming unequal variances) was applied for each gene to investigate the difference between patients and controls in qRT-PCR. The same was done for expression array data. A significance level of 5% was chosen. The percentage of methylated cytosines was obtained from pyrosequencing methylation analysis. The difference means of patients minus means of controls are shown. The same was done for the average beta values.

4.3 RESULTS

4.3.1 MICROARRAY EXPRESSION AND METHYLATION ANALYSIS

To identify changes in the expression level of putative candidate genes, we performed microarray analysis with Affymetrix Human Gene 1.0. Analysis using the ArrayAssist 4.0 software identified 293 transcripts differentially expressed between tissue samples of MRKH patients and controls. Of these transcripts, 161 were upregulated and 132 downregulated with a fold change of at least 1.5 and a p-value of less than 0.05 (Table 3).

TABLE 3: Differential expression of genes and methylation of CpG-sites in MRKH patients compared to controls in numbers

Difference in patients from controls	n
Differential expression, total	293
Downregulated	132
Upregulated	161
Differential methylation, total	194
Hypomethylated	116
Hypermethylated	78
Overlap	9

Pathway analysis revealed genes relevant in the embryological development of the genital tract, including *HOXA* genes and hormone receptors.

The delineation of regional DNA methylation patterns has important implications for understanding why certain regions of the genome can be expressed in specific developmental contexts and how epigenetic changes

TABLE 4: Overlap genes: names of differentially expressed genes that contain differentially methylated CpG-sites

Probe set ID, human 1.0 genechip array	Probe set ID, 27human methylation	Gene title	Gene symbol	Fold change human 1.0 genechip array	p-value	Diff methyl 27human methylation array	p-value
8138735	cg02248486	homeobox A5	HOXA5	1.9	0.00036	-0.33	0.00015
8138749	cg26521404	homeobox A9	HOXA9	1.5	na	-0.23	0.00047
8062864	cg03562120	WNT1-inducible signaling pathway protein 2	WISP2	-1.7	0.00148	0.14	0.00096
7996264	cg22319147	cadherin 5, type 2, VE-cadherin (vascular epithelium)	CDH5	-1.6	0.00503	-0.12	0.00598
8134339	cg19107595	paternally expressed 10	PEG10	1.8	0.00290	-0.12	0.01596
7960919	cg15815843	Microfibrillar-associated protein 5	MFAP5	-2.1	0.04635	0.16	0.02451
7950555	cg20899321	Leucine-rich repeat containing 32	LRRC32	-1.6	0.00435	0.12	0.00045
7907657	cg10559803	Ral GEF with PH domain and SH3 binding motif 2	RALGPS2	2.0	0.00385	-0.11	0.00345
8002249	cg17217677	sphingomyelin phosphodiesterase 3, neutral membrane (neutral sphingomyelinase II)	SMPD3	1.6	0.00001	-0.10	0.01602

might enable aberrant expression patterns and disease [27]. We therefore decided to compare whole-genome expression and methylation patterns in uterine rudiments of MRKH patients compared to control uteri. To achieve this, we performed Illumina HumanMethylation27 BeadArrays and overlaid both datasets. The analysis using the BeadStudio software identified 194 differentially methylated CpG sites in specific CpG islands. Of these sites, 78 were hypermethylated and 116 hypomethylated (Table 3).

Nine genes were detected in both datasets (*HOXA5, HOXA9, WISP2, CDH5, PEG10, MFAP5, LRRC32, RALGPS2, SMPD3*); these are termed "overlap genes" (Table 4). CpG sites within these genes were either hypermethylated and the genes underexpressed or hypomethylated and overexpressed, except for one gene.

Of the nine overlap genes, six (*CDH5, MFAP5, WISP2, HOXA5, PEG10, HOXA9*) were included in the subsequent analyses and experiments as they are known to be relevant to the embryological development of the female genital tract.

4.3.2 NETWORK AND PATHWAY ANALYSIS

Ingenuity Pathways analysis software (Ingenuity Systems) was used to examine the connection between the differentially methylated CpG sites and differentially expressed genes. As shown in Figures 1 and 2, differentially expressed genes and differentially methylated sites can be assigned to basic functions relevant to cell and tissue development and proliferation, cell-to-cell signaling and interaction, cellular movement, cancer, endocrine and reproductive disorders, and others (Figure 1 and 2).

Figure 3 shows a network of differentially regulated overlap genes and other relevant genes. The network was created by fusing the expression and methylation datasets from the microarray experiments. This specific network was selected because of the known relevance of the genes included during embryological development and during functional changes of the female reproductive tract. Interactions between embryologically relevant genes, including *HOXA* genes and hormone receptors, can be clearly detected. Interacting genes are either differentially expressed, carry differentially methylated CpG sites, or both. The gene regulation network

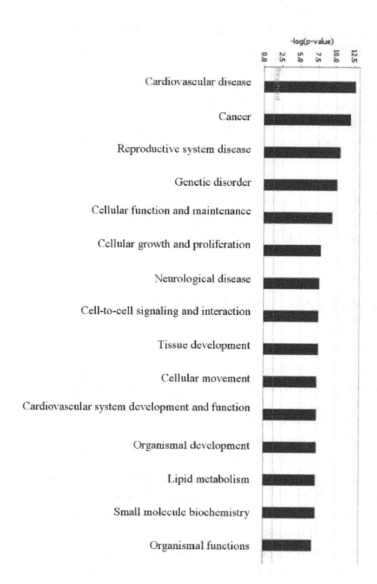

FIGURE 1: Assignment of differentially expressed genes to functional groups. Assignment of all differentially expressed genes to functional groups. The analysis was done with Ingenuity Pathways analysis software. Fischer's exact test was used to test for significance (shown as bars), determining the probability that each biological function assigned to the network is due to chance alone.

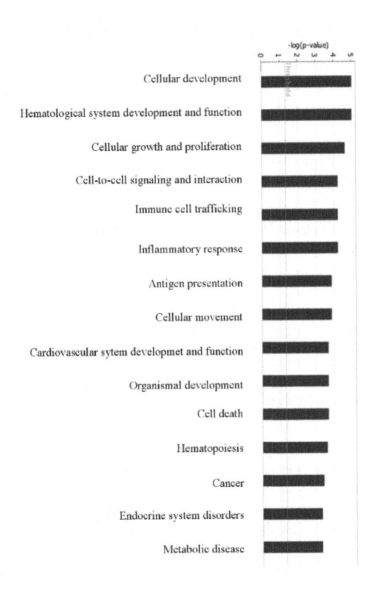

FIGURE 2: Assignment of all genes containing differentially methylated CpG-sites to functional groups. Fischer's exact test was used to test for significance (shown as bars), determining the probability that each biological function assigned to the network is due to chance alone.

contains 15 differentially regulated genes, seven downregulated (green icons), two of these also with hypermethylated CpG sites (dark grey), and seven upregulated (icons), three of these also with hypomethylated CpG sites (light grey). Four genes contained differentially methylated CpG sites without being differentially expressed (three hypo- and one hyper-methylated). Eight genes are supplemented in the network to complete the interactions. Eleven of the transcripts shown were used for qRT-PCR validation and five for pyrosequencing.

Figure 4 shows the relation between expression and methylation in overlap genes later selected for validation. CpG sites in genes were either hypomethylated with genes overexpressed or hypermethylated with genes underexpressed, except for CDH5.

4.3.3 VALIDATION OF EXPRESSION DIFFERENCES BY QRT-PCR

We chose nine key players in the interaction networks for independent verification by qRT-PCR. The genes were selected because of their known relevance during embryological development. Three suitable reference genes (*PDH, SDHA, PGRMC1* or *HISPPD1*) were selected according to their M-values and used for normalization of the qRT-PCR reactions. We were able to validate all nine genes. The results of the qRT-PCR (Figure 5) showed 100% validation efficiency in comparison to the expression data of the microarray experiment, although statistical significance was not always found.

4.3.4 VALIDATION OF METHYLATION DIFFERENCES BY PYROSEQUENCING

Five embryologically important genes were chosen for validation of the methylation array experiments by pyrosequencing. We selected one to five CpG sites within one specific CpG island per gene for analysis (Figure 6). The CpG islands were selected according to the differential methylation in the preceding array experiments. The differential methylation status of the array experiments was confirmed for all five CpG islands within the

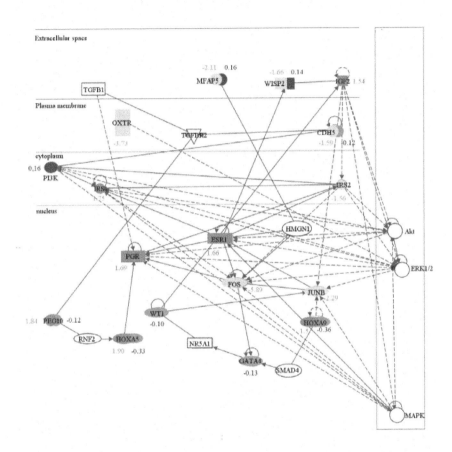

FIGURE 3: Network of differentially expressed genes and genes containing differentially methylated CpG-sites. The fold change of regulation in the microarray analysis, (the p-value of the significance analysis) and the percentage of differential methylation are listed below the symbols. For the purposes of simplification, only selected known gene-to-gene interactions are shown. Continuous arrow lines show direct interactions between genes and broken arrow lines show indirect interactions.

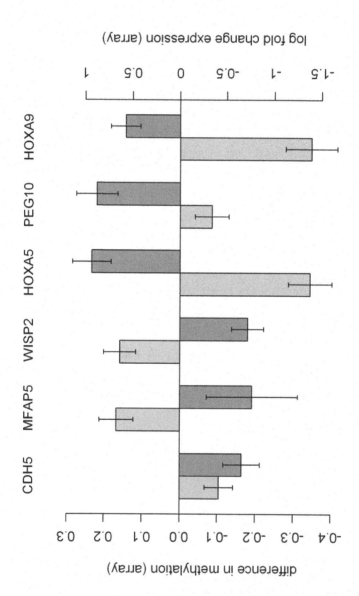

FIGURE 4: Relation between expression and methylation in overlap genes. Methylation (left) and expression (right) of overlap genes in MRKH patients compared to control group. Methylation is shown as difference of average beta of patients minus controls. Expression differences are shown as log fold change of patients divided by controls. Bars indicate the measurement error.

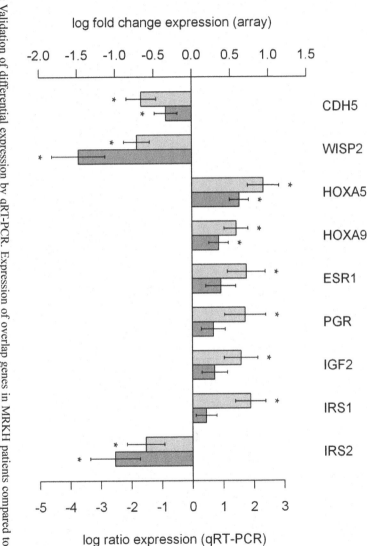

FIGURE 5: Validation of differential expression by qRT-PCR. Expression of overlap genes in MRKH patients compared to control group measured by array (left) and qRT-PCR (right). Array data are shown as log fold change of patients divided by controls, qRT-PCR data are shown as log ratio of patients divided by controls. Bars indicate the measurement error and stars indicate a significant difference between patients and controls (t-test, p-values <0.05).

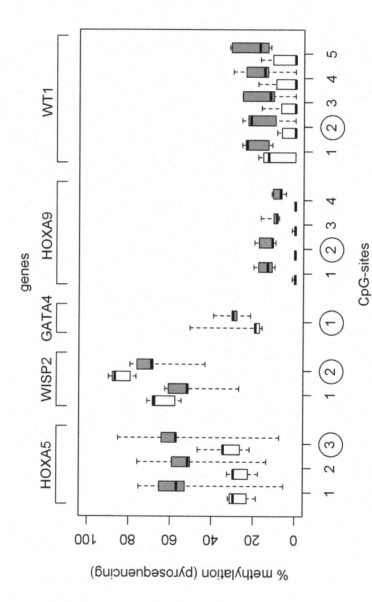

FIGURE 6: Similar methylation in adjacent CpG sites within CpG islands. Degree of methylation within CpG islands: shown are box-and-whisker plots of the percentage of methylated cytosines for patients (white boxes) and contols (grey boxes). The circled CpG sites correspond to the specific sites detected in the array experiments.

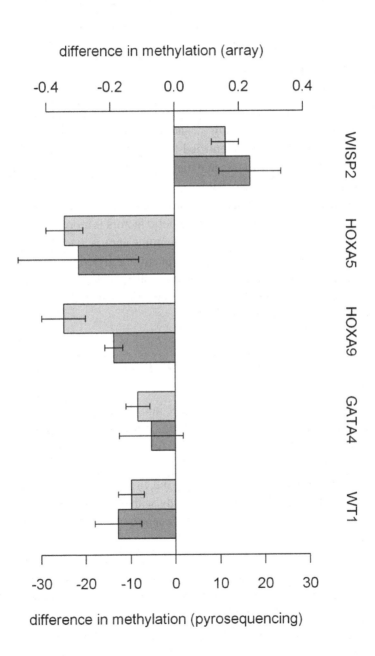

FIGURE 7. Validation of differential methylation by pyrosequencing. Methylation array (left) and pyrosequencing (right) of overlap genes in MRKH patients compared to control group. Both are shown as difference of patients minus controls. Bars indicate the measurement error.

WISP2, HOXA5, HOXA9, GATA4 and *WT1* genes, thus validation efficiency was again 100% (Figure 7).

4.4 DISCUSSION

Although MRKH syndrome is a congenital disorder most patients are not diagnosed until puberty. Using a candidate gene approach, the underlying cause has so far not been identified [5]. Recently, a high incidence of recurrent copy number variants in patients with isolated and syndromic Müllerian aplasia has been described, but none of them was consistently found in a larger group of patients [25]. Cases of discordant monozygotic twins suggest that the involvement of epigenetic factors is more likely. The present study was the first to use a whole-genome approach to identify relevant genes, including differential expression and methylation. This allowed us to create a complex network of genes, which provided insight into possible mechanisms underlying MRKH syndrome. Our data indicate that different potential mechanisms are possible.

4.4.1 DEFICIENCY OF HORMONE RECEPTORS

The overexpression of ESR1 and PGR in rudimentary uterine tissue from MRKH patients could be explained by a deficiency of these hormone receptors. The local overexpression may be the result of a positive feedback mechanism well known from other hormonal regulatory loops. Similar hypotheses have been postulated before but firm scientific evidence has not yet been obtained. This is the first study with an experimental setting that supports the hypothesis of locally deficient hormone receptors in MRKH syndrome.

As early as 1910, Küster explained the MRKH syndrome by regression of the Müllerian duct (MD) [34]. According to Ludwig, the MRKH syndrome results from non-fusion of the MD with the Wolffian duct (WD) [35,36]. Because the embryo is under the influence of maternal hormones, he suggested that both the non-fusion of the MD with the WD and rudimentary development of the vagina are caused by a deficiency of gestagen or estrogen receptors [35,36]. Estrogens are necessary for the embryonic development of the female reproductive tract. The special role of ESR1 in female reproductive tract development has been demonstrated by disrupting the corresponding gene in the mouse, resulting in hypoplastic uterine and vaginal tissue [37].

4.4.2 INFLUENCE OF ESTROGEN ON AMH AND ITS RECEPTOR

One of the first hypotheses for the underlying cause of MRKH syndrome was an activating mutation of either the gene for the AMH receptor (AMHR), resulting in the inappropriate production of AMH, or the receptor itself. Schmid-Tannwald and Hauser proposed the regression of the MD due to a temporary secretion of AMH during the first fetal weeks [38]. Depending upon the amount secreted, a greater or lesser portion of the MD regressed. Nevertheless, mutation analyses of the AMH gene did not support a link between the MRKH syndrome and AMH at the genome level. Also, AMH protein levels in plasma and peritoneal fluid from MRKH patients were equivalent to control individuals [18,23]. Our study confirmed the data given, as we did not see any persistent differential expression or methylation patterns in the AMH or AMHR genes in adolescent MRKH patients. However, low or baseline AMH levels in a female adolescent may not necessarily be correlated with the patient's early embryonic exposure to AMH signaling [23].

It has been reported that estrogen regulates AMH expression [39]. The constant overexpression of ESR1 found in the rudimentary uterine tissue in our patients or the in utero exposure to abnormally high maternal levels of E2 could lead to an increasing AMH promoter activity during embryological development of the female genital tract causing uterine and vaginal aplasia.

Transcription factors involved in primary sex determination are also recruited as important regulators of AMH transcription. A common regulatory factor important for transcription of *AMH* genes is WT-1. WT-1 is essential for the embryonic development of the kidneys and gonads. GATA4 appears to play a predominant role in sex determination and sex differentiation via *AMH* gene regulation [40]. In our study CpG sites within *WT1* and *GATA4* were both hypomethylated compared to the control tissue. This could be a sign of stable activation leading, at least during embryological development, to activation of the *AMH* gene and thus partial regression of the MD.

4.4.3 INFLUENCE OF ENDOCRINE DISRUPTORS ON THE MbLLERIAN DUCT AND ON THE EXPRESSION OF HOX GENES

Chemical compounds homologous to steroids can act as agonists or antagonists in fetuses exposed to them [37]. The involvement of ED with estrogen-like functions would be an explanation for the findings in MRKH syndrome, although the analyses of pregnancy histories available in all our cases so far failed to identify any clear association with drug use, illness or exposure to known substances.

Several examples of a negative impact of estrogens on uterine development are known. Transient exposure of the neonatal ewe to estrogens during critical periods specifically perturbs normal development of the uterus [41]. Estrogen inhibited caudal progression of developing MD in the turtle. It has been shown to block development of the MD when applied before the start of differentiation, and the length of the MD varied with the time point treatment was given [42].

Epithelial-mesenchymal differentiation in the murine MD is regulated by *WNT* signaling correlated with expression of *HOX* genes. Several nuclear hormonal receptors regulate the expression of multiple *HOX* genes. When a *HOX* gene is mutated, the body segment where it is normally expressed typically develops characteristics of the segment anterior to it, an effect known as anterior transformation. In contrast to *Drosophila*, in vertebrates, targeted mutation in a single *HOX* gene usually causes only a subtle transformation. This is because of genetic duplication and functional redundancy of adjacent genes [11]. The hypomethylation of specific CpG sites and corresponding overexpression of *HOXA9* could be due to either exposure to a substance similar to diethylstilbestrol (DES) in utero or a deficient *HOXA10* causing anterior transformation.

It is known that HOXA9 is expressed at high levels in areas destined to become the fallopian tube, HOXA10 is expressed in the developing uterus, HOXA11 is expressed in the primordia of the lower uterine segment and cervix, and that HOXA13 is expressed in the ectocervix and upper vagina. This expression pattern has been preserved in mice and humans [43]. Microarray analysis has shown organ-specific changes in gene expression profiles in the oviduct, uterus, and vagina after DES exposure. Changes in *HOX* and *WNT* expression might lead to abnormalities of segment-related positional identity in the upper part of the MD after DES exposure [43,44]. Sex steroids have been investigated in the regulation of the *HOX* genes at the 5'end of the cluster that determine posterior development, including development of the reproductive tract [45-48]. Both, *HOXA10* and *HOXA11* expression, is upregulated by 17ß-estradiol and progesterone. Changes in *HOX* gene expression are a potential marker for the effects of in utero drug use that may become apparent only at late stages of development [12]. In utero, DES exposure shifts *HOXA9* expression from the oviducts to the uterus and decreases *HOXA10* as well as *HOXA11* expression of the uterus causing a "T-shaped" uterus with a tube-like phenotype [47]. In human uterine and cervical cell cultures, DES has induced *HOXA9* or *HOXA10* gene expression [12].

Continued *HOX* gene expression in the adult has been described in the reproductive tract and may be a mechanism to retain developmental plasticity [49]. Specifically *HOXA10* and *11* are expressed in the endometrium and their expression varies in a menstrual cycle-dependent manner. Although no women with mutations in *HOXA10* and *HOXA11* have been described, patients with lower implantation rates have lower *HOXA10* and *HOXA11* expression in the secretory phase [43].

In addition to *HOXA9*, specific CpG sites in *HOXA5* were hypomethylated and the gene overexpressed. This gene has a crucial role in the specification of the cervical and upper thoracic region of the skeleton. Its correct expression is important for the proper patterning of the embryo. It has been shown that ectopic *HOXA5* expression results in abnormal differentiation [50]. In a similar manner, ectopic *HOXA5* expression at the 5'end of the cluster might prevent normal differentiation of the MD or even regression. *HOXA5* is known as a transcriptional regulator of multiple target genes, two of which are *p53* and the progesterone receptor (PGR). The overexpression of PGR in patients may be induced directly by the overexpression of *HOXA5* [51].

Finally, neonatal DES exposure is also known to cause overexpression of IRS-1 and IGF2, both of which are included in our network [52].

4.4.4 IMPACT OF WNT GENES ON UTERINE DEVELOPMENT

The *WNT* genes and products form the WNT signaling pathway which controls developmental processes. Only the *WNT4* gene has been clearly implicated in atypical MRKH syndrome before [9]. The phenotype of *WNT9b* mutants can be rescued by activation of *WNT1* in the WD, identifying the canonical WNT pathway as a determinant signaling process in MD elongation [37]. A recent study excluded mutations in the coding sequences of *WNT4, WNT5A, WNT7A* and *WNT9B* in 11 MRKH patients [6]. In our study, CpG sites within the *WISP2* (WNT1 inducible signaling pathway protein 2) gene were hypermethylated and the gene underexpressed in rudimentary uterine tissue, thus the relevance is not clear yet. *WISP2* (CCN5), a gene that is important in smooth muscle cell proliferation and migration, is an estrogen-induced gene in the uterus [53].

4.5 CONCLUSION

We were able to draw important conclusions from our study, the first to compare rudimentary uterine tissue from MRKH patients and uterine tissue from healthy controls. *GATA4, WT1* and constant overexpression of *ESR1* might increase AMH promoter activity during embryological development, resulting in partial regression of the MD. Involvement of endocrine disruptors (ED) with estrogen-like functions might mimic this effect. The deficiency of hormone receptors may result in their overexpression and cause both the non-fusion of the MD with the WD and rudimentary development of the vagina.

The hypomethylation of specific CpG sites and the corresponding overexpression of *HOXA9* may be due to either exposure to a substance similar to DES in utero or deficient *HOXA10* causing anterior transformation.

Ectopic *HOXA5* expression at the 5'end of the cluster might prevent normal differentiation of the MD.

Using the synergetic approach of transcriptional and epigenetic regulation, our study has, for the first time, provided a deeper insight into the etiology of congenital vaginal and uterine aplasia, and has significantly advanced the explanation of MRKH syndrome. Further investigations will show which of our hypotheses is correct, but it is already clear that hormone receptors and HOX genes appear to play a major role and should be in focus of further examinations.

REFERENCES

1. Folch M, Pigem I, Konje JC: Müllerian agenesis: etiology, diagnosis, and management. Obstet Gynecol Surv 2000, 55(10):644-9.
2. Ledig S, Schippert C, Strick R, Beckmann MW, Oppelt PG, Wieacker P: Recurrent aberrations identified by array-CGH in patients with Mayer-Rokitansky-Küster-Hauser syndrome. Fertil Steril 2011, 95(5):1589-94.
3. Wottgen M, Brucker S, Renner SP, Strissel PL, Strick R, Kellermann A, Wallwiener D, Beckmann MW, Oppelt P: Higher incidence of linked malformations in siblings of Mayer-Rokitansky-Küster-Hauser-syndrome patients. Hum Reprod 2008, 23(5):1226-31.
4. Morcel K, Camborieux L, Programme de Recherches sur les Aplasies Müllériennes, Guerrier D: Mayer-Rokitansky-Küster-Hauser (MRKH) syndrome. Orphanet J Rare Dis 2007, 2:13.
5. Sultan C, Biason-Lauber A, Philibert P: Mayer-Rokitansky-Kuster-Hauser syndrome: recent clinical and genetic findings. Gynecol Endocrinol 2009, 25(1):8-11.
6. Ravel C, Lorenço D, Dessolle L, Mandelbaum J, McElreavey K, Darai E, Siffroi JP: Mutational analysis of the WNT gene family in women with Mayer-Rokitansky-Kuster-Hauser syndrome. Fertil Steril 2009, 91(4 Suppl):1604-7.
7. Cheroki C, Krepischi-Santos AC, Rosenberg C, Jehee FS, Mingroni-Netto RC, Pavanello Filho I, Zanforlin Filho S, Kim CA, Bagnoli VR, Mendonça BB, Szuhai K, Otto PA: Report of a del22q11 in a patient with Mayer-Rokitansky-Küster-Hauser (MRKH) anomaly and exclusion of WNT-4, RAR-gamma, and RXR-alpha as major genes determining MRKH anomaly in a study of 25 affected women. Am J Med Genet A 2006, 140(12):1339-42.
8. Cheroki C, Krepischi-Santos AC, Szuhai K, Brenner V, Kim CA, Otto PA, Rosenberg C: Genomic imbalances associated with mullerian aplasia. J Med Genet 2008, 45(4):228-32.
9. Biason-Lauber A, Konrad D: WNT4 and sex development. Sex Dev 2008, 2(4-5):210-8.

10. Philibert P, Biason-Lauber A, Rouzier R, Pienkowski C, Paris F, Konrad D, Schoenle E, Sultan C: Identification and functional analysis of a new WNT4 gene mutation among 28 adolescent girls with primary amenorrhea and müllerian duct abnormalities: a French collaborative study. J Clin Endocrinol Metab 2008, 93(3):895-900.

11. Daftary GS, Taylor HS: Endocrine regulation of HOX genes. Endocr Rev 2006, 27(4):331-55.

12. Block K, Kardana A, Igarashi P, Taylor HS: In utero diethylstilbestrol (DES) exposure alters Hox gene expression in the developing müllerian system. FASEB J 2000, 14(9):1101-8.

13. Guerrier D, Mouchel T, Pasquier L, Pellerin I: The Mayer-Rokitansky-Küster-Hauser syndrome (congenital absence of uterus and vagina)--phenotypic manifestations and genetic approaches. J Negat Results Biomed 2006, 5:1.

14. Mortlock DP, Innis JW: Mutation of HOXA13 in hand-foot-genital syndrome. Nat Genet 1997, 15(2):179-80.

15. Goodman FR, Bacchelli C, Brady AF, Brueton LA, Fryns JP, Mortlock DP, Innis JW, Holmes LB, Donnenfeld AE, Feingold M, Beemer FA, Hennekam RC, Scambler PJ: Novel HOXA13 mutations and the phenotypic spectrum of hand-foot-genital syndrome. Am J Hum Genet 2000, 67(1):197-202.

16. Burel A, Mouchel T, Odent S, Tiker F, Knebelmann B, Pellerin I, Guerrier D: Role of HOXA7 to HOXA13 and PBX1 genes in various forms of MRKH syndrome (congenital absence of uterus and vagina). J Negat Results Biomed 2006, 5:4.

17. Lalwani S, Wu HH, Reindollar RH, Gray MR: HOXA10 mutations in congenital absence of uterus and vagina. Fertil Steril 2008, 89(2):325-30.

18. Oppelt P, Strissel PL, Kellermann A, Seeber S, Humeny A, Beckmann MW, Strick R: DNA sequence variations of the entire anti-Mullerian hormone (AMH) gene promoter and AMH protein expression in patients with the Mayer-Rokitansky-Kuster-Hauser syndrome. Hum Reprod 2005, 20(1):149-57.

19. Visser JA: AMH signaling: from receptor to target gene. Mol Cell Endocrinol 2003, 211(1-2):65-73.

20. Guioli S, Sekido R, Lovell-Badge R: The origin of the Mullerian duct in chick and mouse. Dev Biol 2007, 302(2):389-98.

21. Orvis GD, Behringer RR: Cellular mechanisms of Müllerian duct formation in the mouse. Dev Biol 2007, 306(2):493-504.

22. Josso N, Belville C, di Clemente N, Picard JY: AMH and AMH receptor defects in persistent Müllerian duct syndrome. Hum Reprod Update 2005, 11(4):351-6.

23. Resendes BL, Sohn SH, Stelling JR, Tineo R, Davis AJ, Gray MR, Reindollar RH: Role for anti-Müllerian hormone in congenital absence of the uterus and vagina. Am J Med Genet 2001, 98(2):129-36.

24. Bernardini L, Gimelli S, Gervasini C, Carella M, Baban A, Frontino G, Barbano G, Divizia MT, Fedele L, Novelli A, Béna F, Lalatta F, Miozzo M, Dallapiccola B: Recurrent microdeletion at 17q12 as a cause of Mayer-Rokitansky-Kuster-Hauser (MRKH) syndrome: two case reports. Orphanet J Rare Dis 2009, 4:25.

25. Nik-Zainal S, Strick R, Storer M, Huang N, Rad R, Willatt L, Fitzgerald T, Martin V, Sandford R, Carter NP, Janecke AR, Renner SP, Oppelt PG, Oppelt P, Schulze C, Brucker S, Hurles M, Beckmann MW, Strissel PL, Shaw-Smith C: High incidence

of recurrent copy number variants in patients with isolated and syndromic Müllerian aplasia. J Med Genet 2011.

26. Kaminsky ZA, Tang T, Wang SC, Ptak C, Oh GH, Wong AH, Feldcamp LA, Virtanen C, Halfvarson J, Tysk C, McRae AF, Visscher PM, Montgomery GW, Gottesman II, Martin NG, Petronis A: DNA methylation profiles in monozygotic and dizygotic twins. Nat Genet 2009, 41(2):240-5.

27. Laird PW: Principles and challenges of genome-wide DNA methylation analysis. Nat Rev Genet 2010, 11(3):191-203.

28. Brucker SY, Gegusch M, Zubke W, Rall K, Gauwerky JF, Wallwiener D: Neovagina creation in vaginal agenesis: development of a new laparoscopic Vecchietti-based procedure and optimized instruments in a prospective comparative interventional study in 101 patients. Fertil Steril 2008, 90(5):1940-52.

29. Rasmussen R: Quantification on the LightCycler. In Rapid Cycle Real-time PCR, Methods and Applications. Edited by Meurer S, Wittwer C and Nakagawara K. Springer Press, Heidel; 2001::21-34.

30. Hellemans J, Mortier G, De Paepe A, Speleman F, Vandesompele J: qBase relative quantification framework and software for management and automated analysis of real-time quantitative PCR data. Genome Biol 2007, 8(2):R19.

31. Goossens K, Van Poucke M, Van Soom A, Vandesompele J, Van Zeveren A, Peelman LJ: Selection of reference genes for quantitative real-time PCR in bovine preimplantation embryos. MC Dev Biol 2005, 5:27.

32. Vandesompele J, De Preter K, Pattyn F, Poppe B, Van Roy N, De Paepe A, Speleman F: Accurate normalization of real-time quantitative RT-PCR data by geometric averaging of multiple internal control genes. Genome Biol 2002, 3(7):RESEARCH0034.

33. Weisenberger D, Van Den Berg D, Pan F, Berman B, Laird P: Comprehensive DNA Methylation Analysis on the Illumina®Infinium® Assay Platform. [http:/ / www. illumina.com/ Documents/ products/ appnotes/ appnote_infinium_methylation.pdf]

34. Küster H: Uterus bipartitus solidus rudimentarius cum vagina solida. Z Geburtshilfe Gynakol 1910, 67:692-718.

35. Ludwig KS: The Mayer-Rokitansky-Küster syndrome. An analysis of its morphology and embryology. Part I Morphology. Arch Gynecol Obstet 1998, 262(1-2):1-26.

36. Ludwig KS: The Mayer-Rokitansky-Küster syndrome. An analysis of its morphology and embryology. Part II: Embryology. Arch Gynecol Obstet 1998, 262(1-2):27-42.

37. Massé J, Watrin T, Laurent A, Deschamps S, Guerrier D, Pellerin I: The developing female genital tract: from genetics to epigenetics. Int J Dev Biol 2009, 53(2-3):411-24.

38. Schmid-Tannwald I, Hauser GA: Atypical forms of the Mayer- Rokitansky-Kuster-syndrome. Geburtshilfe Frauenheilkd 1977, 37:386-392.

39. Chen G, Shinka T, Kinoshita K, Yan HT, Iwamoto T, Nakahori Y: Roles of estrogen receptor alpha (ER alpha) in the regulation of the human Müllerian inhibitory substance (MIS) promoter. J Med Invest 2003, 50(3-4):192-8.

40. Miyamoto Y, Taniguchi H, Hamel F, Silversides DW, Viger RS: A GATA4/WT1 cooperation regulates transcription of genes required for mammalian sex determination and differentiation. BMC Mol Biol 2008, 9:44.

41. Hayashi K, Carpenter KD, Spencer TE: Neonatal estrogen exposure disrupts uterine development in the postnatal sheep. Endocrinology 2004, 145(7):3247-57.
42. Dodd KL, Wibbels T: Estrogen inhibits caudal progression but stimulates proliferation of developing müllerian ducts in a turtle with temperature-dependent sex determination. Comp Biochem Physiol A Mol Integr Physiol 2008, 150(3):315-9.
43. Taylor HS: Endocrine disruptors affect developmental programming of HOX gene expression. Fertil Steril 2008, 89(2 Suppl):e57-8.
44. Suzuki A, Urushitani H, Sato T, Kobayashi T, Watanabe H, Ohta Y, Iguchi T: Gene expression change in the Müllerian duct of the mouse fetus exposed to diethylstilbestrol in utero. Exp Biol Med (Maywood) 2007, 232(4):503-14.
45. Cermik D, Karaca M, Taylor HS: HOXA10 expression is repressed by progesterone in the myometrium: differential tissue-specific regulation of HOX gene expression in the reproductive tract. J Clin Endocrinol Metab 2001, 86(7):3387-92.
46. Ma L, Benson GV, Lim H, Dey SK, Maas RL: Abdominal B (AbdB) Hoxa genes: regulation in adult uterus by estrogen and progesterone and repression in müllerian duct by the synthetic estrogen diethylstilbestrol (DES). Dev Biol 1998, 197(2):141-54.
47. Du H, Taylor HS: Molecular regulation of mullerian development by Hox genes. Ann N Y Acad Sci 2004, 1034:152-65.
48. Taylor HS: The role of HOX genes in the development and function of the female reproductive tract. Semin Reprod Med 2000, 18(1):81-9.
49. Morgan R: Hox genes: a continuation of embryonic patterning? Trends Genet 2006, 22(2):67-9.
50. Aubin J, Lemieux M, Tremblay M, Behringer RR, Jeannotte L: Transcriptional interferences at the Hoxa4/Hoxa5 locus: importance of correct Hoxa5 expression for the proper specification of the axial skeleton. Dev Dyn 1998, 212(1):141-56.
51. Sauter CN, McDermid RL, Weinberg AL, Greco TL, Xu X, Murdoch FE, Fritsch MK: Differentiation of murine embryonic stem cells induces progesterone receptor gene expression. Exp Cell Res 2005, 311(2):251-64.
52. McCampbell AS, Walker CL, Broaddus RR, Cook JD, Davies PJ: Developmental reprogramming of IGF signaling and susceptibility to endometrial hyperplasia in the rat. Lab Invest 2008, 88(6):615-26.
53. Mason HR, Lake AC, Wubben JE, Nowak RA, Castellot JJ Jr: The growth arrest-specific gene CCN5 is deficient in human leiomyomas and inhibits the proliferation and motility of cultured human uterine smooth muscle cells. Mol Hum Reprod 2004, 10(3):181-7.

CHAPTER 5

THE ROLE OF DNA METHYLATION IN COMMON SKELETAL DISORDERS

JESÚS DELGADO-CALLE AND JOSÉ A. RIANCHO

5.1 BONE CELLS AND BONE REMODELING IN HEALTH AND DISEASE

Bone is a complex connective tissue composed of a calcified extracellular matrix in which different cell types are embedded. The complexity of bone is particularly evident in the cells present in this tissue and the multifaceted interactions between them [1]. Bone cells belong to two different families: the osteoblastic and the osteoclastic families (see Figure 1) [2,3].

There are several cell types within the osteoblastic lineage, including osteoblasts, osteocytes and lining cells. All of them derive from mesenchymal precursors that differentiate into osteoblasts, which eventually evolve into osteocytes or lining cells [4]. Cells of the osteoblastic lineage modulate the proliferation and differentiation of cells belonging to the osteoclastic lineage, mainly by the RANKL-OPG-RANK signaling pathway [5–7]. Osteocytes derive from some osteoblasts that become embedded and surrounded by bone matrix [8]. These cells are emerging as the responders to mechanical stimuli that regulate bone formation and resorption, as well as key regulators of bone metabolism. Osteocytes modulate bone turnover through the modulation of the Wnt pathway and other pathways that influence the activity of both osteoblasts and osteoclasts [9–11].

This chapter was originally published under the Creative Commons Attribution License. Delgado-Calle J and Riancho JA. The Role of DNA Methylation in Common Skeletal Disorders. Biology 2012, 1 (2012). doi:10.3390/biology1030698.

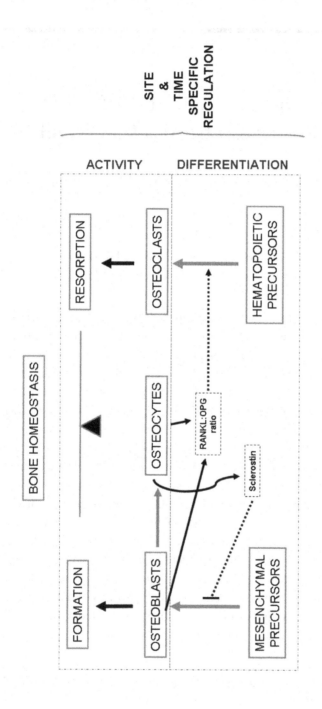

FIGURE 1: Bone is a complex and dynamic organ, which is constantly being remodeled by the balanced and coupled activity of the cells present in this tissue. Osteoblasts derive from mesenchymal precursors and eventually evolve into osteocytes and lining cells. Cells of theosteoblastic lineage are responsible for bone formation. Osteoclasts, derived from hematopoietic cells, are responsible for bone resorption. Interestingly, osteoclast differentiation is influenced by soluble factors secreted by osteoblasts and osteocytes, especially those related to the RANKL-RANK signaling pathway. On the other hand, osteocyte-derived sclerostin negatively modulates bone formation.

Osteoclasts derive from hematopoietic precursors. These cells are formed by the fusion of cells of the monocyte-macrophage lineage and are responsible for bone resorption. As mentioned before, osteoclastogenesis is influenced by osteoblasts and osteocytes, which produce several factors critical for the differentiation of osteoclast precursors, such as the receptor activator of nuclear factor kappa-B ligand (RANKL) and the macrophage colony-stimulating factor (MCS-F) [7]. RANKL interacts with RANK (Receptor activator of nuclear factor kappa-B), present in the membrane of osteoclastic precursors, promoting the activation of the Nuclear factor Kappa B, which induces cell fusion and differentiation to originate multi-nucleated mature osteoclasts [12,13]. It is important to note that osteoblastic cells also express osteoprotegerin (OPG), which acts as a soluble decoy receptor for RANKL, thus impairing the RANKL-RANK interaction [14]. Mature osteoclasts locate on specific surfaces of bone, where they break down and resorb bone matrix, replacing old bone with new bone [12].

Bone is under constant turnover throughout life in order to maintain its properties. It is believed that this process, known as bone remodeling, occurs, in part, randomly. However, sometimes, osteocytes can mark the site where a remodeling cycle must be started in order to repair microcracks, which represent the so called "target remodeling" [15, 16]. Bone remodeling is carried out by the cyclic and coupled activity of osteoclasts and osteoblasts. The process starts when osteoclast precursors are recruited to the bone surface, where they differentiate and remove a small volume of bone. Then osteoclasts undergo apoptosis and osteoblasts arrive to the region to fill up the defect with new bone [17]. Bone mass homeostasis depends on the balance between bone formation and bone resorption. Any disequilibrium between bone formation and bone resorption leads to changes in bone mass. This is the case of osteoporosis and osteoarthritis, two common skeletal diseases that tend to show changes of bone mass in opposite directions [18].

The maintenance of bone mass requires proper cell differentiation and cell activity. Osteoblast and osteoclast differentiation processes are highly organized and driven by deep changes in the gene expression patterns that in turn result in cells with different shapes and functions [3,19]. Since bone remodeling requires the sequential action of osteoclasts and osteoblasts at a given region, the differentiation of both cell types is controlled in a time and site-specific manner, and influenced not only by intrinsic factors, but also by some systemic and environmental factors. Emerging lines of evidence suggest that epigenetic mechanisms play an important role in establishing cellular identities and controlling gene expression. Herein, we summarize the current knowledge about the role of epigenetics, and specifically DNA methylation marks, in bone homeostasis and pathogenesis.

5.2 DNA METHYLATION INFLUENCES GENE EXPRESSION

Presently, epigenetics is defined as, "The study of stable genetic modifications that results in changes in gene expression without a corresponding alteration in DNA sequence [20]." Importantly, epigenetic marks integrate intrinsic and environmental stimuli and confer both lineage commitment and phenotypic plasticity [21]. Thus, epigenetic marks could be considered as a link between genotype, environment, phenotype and disease. Epigenetic mechanisms comprise DNA methylation, post-translational histone modifications and non-coding RNAs [22,23]. Although the mechanisms of epigenetic inheritance during cell division are well established, heritable epigenetic patterns from parents to offspring are starting to be revealed [24,25].

In eukaryotes DNA methylation consists in the covalent addition of methyl groups to cytosines that precede guanines (CpG) [26]. In vertebrate genomes, CpG sites are predominantly methylated [27]. However, the globally methylated pattern is disrupted in regions known as CpG islands. These areas are present in approximately 70% of gene promoters. On average, CpG islands are 1 kb long, have an elevated C + G content and are frequently demethylated [28]. DNA methylation variations do not occur exclusively at CpG islands. Recently, it has been also shown that methylation occurs at a short distance from the CpG islands (at "CpG island"shores)), rather than in the islands themselves [29]. The term CpG island shore refers to regions of lower CpG density that lie in the vicinity (~2 kb) of CpG islands. The addition of methyl groups to cytosines is catalyzed by DNA methyltransferases (DNMTs) [30]. DNMT1 was the first methyltransferase identified in mammals [31]. DNMT1 maintains DNA methylation during cell division by reading and copying the pattern in the hemimethylated strand [31]. Other members of the family are DNMT3A, DNMT3B, responsible for de novo methylation [32], and DNMT2, which has been recently shown to methylate tRNAs [33]. DNA methylation is considered an efficient repressor of transcriptional activity. Until recently, it was commonly thought that methyl groups directly prevent the binding of essential transcription factors to their targets. Although this is true for a specific set of transcription factors, it is not a general phenomenon. In fact, the binding sites for many transcription factors do not have CpGs. Emerging evidences support that the presence of methyl groups models the surrounding chromatin, inducing a DNA conformation less accessible to the transcription machinery. The mechanisms underlying this packing change are not fully understood yet, but many studies have concentrated on nucleosome structure, methyl-binding proteins, such as MECP2, MBD2 and MBD3, and interactions with chromatin remodeling enzymes [34–36]. Whatever the mechanism, on the basis of its potential to silence promoters, DNA methylation is supposed to play an important role in cell commitment and cell-specific gene expression.

How methylation is specifically targeted to a subset of promoters is generating intense debate. Apparently, methylation patterns are established early in the embryo [32,37,38]. Several studies support the idea that the ultimate methylation profile is determined by the underlying DNA sequence. In this sense, it has been shown that local DNA sequence is one of the main determinants for targeting DNA methylation to a specific locus. Thus, sequence variation between individuals might contribute to differential methylation patterns [38,39]. In fact, recent findings suggest that allele-specific methylation (ASM) is a common feature across the genome [40,41]. Notably, most of the ASM is strongly associated with SNPs genotypes [42,43]. Subsequent changes in the methylation pattern, generally of a tissue-specific nature, occur following implantation (i.e., repression of pluripotent genes) [44,45]. It has been proposed that tissue-specific changes occur through mechanisms apparently recruiting molecules needed for de novo methylation and demethylation (see Figure 2). Whereas demethylation may occur by active or repairing mechanisms [46,47], de novo methylation may be mediated by polycomb complexes [48].

5.3 ROLE OF DNA METHYLATION IN ESTABLISHING A BONE CELL PHENOTYPE

An impaired mesenchymal differentiation negatively affects bone mass. Several studies suggest that the osteogenic capacity of mesenchymal cells decrease with aging [49]. However, the contribution of this event to the decline of bone mass associated with aging is not clear yet. Osteogenic differentiation of mesenchymal cells towards osteoprogenitor and osteo-blastic cells is regulated by several mechanisms, including DNA methyla-tion. Kang et al. demonstrated that promoter methylation changes during mesenchymal cell differentiation [50]. Likewise, it has been proposed that active demethylation of gene promoters (i.e., osteocalcin, osterix, or *Runx2*), via GADD45-dependent mechanisms, is involved in the ostegenic differentiation of mesenchymal cells [51]. In fact, as reported by Locklin et al., osteogenic differentiation may be modulated by demethylating agents [52]. DNA methylation marks are not only important in osteoblastogene-sis, but also afterwards in the osteoblast to osteocyte transition. Our group demonstrated that CpG methylation at regulatory regions controls the Bi-ology 2012, 1 702 expression of the alkaline phosphatase and sclerostin genes. We observed that the hypermethylation of *ALPL* and *SOST* promot-ers was inversely correlated with gene expression in osteoblastic cells. Furthermore, we showed that the presence of methyl groups at the proxi-mal promoter of *SOST* markedly decreased the transcriptional activity of this sequence, presumably by impairing the binding of essential transcrip-tion factors to the core promoter. In addition, we demonstrated that the methylation of those promoters changes during osteoblast differentiation towards osteocytes and controls gene expression in a cell-specific man-ner [53,54]. DNA methylation at *ALPL* promoter increased progressively during osteoblast differentiation, silencing *ALPL* expression in osteocytes. DNA methylation represses *SOST* expression in osteoblasts, whereas the physiological demethylation of its promoter favored the expression of this gene in osteocytes (see Figure 2). Consistent with this observa-tion, *SOST* promoter remains methylated in other cell types that do not express sclerostin [53]. The results of other investigators also support that the expression of a number of genes important for osteogenic differentiation

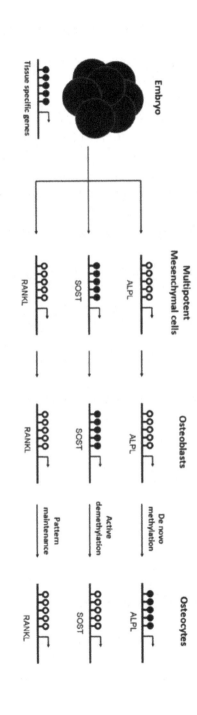

FIGURE 2: Dynamics of tissue-specific DNA methylation of bone cells. DNA methylation is established early in the embryo. Generally, at this stage, pluripotent genes and house-keeping genes are unmethylated, whereas tissue-specific genes are largely methylated. Then, the differentiation to mesenchymal cells promotes not only demethylation of many of these specific cell lineage genes, but also de novo methylation events to silence multipotent-specific genes. During mesenchymal commitment to the osteoblastic lineage, some unmethylated genes undergo de novo methylation to be silenced in osteocytes, such as alkaline phosphatase gene (ALPL). However, other methylated genes are actively demethylated to promote its expression in the late osteocyte [sclerostin (SOST)]. Lastly, other genes already demethylated in mesenchymal cells remain demethylated in differentiated cells, such as the Receptor activator of nuclear factor kappa-B ligand (RANKL). Black and white circles represent DNA methylation and hypomethylation, respectively.

and osteoblast/osteocyte activity (including podoplanin, osteopontin, Brachury transcription factor, estrogen receptor, aromatase, collagen cross-linking enzyme lysyl oxidase or the homeobox protein Dlx-5) is regulated by DNA methylation [55–62].

On the other hand, DNA methylation contributes to regulate self-renewal and differentiation capacity of hematopoietic cells, the early precursors of osteoclasts [63]. The subsequent differentiation of osteoclast precursors towards mature osteoclasts is tightly regulated by soluble factors secreted by osteoblasts and osteocytes, such as RANKL, OPG and MCS-F [7,64]. As first reported by Kitazawa et al., and recently confirmed by our group in human samples, *RANKL* and *OPG* expression is regulated by DNA methylation in osteoblastic cells [65,66]. CpG methylation at the regulatory regions of *RANKL* and *OPG* genes is associated with low transcript levels. In turn, the demethylation of their promoters mediated by 5-azadeoxycitidine, a demethylating agent, induces the expression of both genes. Based upon these evidences, epigenetic mechanisms appear to be important for osteoclast differentiation (reviewed by Yasui et al. [67]). However, it is worth emphasizing that besides DNA methylation, other epigenetic marks, such as microRNAs or chromatin modifiers, are also involved in determining the differentiation and activity of bone cells, recently reviewed by Delgado-Calle et al., Kato S et al. and Earl CS et al. [68–70].

5.4 METHYLATION MARKS AND COMMON SKELETAL DISEASES

5.4.1 OSTEOPOROSIS

Osteoporosis is characterized by reduced bone mass and/or abnormal bone microarchitecture, which decrease bone strength and augment the susceptibility to fracture. Common osteoporotic fractures include those of the vertebral bodies, hip, pelvis, proximal arm and wrist. Any imbalance in the activity of osteoclasts and osteoblasts in a way such that bone formation is smaller than bone resorption results in osteoporosis. In some cases, osteoporosis is secondary to an underlying disease, but quite often it is just an exaggeration of the universal age-associated decrease in bone mass. In part, it is related to the diminished availability of sex steroids taking place in women after menopause and in elderly men [71], but other incompletely known factors associated with aging are likely involved [49,72]. Whatever those mechanisms might be, osteoporosis is the final result of the complex interplay between genetic and acquired factors in which epigenetic marks may also participate.

As discussed above, experimental evidence shows that the methylation of several genes play a major role in the differentiation of bone cells, which is required to sustain a normal bone remodeling. Therefore, it might be hypothesized that DNA methylation is involved in the pathogenesis of osteoporosis, though there is little evidence directly supporting this hypothesis so far. However, it has been recently proposed that reduced Dnmt1 activity decreases bone mineral density and body weight [73]. A number of studies suggest that environmental influences may contribute to shaping the methylation pattern of the individual and that the pattern may change in association with aging [74–78]. Several animal studies have related the environmental factors during early phases of development with DNA methylation and skeletal status. In fact, maternal dietary intake has been shown to influence bone mass of the offspring, both in experimental animals and in humans [79]. In some cases, DNA methylation may be involved. For instance, dietary restriction of pregnant rats induces changes in the methylation of genes that are important for bone cell differentiation and activity, such as the glucocorticoid receptor and the peroxisomal-activated receptor genes [80–83].

5.4.2 OSTEOARTHRITIS

Whereas osteoporosis is primarily a bone disorder, osteoarthritis is the most common form of joint disease. In fact, damage of the articular cartilage is the hallmark of osteoarthritis. However, osteoarthritis involves an abnormal remodeling of other tissues in affected joints, such as the synovium and the subchondral bone [84,85]. Thus, other typical changes in the joints of patients with osteoarthritis (besides the narrowing of joint space secondary to cartilage thinning), include the formation of osteo-phytes (bone excrescences at the periphery of the joints) and sclerosis of the subchondral bone. The extracellular matrix of the articular cartilage contains several types of collagen (II, IX and XI) and proteoglycanes, such as aggrecan. Several investigators have shown an altered homeostasis in the diseased cartilage, with increased expression of catabolic genes, ac-companied by a diminished synthesis of components of the cartilaginous matrix. Matrix metalloproteases (MMPs) and aggrecanases (ADAMTS-4 and 5) are regarded as major enzymes mediating the destructive process of cartilage. The sclerosis of subchondral bone used to be considered a sec-ondary reactive change, but in recent years, the concept is emerging that subchondral bone may play more than a passive role in the pathogenesis of the disease. In line with this concept, it has been postulated that cyto-kines released by bone cells influence the activity of chondrocytes, and vice-versa [86]. Furthermore, subchondral bone influences the overlying cartilage, not only through its biomechanical properties, but also through the synthesis of various humoral factors (see recent reviews [86–90]).

After the seminal work by Roach et al. [91,92], it has been demonstrat-ed that, in some cases, changes in chondrocyte gene expression are associ-ated with inverse changes in DNA methylation. For instance, Zimmerman et al. reported that the induction of type X collagen expression during chondrogenic differentiation of mesenchymal stem cells is associated with the demethylation of specific CpGs in its promoter [93]. However, in adult chondrocytes, the promoter was methylated, which correlated with the absence of gene expression. Inverse correlations between methylation and gene expression have been reported for other genes, including osteo-genic protein 1 (OP-1), interleukin 1 beta, *MMP3, MMP9, MMP13*, leptin and *ADMTS4* [58,94,95]. The exact molecular mechanisms have not been completely elucidated, but in some cases they may include methylation-dependent differences in the ability to recruit transcription factors, such as CREB, to gene regulatory regions [96]. However, gene expression and DNA methylation are not always inversely correlated. Thus, the reduced expression of genes, such as type II collagen or aggrecan reported in dis-eased cartilage, does not seem to be associated with increased methylation of these genes [94,97]. On the other hand, the functional consequences of gene methylation have also been revealed by in vitro experiments, showing that inducing DNA demethylation by 5-azadeoxycitidine modulates the differentiation of articular chondrocytes [98].

Some data suggest that the shape of the bones may also influence osteoarthritis. For instance, epidemiological studies showed that the certain morphological characteristics of the femoral epiphysis and the pelvis determine the risk of hip osteoarthritis [99–101]. This has given support to the hypothesis of a developmental origin of osteoarthritis [102–104]. The importance of developmental factors is also emphasized by recent results from genome-wide association studies [105,106]. Somewhat unexpectedly, these studies have not revealed significant associations between osteoarthritis and genes typically involved in cartilage homeostasis, such as those encoding proteases. Instead, they have shown association between some polymorphisms of genes involved in joint development, such as *GDF5*, and osteoarthritis of the large joints, particularly the knee and the hip [107,108]. It is currently thought that the epigenome is the consequence of environmental factors, genetic features and stochastic variations. In this regard, it is interesting to note that some *GDF5* single nucleotide polymorphisms (SNPs) showed differential allelic expression. Interestingly, the functional effect of these "CpGs SNPs" on gene expression is modulated by DNA methylation [108].

Our group has recently published a genome-wide methylation study in bone samples obtained from patients with severe hip osteoarthritis and compared the results with those obtained in patients with osteoporotic hip fractures [109]. Our results revealed several genes showing differential methylation between osteoporotic and osteoarthritic patients. Somewhat unexpectedly, genes showing differential methylation where not typical bone candidates. However, functional network analysis revealed that epigenetic changes in "upstream" regulator genes may haev downstream influences on well-known bone-related genes. Interestingly, and in tune with the developmental hypothesis, we found that genes showing differential methylation were overrepresented in pathways related to skeletal development, and particularly those of the homeobox family. Globally, DNA methylation correlated negatively with gene expression in both groups of patients. However, as observed in other studies, we found a subset of genes in which there was no inverse correlation between DNA methylation and the abundance of gene transcripts, thus pointing out that factors other than methylation play an important role in the fine tuning of gene expression in adult tissues.

5.4.3 TUMORS AND BONE

Some tumors originate in the skeleton, and many others have a propensity to metastasize in bone. In fact, bone metastases are very common in a variety of advanced cancers and contribute importantly to cancer morbidity. The mechanisms influencing the metastatic potential of tumor cells and their tropism for certain tissues are being actively investigated. They are likely complex and include factors related to the tumor itself and others which depend on the tissue hosting the metastases. In some cases, they may include certain methylation patterns that result in specific gene expression signatures that facilitate the initiation or the growth of the metastases. Prostate cancer cells are among those with a stronger tropism for bone. Saha et al. reported that the hypomethylation of the E-cadherin gene, and the subsequent reduction of gene expression, was associated with metastatic prostate cancer cells in bone [110]. Also, reduced DNA methylation is associated with increased expression of the parathyroid hormone-related protein (PTHrP) by breast cancer cells, which in turn may facilitate osteolysis and the growth of the metastatic niche [111]. On the other hand, the fact that certain tumors have specific gene methylation patterns, different from those of normal tissues, has raised the possibility of using the analysis of DNA remnants present in serum as a biomarker to help in diagnosing specific types of cancer.

5.5 CONCLUDING REMARKS

Common skeletal disorders, such as osteoporosis and osteoarthritis, are the result of a complex interplay of genetic and acquired factors. However, despite tremendous efforts, including several GWAS, the genetic factors so far identified explain less than 10% of the genetic risk. This suggests that mechanisms not related to DNA sequence may be involved in the development of these diseases. This could be the case of DNA methylation

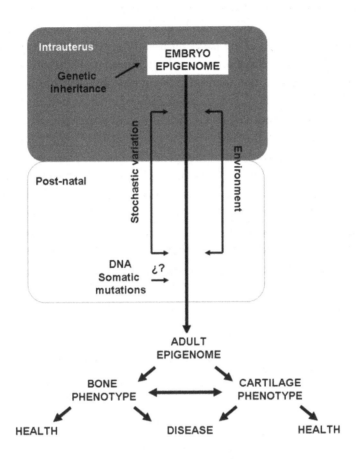

FIGURE 3: Factors involved in epigenetic variability. Epigenetic marks can change throughout life and, thereby, determine the adult phenotypes of the cells present in bone. Several factors (i.e., starving) may influence epigenetic marks at different stages of intrauterus life. For instance, genetic inheritance might influence the de novo methylation that occurs before implantation. Likewise, stochastic variations and environmental cues may also influence the epigenetic pattern. During the post-natal life, epigenetic variability may depend on environmental (i.e., toxic habits, food...) and intrinsic factors (genetic predisposition), as well as on the occurrence of DNA somatic mutations. Epigenetic signatures are directly linked to the control of cell differentiation and gene expression, thus accumulated epigenetic variability can lead to aberrant phenotypes and, consequently, induce skeletal diseases.

and its mediators. DNA methylation marks are heritable, at least through cell divisions, control gene response to environment, change with aging and underlie cell commitment and the spatiotemporal control of gene expression. DNA methylation plays an important role in the differentiation of cells of the osteoblastic and osteoclastic lineages. Therefore, it is tempting to speculate that the aberrant phenotypes observed in bone diseases might be the consequence of a combination of intrinsic and environmental factors, including gene sequence variations and epigenetic signatures (see Figure 3). However, it is important to note that DNA methylation is only one of the mechanisms underlying gene expression. Thus, the integration of knowledge from both epigenenomics and genomics, together with other "omics" (i.e., transcriptomics, proteomics) will be essential for the full understanding of the underlying mechanisms that govern the initiation and progression of bone diseases. Although still a long way to go, further studies in bone epigenetics may open a new door for drug development combining genetic and epigenetic strategies.

REFERENCES

1. Matsuo, K.; Irie, N. Osteoclast-osteoblast communication. Arch. Biochem. Biophys. 2008, 473, 201–209.
2. Jackson, L.; Jones, D.R.; Scotting, P.; Sottile, V. Adult mesenchymal stem cells: Differentiation potential and therapeutic applications. J. Postgrad. Med. 2007, 53, 121–127.
3. Vaananen, H.K.; Zhao, H.; Mulari, M.; Halleen, J.M. The cell biology of osteoclast function. J. Cell. Sci. 2000, 113, 377–381.
4. Dallas, S.L.; Bonewald, L.F. Dynamics of the transition from osteoblast to osteocyte. Ann. NY Acad. Sci. 2010, 1192, 437–443.
5. Boyce, B.F.; Xing, L. Functions of RANKL/RANK/OPG in bone modeling and remodeling. Arch. Biochem. Biophys. 2008, 473, 139–146.
6. Nakashima, T.; Hayashi, M.; Fukunaga, T.; Kurata, K.; Oh-Hora, M.; Feng, J.Q.; Bonewald, L.F.; Kodama, T.; Wutz, A.; et al. Evidence for osteocyte regulation of bone homeostasis through RANKL expression. Nat. Med. 2011, 17, 1231–1234.
7. Xiong, J.; Onal, M.; Jilka, R.L.; Weinstein, R.S.; Manolagas, S.C.; O'Brien, C.A. Matrix-embedded cells control osteoclast formation. Nat. Med. 2011, 17, 1235–1241.
8. Bonewald, L.F. The amazing osteocyte. J. Bone Miner. Res. 2011, 26, 229–238.
9. Zarrinkalam, M.R.; Mulaibrahimovic, A.; Atkins, G.J.; Moore, R.J. Changes in osteocyte density correspond with changes in osteoblast and osteoclast activity in an osteoporotic sheep model. Osteoporos. Int. 2012, 23, 1329–1336.

10. O'Brien, C.A.; Plotkin, L.I.; Galli, C.; Goellner, J.J.; Gortazar, A.R.; Allen, M.R.; Robling, A.G.; Bouxsein, M.; Schipani, E.; Turner, C.H.; et al. Control of bone mass and remodeling by PTH receptor signaling in osteocytes. PLoS One 2008, 3, e2942.

11. Winkler, D.G.; Sutherland, M.K.; Geoghegan, J.C.; Yu, C.; Hayes, T.; Skonier, J.E.; Shpektor, D.; Jonas, M.; Kovacevich, B.R.; Staehling-Hampton, K.; et al. Osteocyte control of bone formation via sclerostin, a novel BMP antagonist. EMBO J. 2003, 22, 6267–6276.

12. Boyle, W.J.; Simonet, W.S.; Lacey, D.L. Osteoclast differentiation and activation. Nature 2003, 423, 337–342.

13. Boyce, B.F.; Xing, L. The RANKL/RANK/OPG pathway. Curr. Osteoporos. Rep. 2007, 5, 98–104.

14. Kong, Y.Y.; Yoshida, H.; Sarosi, I.; Tan, H.L.; Timms, E.; Capparelli, C.; Morony, S.; Oliveirados- Santos, A.J.; van, G.; Itie, A.; et al. OPGL is a key regulator of osteoclastogenesis, lymphocyte development and lymph-node organogenesis. Nature 1999, 397, 315–323.

15. Hadjidakis, D.J.; Androulakis, I.I. Bone remodeling. Ann. NY Acad. Sci. 2006, 1092, 385–396.

16. Sims, N.A.; Gooi, J.H. Bone remodeling: Multiple cellular interactions required for coupling of bone formation and resorption. Semin. Cell Dev. Biol. 2008, 19, 444–451.

17. Raggatt, L.J.; Partridge, N.C. Cellular and molecular mechanisms of bone remodeling. J. Biol. Chem. 2010, 285, 25103–25108.

18. Dequeker, J.; Aerssens, J.; Luyten, F.P. Osteoarthritis and osteoporosis: Clinical and research evidence of inverse relationship. Aging Clin. Exp. Res. 2003, 15, 426–439.

19. Franz-Odendaal, T.A.; Hall, B.K.; Witten, P.E. Buried alive: how osteoblasts become osteocytes. Dev. Dyn. 2006, 235, 176–190.

20. Probst, A.V.; Dunleavy, E.; Almouzni, G. Epigenetic inheritance during the cell cycle. Nat. Rev. Mol. Cell. Biol. 2009, 10, 192–206.

21. Feinberg, A.P. Phenotypic plasticity and the epigenetics of human disease. Nature 2007, 447, 433–440.

22. Esteller, M. Epigenetics in cancer. N. Engl. J. Med. 2008, 358, 1148–1159.

23. Feinberg, A.P.; Tycko, B. The history of cancer epigenetics. Nat. Rev. Cancer 2004, 4, 143–153.

24. Buiting, K.; Barnicoat, A.; Lich, C.; Pembrey, M.; Malcolm, S.; Horsthemke, B. Disruption of the bipartite imprinting center in a family with Angelman syndrome. Am. J. Hum. Genet. 2001, 68, 1290–1294.

25. Buiting, K.; Gross, S.; Lich, C.; Gillessen-Kaesbach, G.; El Maarri, O.; Horsthemke, B. Epimutations in Prader-Willi and Angelman syndromes: A molecular study of 136 patients with an imprinting defect. Am. J. Hum. Genet. 2003, 72, 571–577.

26. Miranda, T.B.; Jones, P.A. DNA methylation: The nuts and bolts of repression. J. Cell. Physiol. 2007, 213, 384–390.

27. Bird, A.P. DNA methylation and the frequency of CpG in animal DNA. Nucleic Acids Res. 1980, 8, 1499–1504.

28. Illingworth, R.S.; Gruenewald-Schneider, U.; Webb, S.; Kerr, A.R.; James, K.D.; Turner, D.J.; Smith, C.; Harrison, D.J.; Andrews, R.; Bird, A.P. Orphan CpG islands

identify numerous conserved promoters in the mammalian genome. PLoS Genet. 2010, 6, e1001134.

29. Irizarry, R.A.; Ladd-Acosta, C.; Wen, B.; Wu, Z.; Montano, C.; Onyango, P.; Cui, H.; Gabo, K.; Rongione, M.; Webster, M.; et al. The human colon cancer methylome shows similar hypo- and hypermethylation at conserved tissue-specific CpG island shores. Nat. Genet. 2009, 41, 178–186.

30. Hermann, A.; Gowher, H.; Jeltsch, A. Biochemistry and biology of mammalian DNA methyltransferases. Cell. Mol. Life. Sci. 2004, 61, 2571–2587.

31. Leonhardt, H.; Page, A.W.; Weier, H.U.; Bestor, T.H. A targeting sequence directs DNA methyltransferase to sites of DNA replication in mammalian nuclei. Cell 1992, 71, 865–873.

32. Okano, M.; Bell, D.W.; Haber, D.A.; Li, E. DNA methyltransferases Dnmt3a and Dnmt3b are essential for de novo methylation and mammalian development. Cell 1999, 99, 247–257.

33. Goll, M.G.; Kirpekar, F.; Maggert, K.A.; Yoder, J.A.; Hsieh, C.L.; Zhang, X.; Golic, K.G.; Jacobsen, S.E.; Bestor, T.H. Methylation of tRNAAsp by the DNA methyltransferase homolog Dnmt2. Science 2006, 311, 395–398.

34. Hashimshony, T.; Zhang, J.; Keshet, I.; Bustin, M.; Cedar, H. The role of DNA methylation in setting up chromatin structure during development. Nat. Genet. 2003, 34, 187–192.

35. Razin, A.; Cedar, H. Distribution of 5-methylcytosine in chromatin. Proc. Natl. Acad. Sci. USA 1977, 74, 2725–2728.

36. Klose, R.J.; Bird, A.P. Genomic DNA methylation: The mark and its mediators. Trends Biochem. Sci. 2006, 31, 89–97.

37. Frank, D.; Keshet, I.; Shani, M.; Levine, A.; Razin, A.; Cedar, H. Demethylation of CpG islands in embryonic cells. Nature 1991, 351, 239–241.

38. Straussman, R.; Nejman, D.; Roberts, D.; Steinfeld, I.; Blum, B.; Benvenisty, N.; Simon, I.; Yakhini, Z.; Cedar, H. Developmental programming of CpG island methylation profiles in the human genome. Nat. Struct. Mol. Biol. 2009, 16, 564–571.

39. Lienert, F.; Wirbelauer, C.; Som, I.; Dean, A.; Mohn, F.; Schubeler, D. Identification of genetic elements that autonomously determine DNA methylation states. Nat. Genet. 2011, 43, 1091–1097.

40. Epsztejn-Litman, S.; Feldman, N.; Abu-Remaileh, M.; Shufaro, Y.; Gerson, A.; Ueda, J.; Deplus, R.; Fuks, F.; Shinkai, Y.; Cedar, H.; et al. De novo DNA methylation promoted by G9a prevents reprogramming of embryonically silenced genes. Nat. Struct. Mol. Biol. 2008, 15, 1176–1183.

41. Feldman, N.; Gerson, A.; Fang, J.; Li, E.; Zhang, Y.; Shinkai, Y.; Cedar, H.; Bergman, Y. G9a-mediated irreversible epigenetic inactivation of Oct-3/4 during early embryogenesis. Nat. Cell. Biol. 2006, 8, 188–194.

42. Niehrs, C.; Schafer, A. Active DNA demethylation by Gadd45 and DNA repair. Trends Cell Biol. 2012, 22, 220–227.

43. Tahiliani, M.; Koh, K.P.; Shen, Y.; Pastor, W.A.; Bandukwala, H.; Brudno, Y.; Agarwal, S.; Iyer, L.M.; Liu, D.R.; Aravind, L.; et al. Conversion of 5-methylcytosine to 5-hydroxymethylcytosine in mammalian DNA by MLL partner TET1. Science 2009, 324, 930–935.

44. Kerkel, K.; Spadola, A.; Yuan, E.; Kosek, J.; Jiang, L.; Hod, E.; Li, K.; Murty, V.V.; Schupf, N.; Vilain, E.; et al. Genomic surveys by methylation-sensitive SNP analysis identify sequence-dependent allele-specific DNA methylation. Nat. Genet. 2008, 40, 904–908.

45. Tycko, B. Allele-specific DNA methylation: Beyond imprinting. Hum. Mol. Genet. 2010, 19, R210–R220.

46. Bell, J.T.; Pai, A.A.; Pickrell, J.K.; Gaffney, D.J.; Pique-Regi, R.; Degner, J.F.; Gilad, Y.; Pritchard, J.K. DNA methylation patterns associate with genetic and gene expression variation in HapMap cell lines. Genome Biol. 2011, 12, R10.

47. Hellman, A.; Chess, A. Extensive sequence-influenced DNA methylation polymorphism in the human genome. Epigenetics Chromatin 2010, 3, 11.

48. Vire, E.; Brenner, C.; Deplus, R.; Blanchon, L.; Fraga, M.; Didelot, C.; Morey, L.; van Eynde, A.; Bernard, D.; Vanderwinden, J.M.; et al. The Polycomb group protein EZH2 directly controls DNA methylation. Nature 2006, 439, 871–874.

49. Jiang, Y.; Mishima, H.; Sakai, S.; Liu, Y.K.; Ohyabu, Y.; Uemura, T. Gene expression analysis of major lineage-defining factors in human bone marrow cells: Effect of aging, gender, and age-related disorders. J. Orthop. Res. 2008, 26, 910–917.

50. Kang, M.I.; Kim, H.S.; Jung, Y.C.; Kim, Y.H.; Hong, S.J.; Kim, M.K.; Baek, K.H.; Kim, C.C.; Rhyu, M.G. Transitional CpG methylation between promoters and retroelements of tissue-specific genes during human mesenchymal cell differentiation. J. Cell. Biochem. 2007, 102, 224–239.

51. Zhang, R.P.; Shao, J.Z.; Xiang, L.X. GADD45A protein plays an essential role in active DNA demethylation during terminal osteogenic differentiation of adipose-derived mesenchymal stem cells. J. Biol. Chem. 2011, 286, 41083–41094.

52. Locklin, R.M.; Oreffo, R.O.; Triffitt, J.T. Modulation of osteogenic differentiation in human skeletal cells in vitro by 5-azacytidine. Cell Biol. Int. 1998, 22, 207–215.

53. Delgado-Calle, J.; Sanudo, C.; Bolado, A.; Fernandez, A.F.; Arozamena, J.; Pascual-Carra, M.A.; Rodriguez-Rey, J.C.; Fraga, M.F.; Bonewald, L.F.; Riancho, J.A. DNA methylation contributes to the regulation of sclerostin expression in human osteocytes. J. Bone Miner. Res. 2012, 27, 926–937.

54. Delgado-Calle, J.; Sanudo, C.; Sanchez-Verde, L.; Garcia-Renedo, R.J.; Arozamena, J.; Riancho, J.A. Epigenetic regulation of alkaline phosphatase in human cells of the osteoblastic lineage. Bone 2011, 49, 830–838.

55. Arnsdorf, E.J.; Tummala, P.; Castillo, A.B.; Zhang, F.; Jacobs, C.R. The epigenetic mechanism of mechanically induced osteogenic differentiation. J. Biomech. 2010, 43, 2881–2886.

56. Villagra, A.; Gutierrez, J.; Paredes, R.; Sierra, J.; Puchi, M.; Imschenetzky, M.; Wijnen, A.A.; Lian, J.; Stein, G.; Stein, J.; et al. Reduced CpG methylation is associated with transcriptional activation of the bone-specific rat osteocalcin gene in osteoblasts. J. Cell Biochem. 2002, 85, 112–122.

57. Dansranjavin, T.; Krehl, S.; Mueller, T.; Mueller, L.P.; Schmoll, H.J.; Dammann, R.H. The role of promoter CpG methylation in the epigenetic control of stem cell related genes during differentiation. Cell Cycle 2009, 8, 916–924.

58. Loeser, R.F.; Im, H.J.; Richardson, B.; Lu, Q.; Chubinskaya, S. Methylation of the OP-1 promoter: Potential role in the age-related decline in OP-1 expression in cartilage. Osteoarthr. Cartil. 2009, 17, 513–517.

59. Lee, J.Y.; Lee, Y.M.; Kim, M.J.; Choi, J.Y.; Park, E.K.; Kim, S.Y.; Lee, S.P.; Yang, J.S.; Kim, D.S. Methylation of the mouse Dlx5 and Osx gene promoters regulates cell type-specific gene expression. Mol. Cells 2006, 22, 182–188.

60. Penolazzi, L.; Lambertini, E.; Giordano, S.; Sollazzo, V.; Traina, G.; del Senno, L.; Piva, R. Methylation analysis of the promoter F of estrogen receptor alpha gene: Effects on the level of transcription on human osteoblastic cells. J. Steroid Biochem. Mol. Biol. 2004, 91, 1–9.

61. Demura, M.; Bulun, S.E. CpG dinucleotide methylation of the CYP19 I.3/II promoter modulates cAMP-stimulated aromatase activity. Mol. Cell Endocrinol. 2008, 283, 127–132.

62. Thaler, R.; Agsten, M.; Spitzer, S.; Paschalis, E.P.; Karlic, H.; Klaushofer, K.; Varga, F. Homocysteine suppresses the expression of the collagen cross-linker lysyl oxidase involving IL-6, Fli1, and epigenetic DNA methylation. J. Biol. Chem. 2011, 286, 5578–5588.

63. Teitell, M.A.; Mikkola, H.K. Transcriptional activators, repressors, and epigenetic modifiers controlling hematopoietic stem cell development. Pediatr. Res. 2006, 59, 33R–39R.

64. Riancho, J.A.; Delgado-Calle, J. Osteoblast-osteoclast interaction mechanisms. Reumatol. Clin. 2011, 7, S1–S4.

65. Delgado-Calle, J.; Sanudo, C.; Fernandez, A.F.; Garcia-Renedo, R.; Fraga, M.F.; Riancho, J.A. Role of DNA methylation in the regulation of the RANKL-OPG system in human bone. Epigenetics 2012, 7, 83–91.

66. Kitazawa, R.; Kitazawa, S. Methylation status of a single CpG locus 3 bases upstream of TATA-box of receptor activator of nuclear factor-kappaB ligand RANKL. Gene promoter modulates cell- and tissue-specific RANKL expression and osteoclastogenesis. Mol. Endocrinol. 2007, 21, 148–158.

67. Yasui, T.; Hirose, J.; Aburatani, H.; Tanaka, S. Epigenetic regulation of osteoclast differentiation. Ann. NY Acad. Sci. 2011, 1240, 7–13.

68. Delgado-Calle, J.; Garmilla, P.; Riancho, J.A. Do epigenetic marks govern bone homeostasis? Curr. Genomics 2012, 13, 252–263.

69. Kato, S.; Inoue, K.; Youn, M.I. Emergence of the osteo-epigenome in bone biology. IBMS BoneKEy 2010, 7, 314–324.

70. Earl, S.C.; Harvey, N.; Cooper, C. The epigenetic regulation of bone mass. IBMS BoneKEy 2010, 7, 54–62.

71. Riggs, B.L.; Khosla, S.; Melton, L.J. Sex steroids and the construction and conservation of the adult skeleton. Endocr. Rev. 2002, 23, 279–302.

72. Manolagas, S.C. From estrogen-centric to aging and oxidative stress: A revised perspective of the pathogenesis of osteoporosis. Endocr. Rev. 2010, 31, 266–300.

73. Liu, L.; van Groen, T.; Kadish, I.; Li, Y.; Wang, D.; James, S.R.; Karpf, A.R.; Tollefsbol, T.O. Insufficient DNA methylation affects healthy aging and promotes age-related health problems. Clin. Epigenetics 2011, 2, 349–360.

74. Rodriguez-Rodero, S.; Fernandez-Morera, J.L.; Fernandez, A.F.; Menendez-Torre, E.; Fraga, M.F. Epigenetic regulation of aging. Discov. Med. 2010, 10, 225–233.

75. Fraga, M.F.; Esteller, M. Epigenetics and aging: The targets and the marks. Trends Genet. 2007, 23, 413–418.

76. Fraga, M.F. Genetic and epigenetic regulation of aging. Curr. Opin. Immunol. 2009, 21, 446–453.
77. Calvanese, V.; Lara, E.; Kahn, A.; Fraga, M.F. The role of epigenetics in aging and age-related diseases. Ageing Res. Rev. 2009, 8, 268–276.
78. Huidobro, C.; Fernandez, A.F.; Fraga, M.F. Aging epigenetics: Causes and consequences. Mol. Asp. Med. 2012, in press.
79. Mahon, P.; Harvey, N.; Crozier, S.; Inskip, H.; Robinson, S.; Arden, N.; Swaminathan, R.; Cooper, C.; Godfrey, K. Low maternal vitamin D status and fetal bone development: Cohort study. J. Bone Miner. Res. 2010, 25, 14–19.
80. Oreffo, R.O.; Lashbrooke, B.; Roach, H.I.; Clarke, N.M.; Cooper, C. Maternal protein deficiency affects mesenchymal stem cell activity in the developing offspring. Bone 2003, 33, 100–107.
81. Lillycrop, K.A.; Phillips, E.S.; Torrens, C.; Hanson, M.A.; Jackson, A.A.; Burdge, G.C. Feeding pregnant rats a protein-restricted diet persistently alters the methylation of specific cytosines in the hepatic PPAR alpha promoter of the offspring. Br. J. Nutr. 2008, 100, 278–282.
82. Lillycrop, K.A.; Slater-Jefferies, J.L.; Hanson, M.A.; Godfrey, K.M.; Jackson, A.A.; Burdge, G.C. Induction of altered epigenetic regulation of the hepatic glucocorticoid receptor in the offspring of rats fed a protein-restricted diet during pregnancy suggests that reduced DNA methyltransferase-1 expression is involved in impaired DNA methylation and changes in histone modifications. Br. J. Nutr. 2007, 97, 1064–1073.
83. Lillycrop, K.A.; Phillips, E.S.; Jackson, A.A.; Hanson, M.A.; Burdge, G.C. Dietary protein restriction of pregnant rats induces and folic acid supplementation prevents epigenetic modification of hepatic gene expression in the offspring. J. Nutr. 2005, 135, 1382–1386.
84. Brandt, K.D.; Dieppe, P.; Radin, E.L. Etiopathogenesis of osteoarthritis. Rheum. Dis. Clin. North Am. 2008, 34, 531–559.
85. Loeser, R.F.; Goldring, S.R.; Scanzello, C.R.; Goldring, M.B. Osteoarthritis: A disease of the joint as an organ. Arthritis Rheum. 2012, 64, 1697–1707.
86. Goldring, S.R. The role of bone in osteoarthritis pathogenesis. Rheum. Dis. Clin. North Am. 2008, 34, 561–571.
87. Bellido, M.; Lugo, L.; Roman-Blas, J.A.; Castaneda, S.; Calvo, E.; Largo, R.; Herrero-Beaumont, G. Improving subchondral bone integrity reduces progression of cartilage damage in experimental osteoarthritis preceded by osteoporosis. Osteoarthr. Cartil. 2011, 19, 1228–1236.
88. Goldring, M.B.; Goldring, S.R. Articular cartilage and subchondral bone in the pathogenesis of osteoarthritis. Ann. NY Acad. Sci. 2010, 1192, 230–237.
89. Herrero-Beaumont, G.; Roman-Blas, J.A.; Largo, R.; Berenbaum, F.; Castaneda, S. Bone mineral density and joint cartilage: Four clinical settings of a complex relationship in osteoarthritis. Ann. Rheum. Dis. 2011, 70, 1523–1525.
90. Suri, S.; Walsh, D.A. Osteochondral alterations in osteoarthritis. Bone 2012, 51, 204–211.
91. Roach, H.I.; Yamada, N.; Cheung, K.S.; Tilley, S.; Clarke, N.M.; Oreffo, R.O.; Kokubun, S.; Bronner, F. Association between the abnormal expression of matrix-

degrading enzymes by human osteoarthritic chondrocytes and demethylation of specific CpG sites in the promoter regions. Arthritis Rheum. 2005, 52, 3110–3124.

92. Roach, H.I.; Aigner, T. DNA methylation in osteoarthritic chondrocytes: A new molecular target. Osteoarthr. Cartil. 2007, 15, 128–137.

93. Zimmermann, P.; Boeuf, S.; Dickhut, A.; Boehmer, S.; Olek, S.; Richter, W. Correlation of COL10A1 induction during chondrogenesis of mesenchymal stem cells with demethylation of two CpG sites in the COL10A1 promoter. Arthritis Rheum. 2008, 589, 2743–2753.

94. Barter, M.J.; Bui, C.; Young, D.A. Epigenetic mechanisms in cartilage and osteoarthritis: DNA methylation, histone modifications and microRNAs. Osteoarthr. Cartil. 2012, 20, 339–349.

95. Goldring, M.B.; Marcu, K.B. Epigenomic and microRNA-mediated regulation in cartilage development, homeostasis, and osteoarthritis. Trends Mol. Med. 2012, 18, 109–118.

96. Bui, C.; Barter, M.J.; Scott, J.L.; Xu, Y.; Galler, M.; Reynard, L.N.; Rowan, A.D.; Young, D.A. cAMP response element-binding CREB recruitment following a specific CpG demethylation leads to the elevated expression of the matrix metalloproteinase 13 in human articular chondrocytes and osteoarthritis. FASEB J. 2012, 26, 3000–3011.

97. Poschl, E.; Fidler, A.; Schmidt, B.; Kallipolitou, A.; Schmid, E.; Aigner, T. DNA methylation is not likely to be responsible for aggrecan down regulation in aged or osteoarthritic cartilage. Ann. Rheum. Dis. 2005, 64, 477–480.

98. Zuscik, M.J.; Baden, J.F.; Wu, Q.; Sheu, T.J.; Schwarz, E.M.; Drissi, H.; O'Keefe, R.J.; Puzas, J.E.; Rosier, R.N. 5-azacytidine alters TGF-beta and BMP signaling and induces maturation in articular chondrocytes. J. Cell Biochem. 2004, 922, 316–331.

99. Javaid, M.K.; Lane, N.E.; Mackey, D.C.; Lui, L.Y.; Arden, N.K.; Beck, T.J.; Hochberg, M.C.; Nevitt, M.C. Changes in proximal femoral mineral geometry precede the onset of radiographic hip osteoarthritis: The study of osteoporotic fractures. Arthritis Rheum. 2009, 60, 2028–2036.

100. Baker-Lepain, J.C.; Lynch, J.A.; Parimi, N.; McCulloch, C.E.; Nevitt, M.C.; Corr, M.; Lane, N.E. Variant alleles of the WNT antagonist FRZB are determinants of hip shape and modify the relationship between hip shape and osteoarthritis. Arthritis Rheum. 2012, 64, 1457–1465.

101. Schiffern, A.N.; Stevenson, D.A.; Carroll, K.L.; Pimentel, R.; Mineau, G.; Viskochil, D.H.; Roach, J.W. Total hip arthroplasty; hip osteoarthritis; total knee arthroplasty; and knee osteoarthritis in patients with developmental dysplasia of the hip and their family members: A kinship analysis report. J. Pediatr. Orthop. 2012, 32, 609–612.

102. Sandell, L.J. Etiology of osteoarthritis: genetics and synovial joint development. Nat. Rev. Rheumatol. 2012, 8, 77–89.

103. Bos, S.D.; Slagboom, P.E.; Meulenbelt, I. New insights into osteoarthritis: Early developmental features of an ageing-related disease. Curr. Opin. Rheumatol. 2008, 20, 553–559.

104. Aspden, R.M. Osteoarthritis: A problem of growth not decay? Rheumatology 2008, 47, 1452–1460.

105. Panoutsopoulou, K.; Southam, L.; Elliott, K.S.; Wrayner, N.; Zhai, G.; Beazley, C.; Thorleifsson, G.; Arden, N.K.; Carr, A.; Chapman, K.; et al. Insights into the genetic

architecture of osteoarthritis from stage 1 of the arcOGEN study. Ann. Rheum. Dis. 2011, 70, 864–867.

106. Arcogen Consortium. Identification of new susceptibility loci for osteoarthritis arcOGEN: A genome-wide association study. Lancet 2012, 380, 815–823.

107. Valdes, A.M.; Spector, T.D. Genetic epidemiology of hip and knee osteoarthritis. Nat. Rev. Rheumatol. 2011, 7, 23–32.

108. Reynard, L.N.; Bui, C.; Canty-Laird, E.G.; Young, D.A.; Loughlin, J. Expression of the osteoarthritis-associated gene GDF5 is modulated epigenetically by DNA methylation. Hum. Mol. Genet. 2011, 20, 3450–3460.

109. Delgado-Calle, J.; Fernandez, A.F.; Sainz, J.; Zarrabeitia, M.T.; Garcia-Renedo, R.J.; Perez-Nunez, M.I.; Garcia-Ibarbia, C.; Fraga, M.F.; Riancho, J.A. Genome-wide profiling of bone reveals differentially methylated regions in osteoporosis and osteoarthritis. Arthritis Rheum. 2012, doi:10.1002/art.37753.

110. Saha, B.; Kaur, P.; Tsao-Wei, D.; Naritoku, W.Y.; Groshen, S.; Datar, R.H.; Jones, L.W.; Imam, S.A. Unmethylated E-cadherin gene expression is significantly associated with metastatic human prostate cancer cells in bone. Prostate 2008, 68, 1681–1688.

111. Tost, J.; Hamzaoui, H.; Busato, F.; Neyret, A.; Mourah, S.; Dupont, JM.; Bouizar, Z. Methylation of specific CpG sites in the P2 promoter of parathyroid hormone-related protein determines the invasive potential of breast cancer cell lines. Epigenetics 2011, 6, 1035–1046.

CHAPTER 6

ENRICHMENT-BASED DNA METHYLATION ANALYSIS USING NEXT-GENERATION SEQUENCING: SAMPLE EXCLUSION, ESTIMATING CHANGES IN GLOBAL METHYLATION, AND THE CONTRIBUTION OF REPLICATE LANES

MICHAEL P. TRIMARCHI, MARK MURPHY,
DAVID FRANKHOUSER, BENJAMIN A.T. RODRIGUEZ,
JOHN CURFMAN, GUIDO MARCUCCI, PEARLLY YAN,
AND RALF BUNDSCHUH

6.1 BACKGROUND

The promise of personalized medicine is that each patient receives customized treatment from a broad base of options rather than a single, generalized standard of care treatment [1]. This is especially important in cancer where each patient's cancer could be viewed as a separate disease

This chapter was originally published under the Creative Commons Attribution License. Trimarchi MP, Murphy M, Frankhouser D, Rodriguez BAT, Curfman J, Marcucci G, Yan P, and Bundschuh R. Enrichment-Based DNA Methylation Analysis Using Next-Generation Sequencing: Sample Exclusion, Estimating Changes in Global Methylation, and the Contribution of Replicate Lanes. BMC Genomics **13 (Suppl 8),***S6 (2012). doi:10.1186/1471-2164-13-S8-S6.*

caused by a unique set of aberrations. The rapidly decreasing cost of Next Generation Sequencing (NGS) is rendering this personalized approach a reality. For diseases with relatively high treatment costs, such as cancer, it is now economically viable to obtain whole genome sequencing data for the affected individual as part of the treatment regimen, and with further decreases in cost more and more diseases will follow suit.

However, the genomic sequence of malignant cells only partially captures the abnormalities that lead to malignancy. Other factors such as gene expression levels and epigenetic signals have to be taken into account when characterizing a specific cancer and deciding on an individual's treatment regimen. One prominent epigenetic signal for which a dysregulation in various types of cancer is already well established [2] is the addition of methyl groups at the 5' carbon of cytosine nucleotides [3,4].

There are several different methods to obtain genome-wide methylation information using NGS. The most reliable method is bisulfite conversion, where the genomic DNA is treated with sodium bisulfite to convert unmethylated cytosines into uracils and subsequently thymines upon PCR amplification [5]. Sequencing of the converted DNA immediately reveals the degree of methylation at any genomic cytosine by counting the number of observed cytosines vs. thymines; however complete methylome profiling using this method requires sequencing depths far beyond what is feasible today on the scale of larger patient cohorts. The sequencing depth requirements can be significantly alleviated by focusing coverage in CpG-rich genomic regions (e.g., using reduced representation bisulfite sequencing [6]), but this comes at the expense of greatly diminished genomic-wide coverage. The method used in our lab, MethylCap-seq [7], instead uses the methyl-binding domain of human MBD2 in order to enrich fragmented genomic DNA based on methylation content. Sequencing the fragments bound to the MBD2 domain provides a genome-wide view of methylation patterns at reasonable sequencing depths.

While the cost aspect of MethylCap-seq is attractive, it has two limitations. First, resolution is at the level of the DNA fragment size, i.e., about 150bp, rather than at the level of the individual CpG. This is not that problematic as long as one is only interested in characterizing the methylation status of extended genomic regions such as CpG islands, promoters, non-coding RNAs, or gene bodies. Second, the number of reads covering a genomic region is only a relative indicator of the amount of methylation in this region, relative to the sample genome as a whole, and thus data normalization is required to compare methylation between samples. This somewhat indirect nature of methylation status determination makes this method prone to data quality issues stemming from poorly prepared libraries. Also, somewhat paradoxically, one of the first parameters one might be interested in knowing, namely the degree of overall methylation of the sample, cannot be directly extracted from the data since relative methylation is encoded in the relative number of reads covering different genomic regions, yet the total number of reads is fixed by the sequencing itself rather than by the actual level of overall methylation in the sample. Here, we first perform a systematic study of the influence of sample quality and the contribution of additional reads (beyond ~13 million unique aligned reads) in MethylCap-seq data. Then, we show experimental evidence that a computational approach for determining overall methylation levels from MethylCap-seq data we recently suggested [8] approximates actual overall methylation levels. These studies underpin the usability of MethylCap-seq as a reliable method to obtain genome-wide methylation information at reasonable cost.

6.2 METHODS

6.2.1 PATIENT SAMPLES

Tissue samples from an endometrial cohort including tumors from 89 endometrial patients and 12 nonmalignant endometrial samples were obtained from Washington University. All studies involving human endometrial cancer samples were approved by the Human Studies Committee at the Washington University and at The Ohio State University.

A subset of 7 ovarian cancer samples from a larger cohort was obtained from TriService General Hospital, Taipei, Taiwan. All studies involving human ovarian cancer samples were approved by the Institutional Review Boards of TriService General Hospital and National Defense Medical Center.

A subset of 14 bone marrow samples from a single-center Phase II trial of patients with acute myeloid leukemia (AML) at The Ohio State University was obtained for this investigation. The study design and the results of the trial for the entire cohort of patients have been reported elsewhere [9]. All studies involving these samples were approved by The Ohio State University Human Studies Committee.

6.2.2 METHYLATED-DNA CAPTURE (METHYLCAP-SEQ)

Enrichment of methylated DNA was performed with the Methyl Miner kit (Invitrogen) according to the manufacturer's protocol as previously described [10]. Briefly, one microgram of sonicated DNA was incubated at room temperature on a rotator mixer in a solution containing 3.5 micrograms of MBD-Biotin Protein coupled to M-280 Streptavidin Dynabeads. Non-captured DNA was removed by collecting beads with bound methylated DNA on a magnetic stand and washing three times with Bind/Wash Buffer. Enriched, methylated DNA was eluted from the bead complex with 1M NaCl and purified by ethanol precipitation. Library generation and 36-bp single-ended sequencing were performed on the Illumina Genome Analyzer IIx according to the manufacturer's standard protocol.

6.2.3 METHYLCAP-SEQ EXPERIMENTAL QUALITY CONTROL AND EXCLUSION CRITERIA

The automated quality control (QC) module was implemented as previously described [10]. Pre-aligned sorted.txt files from the Illumina CASAVA 1.7 pipeline were utilized in the interest of quick turnaround for our users. In brief, duplicate alignments were removed from the aligned sequencing file (a correction for potential PCR artefacts), and the resulting output was loaded into an R workspace. MEDIPS [11] was utilized to perform CpG enrichment, saturation, and CpG coverage analyses.

Sequencing lanes were identified for exclusion using the following thresholds: CpG enrichment < 1.4, saturation < 0.5, CpG 5x coverage <

0.05. These criteria and corresponding thresholds were chosen based on their technical relevance and ability to stratify datasets with known technical issues without a salient bias towards biological groups. Samples were excluded if any of the thresholds were not met. As CpG coverage was assessed qualitatively for analysis of the Endometrial dataset, five lanes of data with borderline 5x CpG coverage were not excluded that would have qualified for exclusion due to this criterion.

For the DMR comparison (Table 1), methylation signal was normalized for each lane and then averaged among replicate lanes for each sample. The "All" group thus contains samples with merged QC pass lanes, samples with merged QC fail lanes, and samples with merged QC pass and QC fail lanes.

For the reproducibility comparison (Additional file 1), Pearson r was calculated using 2 replicate lanes corresponding to each sample represented in the QC pass and QC fail groups. In the case that a sample had more than two replicate lanes in a single group, two lanes were randomly chosen for the analysis. Samples lacking two replicate lanes in either the QC pass or QC fail group were excluded from this analysis. Lanes corresponding to the same sample but generated using different library preparations were also excluded.

We routinely provide sequencing and QC summaries for our users, and the summaries corresponding to the datasets referenced in this manuscript can be viewed in Additional files 2, 3, and 4.

6.2.4 STANDARD SEQUENCE FILE PROCESSING AND ALIGNMENT

Sequence files were processed and aligned as previously described [10]. Briefly, QSEQ files from the Illumina CASAVA1.7 pipeline were converted to FASTA format, duplicate reads removed (to control for PCR bias), and then uniquely aligned with Bowtie to generate SAM files using the following options: -f -t -p 1 -n 3 -l 32 -k 1 -m 1 -S -y --chunkmbs 1024 -max -best [12]. Duplicate alignments (reads aligning to the same genomic position) were removed using SAMtools [13].

6.2.5 STANDARD GLOBAL METHYLATION ANALYSIS WORKFLOW

Aligned sequence files in SAM format were analyzed using our custom analysis workflow as previously described [10]. Briefly, aligned reads were extended to the average fragment length (as determined by BioAnalyzer fragment analysis) and counted in 500 bp bins genome-wide. The resulting count distribution was normalized against the total aligned reads by conversion to reads per million (RPM). These normalized genome-wide count files were then interrogated by genomic feature (e.g., CpG islands, CpG shores, promoters). Differentially methylated regions were identified by summing RPM across the bins for each locus in the genomic feature, then performing a Wilcoxon rank sum test to assess differences in these summed RPMs between sample groups. Results were then adjusted for multiple comparisons by setting a false discovery rate (FDR) cutoff of 0.05.

6.2.6 CALCULATION OF NOISE IN METHYLATION SIGNAL

Noise in methylation signal, representing extended reads falling in regions without CG dinucleotides, was quantified as the summation of reads falling into bins with zero CpG content. In the case that a sample in a given group had multiple lanes of data, noise was computed for each lane individually and averaged among replicate lanes in the group. As a single sample could have a lane that passed QC and a lane that failed QC, the number of samples in each group does not sum to the total number of samples in the study.

6.2.7 CALCULATION OF THE GLOBAL METHYLATION INDICATOR

To assess genome-wide changes in methylation patterns for each sample across a given experiment, a custom parameter termed the global methylation indicator (GMI) was calculated as previously described [8]. Briefly, normalized read counts (in RPM) were classified by CpG density and averaged to construct a methylation distribution. The average RPM were then summed across the distribution (i.e., the estimated area under the methylation distribution curve) to yield the GMI.

6.2.8 ASSESSMENT OF METHYLATED FRAGMENT ENRICHMENT USING AN IN VITRO METHYLATED CONSTRUCT

6.2.8.1 EXPERIMENTAL PROCEDURE

The 5.3 kb plasmid vector pIRES2-EGFP, which contains three CpG islands, was chosen to empirically assess methylated fragment enrichment. The construct was linearized with Nhe I and then in vitro methylated with M.SssI. The methylated spike-in DNA was quantified by Qubit high sensitivity assay and diluted. Plasmid was spiked into genomic DNA at a concentration of 1.5 pg plasmid/1 µg genomic DNA (~2.5 plasmid copies per cell) prior to sonication of genomic DNA for library generation.

6.2.8.2 ANALYSIS

Reads mapping to the construct were identified by converting QSEQ files to FASTA format as described above, then aligning the files with Bowtie using the following options: -q -t -p 1 -n 3 -l 32 -k 1 -S --chunkmbs 1024 --max --best. Duplicate reads were retained for this analysis. To control for variation in construct aligned read counts that might be attributable to fluctuations in lane yield, construct aligned read counts were normalized against the total raw read counts by conversion to reads per million (RPM).

6.3 RESULTS AND DISCUSSION

6.3.1 QUALITY CONTROL EXCLUSION CRITERIA REDUCE NOISE IN METHYLATION SIGNAL AND IMPROVE ANALYTICAL POWER

Our automated quality control (QC) module, which is based on MEDIPS [11], was implemented to identify technical problems in the sequencing data and flag potentially spurious samples. One goal of the QC module was to provide rapid feedback to investigators regarding dataset quality, facilitating protocol optimization prior to committing resources to a larger scale sequencing project. A second goal was to identify samples that should be excluded from analyses due to data validity concerns. The validity of a MethylCap-seq experiment is dependent on enrichment of methylated fragments prior to sequencing. A failure in enrichment invalidates any downstream data, and therefore identifying such failures is vital. Also important is verifying the statistical reproducibility of the data for each sample. As it is often not cost-effective to generate replicate sequencing lanes for each sample to assess experimental reproducibility empirically, addressing this issue computationally is desirable. Similarly, the confidence in methylation calls is related to the breadth and strength of signal at the CpGs in the genome. We assessed enrichment of methylated fragments using the CpG enrichment parameter, which compares the frequency of CpGs in the sequenced sample with the frequency of CpGs in the reference genome. Statistical reproducibility was assessed by calculation of saturation, the Pearson correlation of two random partitions of the sequenced sample [11]. Breadth and strength of methylation signal was assessed using 5X CpG coverage, which represents the fraction of CpG loci that have five or more reads in the sample compared to the total number of CpGs in the reference genome. These QC parameters were calculated for each sample using MEDIPS [11].

Additional file 2 demonstrates the results of the QC module for the Endometrial dataset. 203 lanes of sequencing data were generated for 101

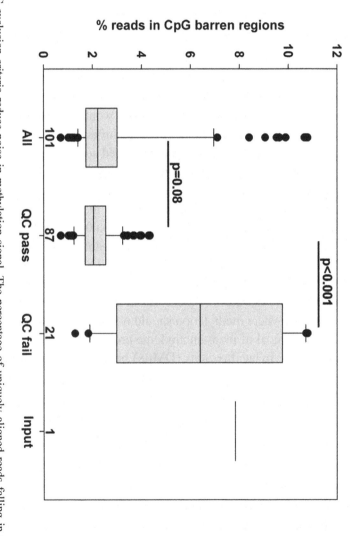

FIGURE 1: QC exclusion criteria reduce noise in methylation signal. The percentage of uniquely aligned reads falling in 500 bp bins containing no CpG dinucleotides pre- and post-QC analysis are plotted as a standard boxplot for samples prior to QC filtering, samples that passed QC, and samples that did not pass QC. An input from a sample that was not subjected to methylation capture is included for reference. The number of samples in each group is included above the baseline. Values for replicate lanes in each group were averaged, and samples were statistically compared using a Wilcoxon rank-sum test. Whiskers indicate 10th and 90th percentiles. 13.5% of 500 bp bins in the genome are classified as CpG barren.

unique samples. 43 lanes failed QC, representing 21 unique samples. To assess how lanes that pass QC might differ from lanes that failed QC, we computed the noise in methylation signal, representing percentage of uniquely aligned extended reads falling in 500 bp bins without CpG dinucleotides (Figure 1). Median noise in samples that failed QC (6.40%) was more than 3-fold greater than in samples that did not fail QC (2.04%, $p < 0.001$), and closely resembled noise in input (7.82%). Excluding QC failed lanes did not significantly decrease median noise levels (2.04 vs. 2.22, $p = 0.08$), but did greatly decrease the variation in noise levels between samples. As the distribution of noise levels is positively skewed and not normal, a small number of outliers would not be expected to significantly shift the median noise level. To investigate whether the additional noise seen in QC failed samples impacted sequencing reproducibility, we computed the Pearson correlation between replicate lanes of samples that passed QC vs. failed QC (Additional file 1). Replicates of samples that passed QC correlated much more highly than replicates of samples that failed QC (average $r = 0.90$ vs. 0.59; $p < 0.001$). Variation in replicate correlation between samples was also noticeably less in the QC pass group (relative standard deviation = 6.7% vs. 27.1%). We surmise that failures in methylation enrichment result in a more random sampling of the fragment distribution regardless of methylation status, resulting in increased signal in regions where methylation should not be detectable.

As the goal of many methylome profiling studies is to identify differentially methylated regions (DMRs) between biological groups, we next assessed whether our QC exclusion criteria might improve our analytical power to detect DMRs. We compared DMRs between 89 endometrial tumors and 12 nonmalignant endometrial tissue samples across several genomic features. Excluding sequencing lanes that failed QC (corresponding to 19 tumor and 2 nonmalignant samples) resulted in more DMRs in every genomic feature assessed (Table 1). The greatest gains were seen in promoters and CpG shores, where the number of DMRs increased 22-fold and 2-fold, respectively, while gains in CpG islands and promoter-associated CpG islands were more modest (1.6-fold and 1.05-fold). These results appear to trend inversely with CpG density, possibly reflecting greater benefit from QC exclusion in regions where coverage is lower. We speculate that the improvements in DMR detection resulting from exclusion of samples that fail QC would be even greater when working with smaller sample sizes or biological groups with more similar methylation patterns.

TABLE 1: Differentially methylated regions, endometrial tumors vs. nonmalignant endometrial tissue

Genomic feature	All samples	Samples passing QC only
CpG islands	4717	7541
Promoter- associated	3806	3980
CpG shores	7515	15371
Promoters	314	6803

6.3.2 THE EFFECT OF ADDITIONAL SEQUENCING LANES ON QUALITY CONTROL METRICS

As a sequencing core, we are frequently asked whether additional lanes of sequencing data are necessary or desirable for MethylCap-seq experiments. To address this issue, we analyzed a large dataset of ovarian tumors, of which 7 samples had been resequenced (using the same genomic library), for a total of 15 lanes (Additional file 3). Before comparing the effect of additional lanes, the degree of correlation between the replicate lanes was analyzed to ensure that additional lanes of data would not introduce excessive variation. As shown in Figure 2, replicate lanes from sequencing the same library twice correlated highly (R^2 value of 0.98; note, that we here specifically address the question of the value of additional sequencing lanes and not of additional technical or biological replicates - the correlation between technical or biological replicates would be expected to be much lower than the correlation between two lanes sequencing the same library shown here). CpG enrichment, saturation, and 5X coverage were then evaluated for individual lanes and combined lanes (Figure 3). CpG enrichment varied somewhat between samples (range: 2.33-3.02), but was extremely similar for replicate lanes (< 1% percent deviation from the combined lane on average). Saturation improved modestly from a median of 0.79 to a median of 0.86. As saturation values for individual lanes of MethylCap-seq data typically range from 0.6 to 0.85 for single lanes in our hands, and we consider a saturation value of 0.6 acceptable for analysis, this improvement may be inconsequential although it is statistically significant. 5X coverage improved noticeably from a median of 0.21 to a median of 0.28, representing an average 38% gain. As 5X coverage represents a minimum signal level needed to reliably differentiate a methylated locus from a locus with no methylation (or the absence of a methylation signal), we speculate that this increase could significantly increase the statistical power to detect DMRs, particularly in small or lightly methylated regions.

6.3.3 GLOBAL METHYLATION INDICATOR CORRELATES INVERSELY WITH AN IN VITRO METHYLATED INDICATOR SEQUENCE

We recently proposed a computational method to compare genome-wide changes in methylation patterns between samples in a given experiment [8]). As MethylCap-seq signal (in reads) is normalized by total aligned read counts to adjust for variability in lane yield, two samples with identically distributed methylation yet different absolute levels of methylation would be expected to yield identical normalized methylation signals at any given loci. The GMI method relies on the observation that in vitro methylated samples display characteristic changes in the methylation signal distribution as quantified in a MethylCap-seq experiment, and these changes are CpG density dependent. Methylation signal shifts from low CpG content regions to high CpG content regions, and this can be quantified by calculating the area under the curve of the average normalized methylation signal plotted across CpG density. The GMI calculation is a potentially powerful tool for capturing changes in global methylation between samples.

In an effort to validate the GMI as a surrogate for global methylation, we developed a complementary analysis utilizing an in vitro methylated construct. This methylated construct was spiked-in to the genomic DNA in the AML samples prior to sonication at a defined concentration and subjected to methylated enrichment along with the genomic DNA. The spike-in was originally intended to verify successful enrichment; if

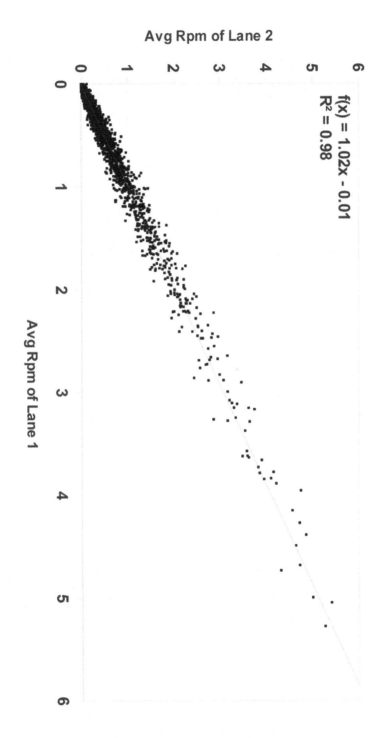

FIGURE 2: Replicate sequencing lanes for MethylCap-seq experiments correlate highly. Replicate lanes for each sample were randomly assigned to two partitions, and the average rpm of 6000 (of 6 M) randomly selected 500 bp bins were compared between partitions.

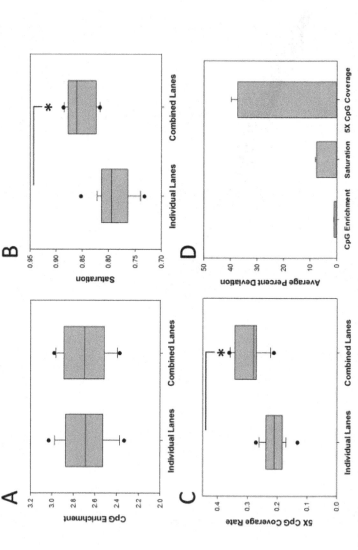

FIGURE 3: Additional lanes of sequencing data moderately increase saturation and greatly increase 5X CpG coverage. Variation in CpG enrichment (A), saturation (B), and 5X coverage (C) was assessed for 15 lanes of data in the ovarian study corresponding to 7 samples by generating plots of individual lanes and combined replicate lanes for each sample. (D) Average percent deviation of the individual lanes from the combined lane for each sample was plotted for each parameter. Error bars for (D) represent standard error. Asterisks represent Student t-test p < 0.05.

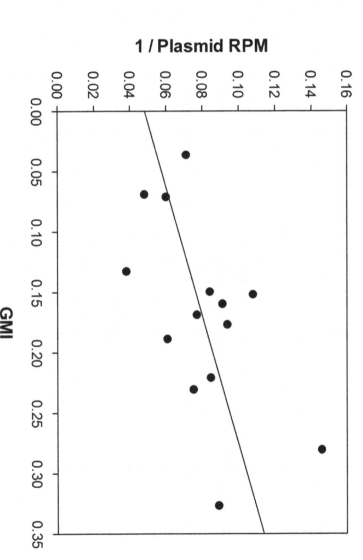

FIGURE 4: Global methylation indicator scales inversely with read counts from a spiked-in in vitro methylated construct. The pIRES2-EGFP plasmid was in vitro methylated and spiked-in at a set concentration into each of 14 samples from the decitabine study prior to sequencing. After sequencing, GMI was calculated and plotted against the inverse of the number of normalized reads aligning to the plasmid, and a linear best fit drawn through the points (p = 0.036, R2 = 0.318).

enrichment occurred, PCR for the methylated plasmid would show increased copy number after enrichment. However, this spike-in is also a way to determine global methylation levels since the methylated plasmid competes with the natively methylated genomic DNA fragments for binding to the MBD protein. When the proportion of methylated to unmethylated genomic fragments is high prior to enrichment, the methylated plasmid gets enriched relatively less, and vice versa. Indeed, we found that read counts aligned to the plasmid correlate inversely with GMI (Figure 4, Additional file 4). This result provides empirical evidence that GMI can capture changes in absolute global methylation levels for MethylCap-seq experiments. Such a metric might be useful for gauging response to treatments that are known or expected to globally alter the methylome.

6.4 CONCLUSIONS

We show that post-sequencing QC metrics can be used to exclude poor quality samples from analysis, resulting in decreased noise in methylation signal and improved power to detect DMRs. Furthermore, we show that resequenced lanes from the same library correlate very well, and that additional lanes of data have a small impact on saturation (data reproducibility) and a large impact on 5X CpG coverage (confidence in methylation calls at a given locus). Finally, we demonstrate that our computational indicator of global methylation correlates with an unrelated method that utilizes spike-in of DNA with known methylation status. These findings verify that with appropriate quality control MethylCap-seq is a reliable tool that provides reproducible relative methylation information on a feature by feature basis, provides information about the global level of methylation, and can be applied to entire patient cohorts of hundreds of patients.

REFERENCES

1.   Hurd PJ, Nelson CJ: Advantages of next-generation sequencing versus the microarray in epigenetic research. Brief Funct Genomic Proteomic 2009, 8:174-183.
2.   Esteller M: Epigenetics in cancer. N Engl J Med 2008, 358:1148-1159.

3. Bird A: DNA methylation patterns and epigenetic memory. Genes Dev 2002, 16:6-21.
4. Rodriguez-Paredes M, Esteller M: Cancer epigenetics reaches mainstream oncology. Nat Med 2011, 17:330-339.
5. Frommer M, McDonald LE, Millar DS, Collis CM, Watt F, Grigg GW, Molloy PL, Paul CL: A genomic sequencing protocol that yields a positive display of 5-methylcytosine residues in individual DNA strands. Proc Natl Acad Sci USA 1992, 89:1827-1831.
6. Meissner A, Gnirke A, Bell GW, Ramsahoye B, Lander ES, Jaenisch R: Reduced representation bisulfite sequencing for comparative high-resolution DNA methylation analysis. Nucleic Acids Res 2005, 33:5868-5877.
7. Brinkman AB, Simmer F, Ma K, Kaan A, Zhu J, Stunnenberg HG: Whole-genome DNA methylation profiling using MethylCap-seq. Methods 2010, 52:232-236.
8. Rodriguez B, Frankhouser D, Murphy M, Trimarchi M, Tam HH, Curfman J, Huang R, Chan MW, C LH, Parikh D, et al.: A Scalable, Flexible Workflow for MethylCap-Seq Data Analysis. BMC Genomics 2012., 13
9. Blum W, Garzon R, Klisovic RB, Schwind S, Walker A, Geyer S, Liu S, Havelange V, Becker H, Schaaf L, et al.: Clinical response and miR-29b predictive significance in older AML patients treated with a 10-day schedule of decitabine. Proc Natl Acad Sci USA 2010, 107:7473-7478.
10. Rodriguez B, Tam HH, Frankhouser D, Trimarchi M, Murphy M, Kuo C, Parikh D, Ball B, Schwind S, Curfman J, et al.: A Scalable, Flexible Workflow for MethylCap-Seq Data Analysis. IEEE Int Workshop Genomic Signal Process Stat 2011, :1-4.
11. Chavez L, Jozefczuk J, Grimm C, Dietrich J, Timmermann B, Lehrach H, Herwig R, Adjaye J: Computational analysis of genome-wide DNA methylation during the differentiation of human embryonic stem cells along the endodermal lineage. Genome Res 2010, 20:1441-1450.
12. Langmead B, Trapnell C, Pop M, Salzberg SL: Ultrafast and memory-efficient alignment of short DNA sequences to the human genome. Genome Biol 2009, 10:R25.
13. Li H, Handsaker B, Wysoker A, Fennell T, Ruan J, Homer N, Marth G, Abecasis G, Durbin R: The Sequence Alignment/Map format and SAMtools. Bioinformatics 2009, 25:2078-2079.

PART II

INTEGRATING GENOMIC MEDICINE
INTO THE CLINICAL PRACTICE

ASSESSING CAUSAL RELATIONSHIPS IN GENOMICS: FROM BRADFORD-HILL CRITERIA TO COMPLEX GENE-ENVIRONMENT INTERACTIONS AND DIRECTED ACYCLIC GRAPHS

SARA GENELETTI, VALENTINA GALLO, MIQUEL PORTA, MUIN J. KHOURY, AND PAOLO VINEIS

7.1 INTRODUCTION

Observational studies of human health and disease (basic, clinical and epidemiological) are vulnerable to methodological problems—such as selection bias and confounding—that make causal inferences problematic. Gene-disease associations are no exception, as they are commonly investigated using observational designs. However, as compared to studies of environmental exposures, in genetic studies it is less likely that selection of subjects (e.g., cases and controls in a case-control study) is affected by genetic variants. Confounding is also less likely, with the exception of linkage disequilibrium (i.e., the attribution of a genetic effect to a specific gene rather than to an adjacent one) and population stratification (when cases and controls are drawn from different ethnic populations). There is in fact some empirical evidence suggesting that gene-disease associations

This chapter was originally published under the Creative Commons Attribution License. Geneletti S, Gallo V, Porta M, Khoury MJ, and Vineis P. Assessing causal relationships in genomics: From Bradford-Hill Criteria to Complex Gene-Environment Interactions and Directed Acyclic Graphs. Emerging Themes in Epidemiology *8,5 (2011). doi:10.1186/1742-7622-8-5.*

are less prone to confounding (e.g., by socio-economic status) than associations between genes and environmental and lifestyle variables [1]. There are some well known methodological challenges in interpreting the causal significance of gene-disease associations; they include epistasis, linkage disequilibrium, and gene-environment interactions (GEI) [2].

A rich body of knowledge exists in medicine and epidemiology on assessment of causal relationships involving personal and environmental causes of disease; it includes seminal causal criteria developed by Austin Bradford Hill and more recently applied directed acyclic graphs (DAGs). Perhaps unsurprisingly, such knowledge has seldom been applied to assess causal relationships in clinical genetics and genomics, even when studies aimed at making inferences relevant for human health. Conversely, incorporating genetic causal knowledge into clinical and epidemiological causal reasoning is still a largely unexplored task.

In this paper, we first state our main aim; secondly, we propose applications of Hill's criteria to genetic problems and genetic epidemiology; thirdly, we use graphical methods to formulate and assess causal hypotheses involving genes; finally, we use a case study of Parkinson's disease to apply the combined Hill / DAGs approach to untangling the underlying GEIs.

7.2 AIM OF THE PAPER

The main aim of this paper is to propose a conceptual framework to assess causal relationships in clinical genomics and, particularly, for evaluating the etiopathogenic significance of gene-disease associations and gene-environment interactions; i.e., a framework to assess the validity and significance of such environment-host-gene relationships in the etiology of human diseases. The framework includes a two-step approach that combines the causal criteria of Austin Bradford Hill with graphical models such as directed acyclic graphs (DAGs). The approach we propose thus helps, first, to untangle the web of interactions amongst several exposures and characteristics (environmental, clinical and genetic) and a disease. Once these relationships have been specified, they are analyzed using criteria to assess causality that have long been used in clinical and epidemiological research. More generally, the present paper is an example of integrative research, i.e., research that integrates knowledge, data, methods, techniques, and reasoning from multiple disciplines, approaches and levels of analysis to generate knowledge that no discipline alone may achieve [3].

7.3 APPLYING CAUSAL GUIDELINES TO GENETIC STUDIES

For several decades, guidelines to assess causality have been a powerful tool in clinical and epidemiological research, as well as in the professional practice of medicine and epidemiology outside academia [4-7]. Causal guidelines usually include a series of criteria that help assess which observed associations are potentially causal. They were introduced initially by Bradford-Hill in the debate about the role of smoking in the aetiology of lung cancer; given the issue, they were meant for observational studies only, but many of the criteria can be applied to clinical trials and other experimental studies as well [8]. Although Hill did not have genetic epidemiology in mind at the time, today his criteria remain relevant to causal assessment in this field and, as we will show, to many areas of human genetics as well.

Hill's approach is based on nine criteria: 1) Strength of association; 2) Consistency; 3) Specificity of association; 4) Temporality; 5) Biological gradient (dose-response relationship); 6) Biological plausibility; 7) Coherence; 8) Experimental evidence (e.g. reproducibility in animal models); and 9) Analogy. Statistical significance was not listed but discussed separately by Hill [8].

One major criticism leveled at Hill's approach is that it considers one causal factor at a time and is not intended to tackle complex relationships and interactions, such as those encountered in modern molecular medicine and genomics, which deal with chains of mediators and not only directly acting exposures. However, even complex situations can often be decomposed into simpler constituents, and in such case Hill's criteria can be applied fruitfully. This is a main motivation behind the present work.

In 2006, a Human Genome Epidemiology Network (HuGENet) workshop in Venice was devoted to the development of standardized criteria for the assessment of the credibility of cumulative evidence on gene-disease associations. This led to synopses on various topics in genetic epidemiology;

e.g., on DNA repair [9], and on Parkinson's disease [10]. Briefly, according to the Venice guidelines [2] each gene-disease association is graded on the basis of the amount of evidence, replication, and protection from bias. These guidelines contributed to modifying the approach to genetic inferences using Hill's criteria that we adopt here.

Main theoretical issues underlying the application of Hill's criteria in genetics and genomics are shown in Appendix 1 [11-29]; below we will show how these criteria can be applied to an example of gene-environment interaction. Interactions here are defined as "the interdependent operation of two or more causes to produce, prevent, or control an effect" [2].

In summary, Hill's causal criteria and related logical tools that have long been applied fruitfully to clinical and epidemiological research may also be applied productively to research in genetics. However, genetic research has fundamental differences from clinical and epidemiological research. For example, in genetics confounding can be the consequence of events that may not be directly addressed at the other levels, including haplotype blocks, allelic heterogeneity, overdominance, and epistasis [15]. Selection bias is more easily measurable in genomic studies, because we have the null hypothesis represented by Hardy-Weinberg equilibrium (HWE); i.e., we expect independent assortment of alleles in the population, whereas a similar reasoning cannot be applied to daily life exposures. Hardy-Weinberg equilibrium is based on assumptions of population genetics related to the lack of selection, inbreeding, migration; departure from HWE can thus point towards the possibility of gross bias (such as genotyping errors or selection bias).

Explicit guidelines for causal assessment are more popular in clinical and epidemiological research than in genetics [3,30]. The reasons for that have seldom been addressed. They are probably related to the different nature of the objects, factors, mechanisms and processes that we study at each level. However, genetic guidelines on causality do exist and, in fact, have interesting similarities with Hill's criteria: (a) linkage to a particular region of the human genome (LOD>3); (b) one or more independent mutations that are concordant with disease status in affected families (specificity, strength of association); (c) defects that lead to macrochanges in the protein (specificity, coherence); (d) putative mutations that are not present in a sample from a control population (specificity); or (e) presence of some other line of biological evidence (including expression, knockout data, etc.) [15]. Criteria (a), (b) and (c) refer to background knowledge. But it is in particular criterion (e) that supports the causal association by conferring coherence with previous knowledge [3,15].

7.4 DIRECTED ACYCLIC GRAPHS AS TOOLS TO CLARIFY ASSOCIATIONS AND COMPLEX CAUSAL RELATIONSHIPS

Directed acyclic graphs (DAGs) have a long tradition in science. They are a rigorous way of visualising complex systems, clarifying ideas, complementing the formulation of hypotheses, and guiding quantitative analyses. There has been much debate on the exact nature and roles of DAGs in the biomedical literature. The most widespread approach in the health sciences is the causal DAG approach promoted by Greenland, Robins, Hernán and colleagues [31-33], and the equivalent mathematical framework of counterfactuals [34]. In causal DAG approaches, the directed edges in a DAG represent causal relationships. Whilst the causal DAG framework is appealing and intuitive, we wish to draw attention to an alternative approach to causal inference, the Decision Theoretic Framework (DTF), which is based on a formal treatment of conditional independences (a non-graphical version of the 'd-separation criteria') [35]. Appendix 2 provides additional details on statistics and assumptions underlying the DTF [36-38]. This approach has recently become increasingly popular in epidemiology, in particular to assess the role of genes as instrumental variables for causal inference [39]. DTF retains the advantages of the causal DAG approach but overcomes some of its limitations. In particular, as DTF uses DAGs to describe the relationships between variables, it retains the capacity of DAGs to clearly and formally visualise complex systems. In contrast to the causal DAG approach where all directed edges are assumed to represent causal relationships, DTF takes a more conservative view where the edges represent statistical associations (and the lack of edges represents independence). Causality in DTF is viewed as external knowledge that can be added to the DAGs and allows some of the edges to be interpreted as causal. There are three reasons for this conservative viewpoint. The first is that it entails fewer assumptions about the existence and direction of causal relationships between variables. The second is that it is not necessary to include all possible causes or covariates in a DAG, only the variables of interest, making DTF more flexible than the causal DAG approach. The third is that when we perform a statistical analysis of observational data, we obtain measures of association (not causation) between variables. We explain this concept in more detail below.

A main problem when making causal inferences in clinical and epidemiological research is that most data are observational. This is also true for a substantial part of basic biomedical research. It is certainly an issue in human genetics, where there is usually no randomization (except in circumstances where Mendelian randomization can be applied [1,3,39,40]), and knowledge of the genetic pathways is tenuous or incomplete. In such circumstances we must be careful to distinguish causal relationships from associations resulting from unobserved biases or chance.

DAGs can still be used to make causal inference, but the causal element is an external assumption that needs to be explicitly incorporated into the DAG rather than implicit in the direction of an edge. We use a DAG to visualise complex associations, but when we only have observational data at our disposal, we must find other ways to assess a) whether a particular association is causal and not due to confounding or other bias, and b) what the direction of this association is.

The problem of inferring causality from observational data in the presence of unobserved confounding is simply described in the DAGs in Figure 1.

In the DAG on the left hand side X is the putative cause -e.g., a particular environmental exposure such as urban pollution-, Y is the disease outcome under investigation, and U a set of confounders, many of which will typically be unobserved. Epidemiologists are interested in the existence, direction and strength of the X-Y association and whether this can be considered causal. (They are not necessarily interested in whether the other relationships in the DAG are causal). However, they are often unable to capture all this information from observational studies due to the presence of unobserved confounders U. Even when there is no direct association— i.e., there is no edge between X and Y as in the DAG on the right hand side of the Figure 1—the presence of U (this time as a common parent) will result in a statistical association between the two. Again, the question is, how do we distinguish a causal association from a statistical association when only observational data are available?

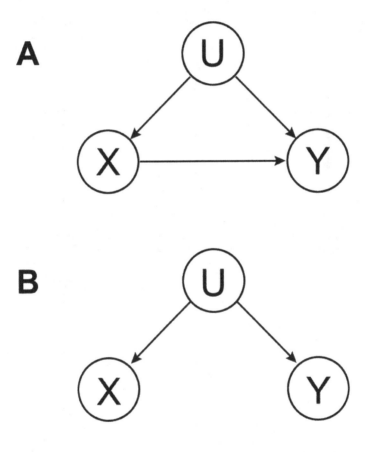

FIGURE 1: DAG demonstrating the ideas of confounding. A: U is an unobserved confounder for the association between X and Y and X is a cause of Y. B: U is an unobserved confounder for the association between X and Y but X is not a cause of Y. From purely observational data these two situations cannot be separated.

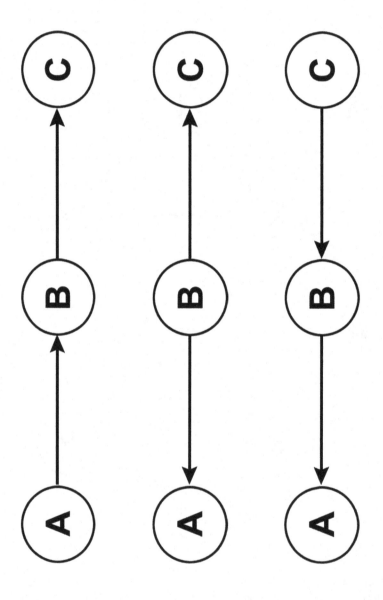

FIGURE 2: Three DAGs exhibiting the same conditional independence but with different causal interpretations.

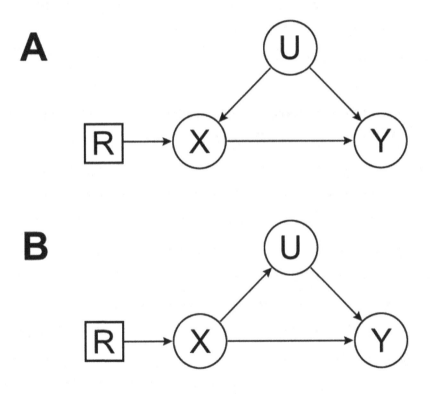

FIGURE 3: DAG with a randomisation node R. R indicates whether X is randomised or allowed to arise naturally. A: U is a confounder. B: U is a mediator. Randomisation allows us to distinguish between these situations.

One way to answer this question is by incorporating prior knowledge in Hill's scheme (or similar criteria) with DAGs to determine which edges can be considered causal. This is the approach we propose in this paper and that we describe in detail below. Another way of introducing causality is by adding so called intervention or randomisation variables to a DAG and to the corresponding probability statements. A more detailed description of such variables is given in Appendix 2. As a thorough explanation is beyond the scope of this paper we refer the interested reader to Dawid [41], Didelez [42], Geneletti [43], and Lauritzen [44].

For the remainder of this paper, the DAGs we use can be viewed as heuristic tools to understand gene-environment relationships.

7.5 PARKINSON'S DISEASE: PESTICIDES, AND GENE-ENVIRONMENT INTERACTIONS

In order to illustrate our methods, we present a case study based on Parkinson's disease. First we present a short description of the disease and a summary literature review of its genetic component; we focus in particular on a recently identified genetic form. Second, we use graphical methods to propose and assess hypotheses on how the risk factors might interact. Third, we apply Hill's criteria to each of the hypothesised associations to assess causality in light of the available evidence.

Parkinson's disease is the most common neurodegenerative disorder after Alzheimer's disease, affecting 16-19 new individuals per 100,000 persons each year in developed countries [45]. Characterized by bradykinesia, resting tremor, rigidity and postural instability, it is also one of the most common late-life movement disorders. The pathological characteristic of the disease is a selective loss of pigmented neurons, most prominently in the substantia nigra (one of the brain basal ganglia) accompanied by a characteristic α-synuclein-positive inclusion bodies in neurons (Lewy bodies) [45]. While the causes of Parkinson's disease remain unknown, significant progress is being made in elucidating genetic and environmental risk factors and the neurodegenerative process underlying the disease. Appendix 3 summaries the key evidences to date on environmental and genetic risk factors for Parkinson's disease [46-49].

A deletion of the *DJ-1* gene in a Dutch family and a mutation conferring a functionally inactive form in an Italian family associated with early onset PD were first observed in 2001 [50], and confirmed in 2003 [51] (as is convention, we use italics to indicate the gene and non-italics to indicate the protein; thus, *DJ-1* means the gene, and DJ-1 means the protein). DJ-1 is involved in many cell processes including oncogenic transformation, gene expression and chaperon activity, and it mediates oxidative stress responses [52]. A recent meta-analysis of the association between pesticides and Parkinson's disease [53] concludes that the epidemiologic evidence suggests a fairly consistent association between exposure to pesticides and risk of developing Parkinson's disease. In particular, among the herbicides, paraquat has been found to be most strongly associated with the risk of the disease (with odds ratios ranging from 1.25 to 3.22). Toxicological evidence suggests that both paraquat and rotenone exert a neurotoxic action that might play a role in the etiopathogenic process of Parkinson's disease. Moreover, clinical symptoms of Parkinson's disease have been reproduced in rats by chronic administration of paraquat [54]. Evidence from animal experiments shows that knockout models of *Drosophila melanogaster* (fruit fly) lacking DJ-1 function, display a marked and selective sensitivity to the environmental oxidative insults exerted by both paraquat and rotenone [54]; this suggests that there is an interaction between these toxicants and the *DJ-1* genotype [3]. On the basis of these data, it is sensible to hypothesise an interaction between *DJ-1,* exposure to some pesticides, and risk of Parkinson's disease in humans as well. Using Hill's criteria we can say that the hypothesis has biological plausibility; also, testing the hypothesis entails testing Hill's criterion of analogy (i.e., testing that there are analogous causal mechanisms in certain animal models and in humans). To test the hypothesis, further investigation is needed in order to estimate the effect of the interaction between *DJ-1* and exposure to specific pesticides in humans on the risk of developing Parkinson's disease. We can construct a logic framework displaying (a) the association of paraquat (P) with Parkinson's disease (Y); (b) the association of *DJ-1* with Parkinson's diseases; and (c) the interaction of *DJ-1* with exposure to paraquat. We can also assume the existence of confounding between the exposure to paraquat and the disease outcome (Cp), and between *DJ-1* and disease outcome (Cd) (Figure 4). First we are going to propose a graphical method to untangle the relationship between these two risk factors and Parkinson's disease; in a second step we will evaluate the associations from a more strictly causal point of view.

7.6 CASE STUDY: THE DJ-1 GENE, EXPOSURE TO PARAQUAT AND RISK OF PARKINSON'S DISEASE

The process we describe in this section has two components. The first uses DAGs as a visual tool to explore a range of possible interaction scenarios. The second uses DAGs as a formal tool to describe the formal dependence among the variables in the problem. These two components go hand in hand, as intuition about the problem will generally guide the first whilst the second will reflect information in the observed data as well as considerations about what is biologically plausible. In a second instance, which is beyond the scope of this paper, the interaction quantitative effects can be estimated. How the latter step is done will depend both on the nature of the data available and crucially on the model for interaction. We assume an additive interaction model for simplicity; however, the DAGs work equally well with a multiplicative model as they describe associations rather than their exact mathematical nature.

We consider first the case study of gene-environment interactions (GEI) involving risk of Parkinson's disease, the DJ-1 gene and exposure to paraquat described above. To do this we use simplified versions of models proposed by Khoury et al. [55] and Ottman [56]. Subsequently, we consider fruit fly experiments where the associations between Parkinson's, DJ-1 and paraquat have been ascertained, and we present this as the ideal situation to make causal inference. The approach we are proposing can be also used to tackle a range of other complex problems.

In order to look at possible GEI scenarios we need to introduce some simple notation:

gene
: *DJ-1* = d* variant (deletion as in the Dutch families or inactivity as in the Italian families); *DJ-1* = d wild type

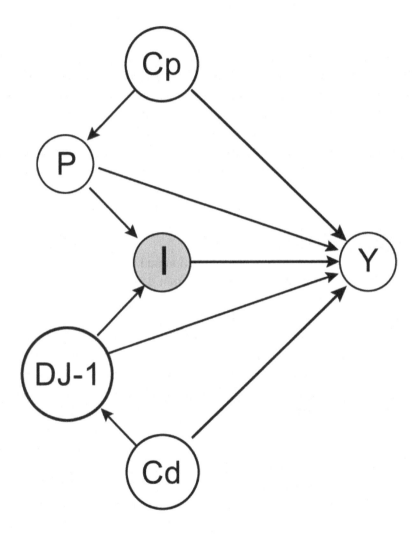

FIGURE 4: DAG showing all possible one way relationships for gene-environment interactions based on the observed variables.

pesticides
: P = p* exposed; P = p unexposed

disease
: Y = 1 with Parkinson's disease; Y = 0 without Parkinson's disease

The crux of this approach is the introduction of an interaction variable I. It is determined by the values of the genetic and environmental exposure variables. In simple terms, it acts like a switch and is turned "on" when the parents (a parent P of another variable X has an edge pointing into X, and X is a child of P) take on some values, and "off" when the parents have other values. In the current context this is typically the presence of the genetic exposure (i.e., the genetic variant) and/or the environmental exposure that leads to an increase in disease risk which turns the interaction "on". Thus, in addition to the above variables, we also define:

interaction
: I = 1 ("on") if there is an interaction and I = 0 ("off") if there isn't. The exact nature of the interaction depends on the contexts sketched below.

For the sake of simplicity, we assume that I is a deterministic variable. What we mean by this is that unlike the other variables in the problem, I is not random. Once the value of its parents is known, then so is the value of I. This might be considered unduly restrictive if there are other potential parents in the interaction which are suspected but unobserved. It is possible in these cases to view I as a random variable, where its variability is associated with that of the unobserved interactant. However, in the paper we focus on the simplest case and thus we make the following assumption:

1. *DJ-1* and P are the only parents of the interaction variable I. Another assumption that is generally plausible, provided that the exposure does not modify the genetic structure (e.g., the exposure does not cause somatic mutations) is that:

2. There is no a priori association between the gene and the external exposure; this is represented by the absence of a directed edge between *DJ-1* and P in the DAGs below.

Generally, this is a plausible assumption provided that the exposure does not modify the genetic structure [57]. In this specific example, this assumption is likely to be true. However, with other environmental exposures this assumption does not hold. For example, the association of some lifestyle factors with genotypes predisposing (or causing) Parkinson's disease is possible as the dopaminergic system is involved in rewarding mechanisms and it is hypothesized to influence some seeking behaviours and addiction (i.e., smoking or alcohol drinking) [58].

The idea of I as a variable to represent interaction is similar to the sufficient component cause (SCC) variables in VanderWeele and Robins [59]. We feel however that our approach presents a few advantages over the SCC framework. As we do not need to incorporate all the sufficient causes (we are not using a causal DAG), the structure of our DAGs is less cumbersome. Also, although for the sake of simplicity we have defined I in terms of binary exposures, we can easily extend it if we are considering multi-valued or continuous exposures. The DAG in Figure 4 shows a complex situation we can imagine, given assumptions 1 and 2, in which there is confounding between both the exposure to paraquat and the disease outcome (Cp) as well as confounding between *DJ-1* and the disease (Cd), and no other variables are postulated. Confounding between both exposure to paraquat and the disease might be due, for example, to the fact that people exposed to paraquat may also be more likely to smoke, a factor that is negatively associated with the risk of Parkinson's disease [60]. Confounding between *DJ-1* and the disease might be due to the involvement of the dopamine-mediated rewarding system [58]. Any observational study -any study of these issues in humans- is unlikely to observe all potential confounders. Nevertheless, just to simplify our model, we also assume that:

3. There are no further confounders between either the gene and the outcome or the exposure and the outcome. This is represented by

the absence of additional variables and corresponding directed edges in the DAGs below.

Now we turn our attention to looking at the case by evaluating the plausibility of a few different GEI scenarios. As mentioned above, these are loosely based on Khoury et al. [55]. For each of the models that we consider below, we present a more formal description in Appendix 4.

7.6.1 MODEL I

Both exposure and genotype are required to increase risk as in Figure 5. Here, if I is "on" then there is an association between the disease and the genetic exposure and the environmental exposure to pesticides when both are present. If on the other hand I is "off" then there is no association -in other words, Parkinson's is only associated with *DJ-1* and paraquat exposure through the interaction itself. This is an extreme form of interaction that is unlikely to occur in the pathogenesis of common diseases. Does this model describe the relationship between *DJ-1*, exposure to pesticides and Parkinson's disease? For this to be the case, all the Dutch and Italian families with the variant *DJ-1* and Parkinson's would also have to have been exposed to pesticides. Further, the incidence of Parkinson's amongst the families with the gene variant would have to be the same on average as that of those without the gene variant (if unexposed to pesticides). Similarly, those exposed to pesticides would have to have the same incidence as those not exposed to the pesticides without the *DJ-1* variant. This is clearly not the case.

7.6.2 MODEL II

The exposure to pesticides increases the risk of disease but the presence of the gene variant alone does not increase the risk of disease, although the variant further increases the risk of disease in the exposed population (Figure 6). In this model, I is switched on and off by P. When $P = p^*$ (exposure to pesticides) $I = 1$, indicating that the interaction is switched "on" and the

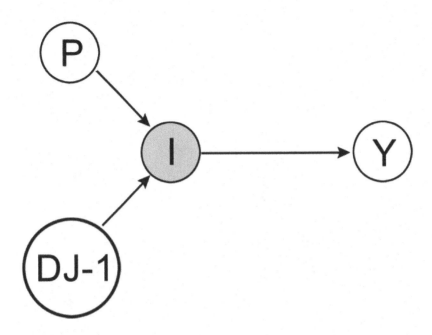

FIGURE 5: Both *DJ-1* gene and pesticide exposure need to be present to activate the interaction.

presence of the variant in *DJ-1* and Parkinson's is influential. When P = p then I = 0 and whether *DJ-1* is the variant or wild-type form makes no difference to the outcome Y. It is possible that in some cases exposure to P is protective; i.e., I would take the opposite value of P in a binary situation. In more complex situations, the effect of P might be such that only certain values of P result in interactions and in these cases the values of I and P would not be the same. In this instance, we have that Y depends directly on exposure P; however, Y depends on *DJ-1* only through the interaction and the exposure when this is present -i.e. when P = p*.

This model is also not a plausible description of the relationship between the three variables based on the evidence at hand, as it would mean that all the families with the variant and Parkinson's would have to also have been exposed to pesticides.

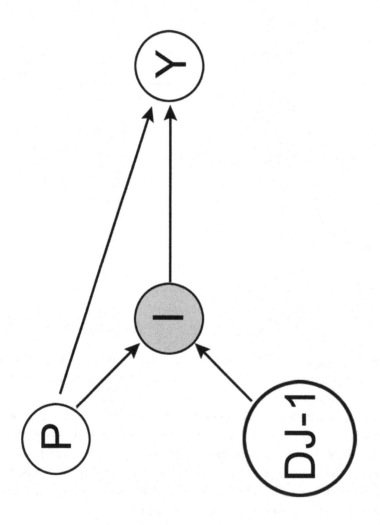

FIGURE 6: Pesticide has an effect but DJ-1 only has an effect if pesticide exposure is present.

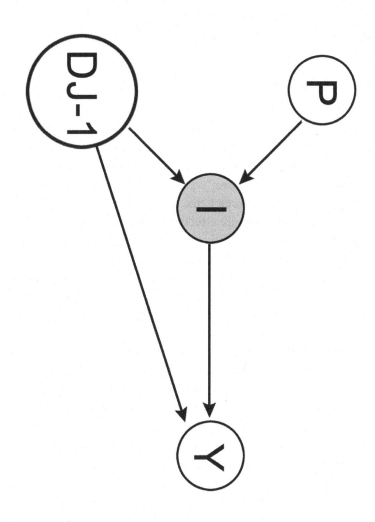

FIGURE 7: DJ-1 has an effect but pesticide only has an effect if the gene mutation is present.

7.6.3 MODEL III

Exposure to pesticides exacerbates the effect of the gene variant but has no effect on persons with the normal genotype. In this model, I is switched on and off by *DJ-1*. The model does not provide either a plausible explanation of the available evidence (Figure 7).

7.6.4 MODEL IV

The environmental exposure and the gene variant both have some effect of their own but together they further modify the effect of the other. Here I is a function of both P and *DJ-1* and is defined as follows: I is "on" if and only if both P and *DJ-1* are "on" otherwise I is "off". Here there are also direct associations between P and Y and *DJ-1* and Y other than through I; this indicates that there are effects of P on Y irrespective of *DJ-1*, and effects of *DJ-1* on Y irrespective of P. From the data we cannot distinguish between DAGs A and B in Figure 8.

A core issue with these models is that I is essentially unobservable in humans living under normal conditions; these biological interactions can only be tested in animal experiments. Thus, in humans we cannot disentangle the two DAGs above apart without further information (VanderWeele and Robins [61] provide some tests to determine which individuals present Y only when the interaction I is "on" provided there is no unmeasured confounding). In order to be able to fully tell them apart, an experiment can be conducted or the relative risks can be compared (see Appendix 1).

In light of the evidence on Parkinson's disease, we have to favour one of the two models IV above the other three, as it would appear that both the genetic and the environmental exposure have separate (independent) effects on the risk of Parkinson's. However, from the data on humans we cannot distinguish between the two "type IV" models until we run a study to determine the presence of an interaction. In the case of the *Drosophila* experiments (see section below) the interaction model on the left-hand side provides a better explanation, as flies with the mutation that have been exposed demonstrate further sensitivity to exposure to pesticides than those who do not have the mutation.

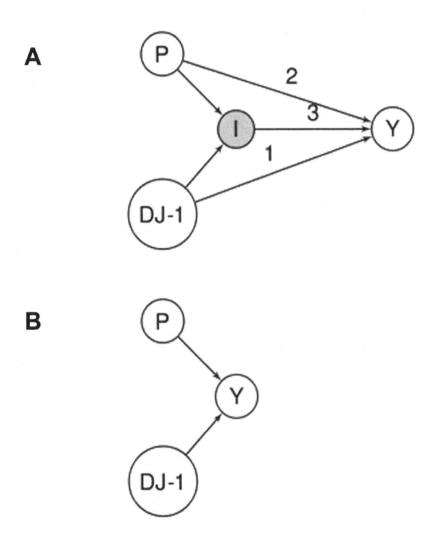

FIGURE 8: Both DJ-1 and the pesticide have an effect and there is a possible interaction in A but not in.

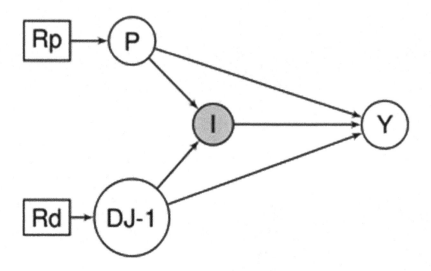

FIGURE 9: DAG representing the fruit-fly experiment where interventions were performed both on the genetic make-up and the pesticide exposure. The interaction can therefore be identified.

The example we have shown exemplifies, we think, a common situation concerning the interaction between metabolic genes and environmental exposures (e.g. arylamines and *NAT2*, *PAH* and *GSTM1* and many others) but has the peculiarity that experiments in *Drosophila* have been done (see below).

7.6.5 EXPERIMENTAL EVIDENCE: THE CASE OF THE DROSOPHILA

The DAGs above alone cannot be directly used for causal inference unless additional assumptions are made or experiments conducted. The reason is the limited information on potential confounders (and intermediate variables, etc.) that can influence the relationship between the three observed variables. For the sake of making the DAGs clear, we have assumed that there are no confounders; however this is unlikely to be the case in practice as Parkinson's is a multifactorial disease. The method we have proposed can however be extended to include confounders and intermediate variables.

In the case of *Drosophila* the situation is simpler. Meulener et al. [49] show that both exposure to pesticides and the mutation of *DJ-1* may be associated with increased risk of neural degeneration. Further, the combination of the two has also been demonstrated to aggravate the condition, as the flies which had the *DJ-1* gene knocked out exhibited a ten-fold increase in sensitivity to paraquat (which would indicate a supra-multiplicative interaction).

As in this case both the genetic make-up and the exposure status of the flies have been intervened upon under controlled conditions, we can make causal inference based on this data by introducing randomisation variables into our DAG. The DAG in Figure 9 is an augmented DAG [38] that includes randomisation variables Rp and Rd. These tell us whether P or *DJ-1* are being randomised or not and allow us to make inferences about interventions and, hence, causality using DAGs. For a more detailed discussion see Appendix 2.

The DAG in Figure 9 implied that for the *Drosophila* at least we can state that exposure to pesticides causes an increased risk of neural damage, as does the presence of the mutated *DJ-1* gene. Also as the combined presence of the mutation and paraquat further increases the risk of neural damage, we can ascertain the presence of an interaction. It should be noted that DAGs do not specify or constrain the model of statistical interaction, which can follow either an additive or a multiplicative null hypothesis model.

In the case of humans, we cannot assume such randomisation variables exist (except in Mendelian randomisation which, however, applies to gene variants only, and not to exposure); thus, we cannot expand the DAG in Figure 6. On the other hand, etiologic factors and clinical phenotypes are usually more diverse in human diseases than in animal models; inferences to human diseases from relatively simple animal experiments have well known limitations. An avenue for progress lies in integrating DAGs with the inductive reasoning implicit in Hill's guidelines.

7.6.6 APPLICATION OF CAUSAL GUIDELINES TO DJ-1 AND EXPOSURE TO PARAQUAT FOR PARKINSON'S DISEASE

Following the DAG approach, we established the relationship between genes and some environment exposures in promoting Parkinson's disease, and we proposed different interaction models between *DJ-1*, pesticides and Parkinson's disease. In order to apply Hill's causal guidelines to the DAGs we are going to work with (Figure 6A), we need to label each of the edges. Throughout the rest of this section we use the following labels:

- The edge between *DJ-1* and Parkinson's disease is referred to as [edge 1],
- The edge between exposure to pesticides and Parkinson's disease is referred to as [edge 2],
- The interaction between *DJ-1* and the exposure to pesticides in causing Parkinson's disease is called [edge 3].

Hill's guidelines are discussed in a slightly different order than in the original version and statistical significance is omitted because it refers to the contingent evaluation of each study and does not require a specific discussion in relation to genomics.

1. Strength of association. *DJ-1* has been seen to be lacking in Dutch families with Parkinson's disease, and to be functionally inactive because of a point mutation in the Italian families studied by Bonifati and cols [51]. The deletion showed complete cosegregation with the disease allele in the Dutch family [51]; also in the Italian family the homozygous mutation showed complete cosegregation with the disease haplotype, and absence from large numbers of control chromosomes [62]. Although the function of the DJ-1 protein is unknown, these data suggest a strong association between the *DJ-1* gene and the occurrence of Parkinson's disease in certain families [edge 1]. To establish the strength of the association between specific environmental factors and a disease is far more complicated, mainly due to the quality of exposure assessment, the latency period, and body concentrations during the lifecourse. A meta-analysis of the association of pesticides and Parkinson's disease points out that both pesticide exposure in general and

selective exposure to paraquat seem to be associated with Parkinson's disease, with odds ratios ranging from 1.25 (95% C.I.: 0.34 - 4.36) to 3.22 (95% C.I.: 2.41 to 4.31) [53] [edge 2]. With respect to the interaction parameter, there is as yet no epidemiological study that has tested whether there is an interaction between *DJ-1* and pesticides; thus neither the existence nor the strength of such an association are known. However, knockout models of *Drosophila melanogaster* (fruit fly) lacking *DJ-1* function, display a marked and selective sensitivity to the environmental oxidative insults exerted by both paraquat and rotenone [49], suggesting an interaction between these toxicants and the *DJ-1* genotype [edge 3] in animal models and, consequently, that in humans the interaction between the chemicals and *DJ-1* is biologically plausible (as can be seen, Hill's criteria often "interact", i.e., they are often related to each other, as in this paragraph the strength of association is related to the biological plausibility).

2. Consistency of the association. After the first variants described, different variants of the *DJ-1* gene associated with the same Parkinson's disease phenotype have been found in patients of Ashkenazi Jewish and Afro-Caribbean origins [63,64] [edge 1]. The association of paraquat and rotenone with Parkinson's disease is more consistent in animals (in which these two toxicants are often used to produce animal models of the disease) [54] than in humans. In environmental epidemiological studies in humans, the association has been found substantially consistent across studies, although some associations did not reach statistical significance, mainly due to limited sample size. In a study in Taiwan, where paraquat is routinely used in rice fields, a strong association between paraquat exposure and Parkinson's disease was found; the hazard increased by more than six times in subjects exposed for more than 20 years [64]. A dose-response curve with length of exposure was also observed in plantation workers in Hawaii [65], and British Columbia [66]. In a population-based case-control study in Calgary, occupational herbicide use was the only significant predictor of Parkinson's disease in multivariable analysis [67]. However, in another population-based case-control study in Washington, the odds ratio

of 1.67 did not reach statistical significance (95% CI: 0.22-12.76) [68] [edge 2]. There is yet no evidence from human studies to confirm the consistency of GEIs in the causation of Parkinson's disease [edge 3]. Furthermore, genes other than DJ-1 may be involved in the etiopathogenic process, and so may be exposures other than pesticides, and other GEIs. Since environmental conditions vary substantially across the globe, and the role of one gene, one exposure or one GEI is often dependent on other genes, exposures and GEIs, lack of consistency is to be expected in studies conducted in different settings, and in particular when studies focus only on a few GEIs and overlook other interactions.

3. Specificity of the association. The specificity of the association between *DJ-1* gene mutations and Parkinson's disease [edge 1] will be clearer once the data on the pathological features of the *DJ-1* patients will be available (see Appendix 3). Chronic systemic exposure to rotenone has been demonstrated to cause highly selective nigrostriatal dopaminergic degeneration associated with characteristic movement disorders in rats [54] [edge 2]. Similarly, paraquat caused a significant loss of nigral dopaminergic neurons in mice compared to controls [69] [edge 2]. Once an appropriate epidemiological study is set up aimed at studying GEIs in this context, results from the pathological analysis of the sample subjects will help to answer important questions regarding the aetiological pathway of the disease [edge 3].

4. Temporality. This criterion does not apply directly to genotype, as it is determined at conception and it remains constant over time (see Appendix 1) [edge 1]. However, temporality is crucial if we go beyond genetic effects and consider epigenetic mechanisms; e.g., gene regulation by environmental factors [14,16-18]. This problem goes beyond the present contribution, but is worth mentioning. Concerning pesticides, temporality might be a concern given that all studies on GEI in Parkinson's disease are case-control studies, which are particularly prone to selection bias, disease progression bias, and so-called "reverse causality" [3,70,71]. In this case, while it is unlikely that suffering from Parkinson's disease would have influenced past exposure to pesticides or their metabolism, it could

have influenced recall. The observed dose-response relationship, with 20 years of exposure required [53], favours the existence of a true association, and is compatible with disease characteristics of neurodegeneration, making the temporality pattern suggestive of a causal role [edge 2].

5. Biological gradient. This criterion does not apply since we are dealing with a recessive model of inheritance. Nonetheless, a co-dominant model should not be completely ruled out as a careful neurological evaluation of heterozygote subjects might point out some sub-clinical changes [edge 1]. A dose-response relationship between toxicant exposure and neural loss in animal experiments has been observed [72]. In addition, several studies observed a positive correlation with duration of exposure to, and high dose of, herbicides and insecticides in humans [53] [edge 2].

6. Biological plausibility. Biological plausibility of the *DJ-1* mutation awaits the discovery and characterisation of the encoded protein [edge 1]; the capability of some toxicants to induce a progressive cellular loss in the substantia nigra and to be responsible for a progressive clinical syndrome with an intervening latent period has been hypothesized [54] [edge 2]. It is, therefore, plausible that these two factors may interact during the course of life producing Parkinson's symptoms in genetically susceptible individuals [edge 3].

7. Coherence with previous knowledge. Confirmation of the presence of different mutations on the same *DJ-1* gene in families with other background origins but manifesting the same symptoms supports the involvement of the gene in the disease [63,64] [edge 1]. A role of herbicides in neurodegeneration has also been studied with generally confirmatory results [edge 2].

All these considerations taken together suggest that there may be a potential interaction between exposure to certain pesticides and the DJ-1 mutation in the risk of developing Parkinson's disease. However, as no studies on humans have yet been specifically conducted to investigate this issue, we can use the evidence only as a reason to further explore this interaction, perhaps by conducting a more targeted study. As mentioned, it is likely that other factors (both genetic and environmental) also contribute to the final development of the disease.

In the example above we have shown that the DAG approach can be complemented by the use of Hill's guidelines when no experimental evidence can be brought to bear on a particular gene-environment interaction.

7.7 CONCLUSIONS

While medical and epidemiologic evidence is routinely assessed to determine the causal nature of relationships involving personal and environmental causes of disease, genetic associations have so far not undergone similar scrutiny. However, like epidemiologic studies, genetic studies are also commonly based on observational studies, and may thus be affected by similar weaknesses. As the contribution of genetics to the understanding of disease etiology becomes more important, causal assessment of genetic and genomic evidence will become a key issue [73].

We have explored two complementary ways to tackle causality in gene-environment interactions. The application of causal guidelines to genetics is not straightforward, and it becomes very complex, in particular, if one wants to study gene-environment interactions, as we have illustrated with Parkinson's disease. Hill's criteria were developed to examine one factor at a time and have seldom been applied to evaluate the causal nature of complex relationships involving several exposures. On the other hand, graphical approaches like DAGs are effective in making potential causal networks explicit, but are insufficient to establish the strength of evidence (e.g., edges cannot be interpreted as causal without some kind of additional external support). This seems to be a general problem of causal networks, not only gene-environment interactions.

The graphical approach is useful in particular for clarifying complex causal pathways. We have applied it to a simple example where the inner workings (i.e., the detailed biological mechanisms in animal models) of the interaction are not completely known. The approach we propose uses the statistically formal representation of DAG models. This is in contrast to Weinberg's paper [74] which, although invaluable in highlighting the pros and cons of DAG models, does not actually use DAGs, but heuristic diagrams not dissimilar to those proposed by Ottman [56] and, over 35 years ago, Susser [75]. In the approach advocated by VanderWeele and Robins [76], DAGs are considered implicitly causal. We feel that this can be overly confident when the bases for inference are observational studies, which is generally the case in human genetic studies. Thus, we propose a more conservative approach that involves assessing the causal properties of each individual relationship.

A final caveat to interpreting DAGs involving genes as causal is whether genetic variants can be considered causes of diseases [30]; in a strict sense this issue is unresolved. It is generally accepted that the causal nature of a relationship can be assured when interventions (such as those performed in experiments) take place. This is because controlled interventions usually (and more easily) guarantee that the association investigated is not confounded (but this is not an absolute rule). VanderWeele and Robins [61,76] assume that genes can be considered causes of diseases, without discussing the implications or bringing additional information such as Hill's criteria into play; we believe that this is a strong assumption: knowledge on the mechanisms that govern the subclinical development and clinical course of complex diseases is rather limited.

In summary, we believe that the DAG and causal criteria-based approaches can complement one another, as one helps to assess the strength of evidence, while the other disentangles -in a visual but also formal way- the role played by genes, environmental exposures, and their interactions. The method we suggest can easily be extended to more complex situations and in particular to the understanding of gene-gene associations and interaction. The problems we raise are likely to become more relevant as genome-wide association studies provide new candidate genes for a variety of diseases, Mendelian randomization is used to assess exposure-disease associations, and gene-environment interactions are further investigated in genetics and epigenetics.

7.A1 APPENDIX 1: USING AUSTIN BRADFORD HILL'S GUIDELINES IN GENETICS AND GENOMICS

There are some general aspects to consider when tackling cause-effect relationships in genetics. First, most associations for individual genetic variants and common chronic diseases have weak to modest effects. Empirical findings show that even for fairly well established associations, the effect sizes are weak to modest; i.e., relative risks are usually under 2, and often between 1.2 and 1.6) [11]. Generally speaking, the stronger the association between a risk factor and a disease, the more likely it is that the association is causal, because confounding and other biases are unlikely to explain it away. However, in genetics the penetrance of an individual genetic variant associated with a disease depends on the interactions of the variant with external exposures, the internal environment, or other genetic variants. In spite of the etiologic complexity of common diseases and the resulting weak effects of individual genetic variants, theoretical work suggests that the combination of as few as 20 common variants with weak to moderate effect sizes, when put together as a system of variants (or genomic profiles), can account for a substantial attributable fraction of the disease in the population [12]. On the other hand, a large number of rare variants each contributing (or causing) a strong disease risk may also be a plausible explanation. The potential rarity of highly-penetrant variants, the weakness of common associations, and the frequency of complex gene-environment interactions pose severe challenges to the statistical power to find marginal effects of single gene variants on risks for common diseases. In fact, the strength of the association with the gene (main effect) may be low while the gene-exposure interaction is strong. This may be more convincing evidence of the truly causal nature of the association, given the available biological knowledge on environmental influences on gene expression.

Consistency in genetic studies was traditionally poor in the "candidate gene" era, with few associations confirmed in more than one study [13], but this has changed rapidly with genome-wide association studies (GWAs). More than 600 stable replicated hits have been reported in 2007 and 2008 from GWAs, due to an in-built, strong process of replication of findings. One advantage of GWAs is that they are published only if the results are replicated in 3-4 or more independent studies. As a result in genetic epidemiology there is now a widely accepted requirement for "internal" consistency. A similar approach would be invaluable in non-genetic epidemiology but is currently not practiced. Poor replication for candidate genes is related to multiple factors, including type 1 errors ("false positives") and publication bias, as well as to methodological issues as biases in the selection of cases and controls, exposure assessment errors, and confounding.

In addition, the expression of genes is so dependent on the surrounding circumstances (other genes, internal environment -e.g., immunological and nutritional status [14]-, external physical environment, gene expression), that the same main clinical effect of a gene variant is difficult to capture in different studies conducted under different conditions. In fact, such main effects may not be identical in different studies that are conducted in actual -sometimes, very different- human contexts; a genuine heterogeneity of human genetic effects across population groups -and individuals- is to be expected on the basis of knowledge on how biological, clinical and environmental processes jointly cause disease in humans. An example of the influence of study design is the investigation of gene-disease associations in founder populations, in which the effect of a genetic variant is likely to be higher than the average across all populations [15]. Another example is familial aggregation studies, where familial disease risks are influenced not only by the genetic mutations or variants of interest, but also by other genetic and epigenetic processes; if the latter are overlooked, the penetrance of the former may be overestimated [16-18].

To some extent it is reasonable to hope that genetic associations are specific, thus facilitating causal inference. For example, 5-HTT variants have been associated specifically with bipolar disorder, probably because of the role of the gene in serotonin metabolism [19]. But expectations of specificity may disregard biological knowledge (e.g., on cofactors, multiple causes and effects) that makes unspecificity more plausible. A potential problem in the use of specificity as a criterion for causality is that many genetic variants belong to metabolic, inflammatory, homeostatic and other pathways that could influence multiple disease processes. This is an extension of the concept of pleiotropy that we see in single gene disorders. For example, MTHFR variation involves folic acid and methylation pathways that may have potential relevance to the genesis of many disease outcomes, as birth defects, cardiovascular disease and cancer [20]. The same is likely to be true for DNA repair genes [21]. This issue has long been observed in non genetic epidemiology in relation to some common risk factors, such as socio-economic status or cigarette smoking, which are associated with many disease outcomes. The value of specificity increases with increasing knowledge about the constituents of the exposure (e.g., PAHs and other carcinogens for cigarette smoking), and of its biological or environmental effects. For example, on the basis of functional knowledge, only bladder cancer, and perhaps colon cancer, may be expected to be associated with NAT2 variants [22-24]. Such postulated associations are biologically plausible because there is evidence that aromatic amines or heterocyclic aromatic amines, which are metabolised by NAT2, are involved in bladder or colon carcinogenesis. Nevertheless, NAT2 associations are also observed with breast and lung cancer and mesothelioma [25,26], without evidence of biological plausibility. This unexpected non-specificity may be true and due, for instance, to a pleiotropic effect of the exposure; or the apparent association with the outcome (in this case, other than bladder cancer) may be confounded by yet unknown factors. Similar situations are encountered in clinical medicine and non genetic epidemiology; for example, the early observation of an inverse association between hormone replacement therapy (HRT) and mortality due to accidents and violence, which was of the same magnitude as that originally found for cardiovascular mortality [27]. This prompted a debate on the causal nature of the association between HRT and cardiovascular mortality, as no plausible biological reason for the protective effect of HRT on violent death could be argued.

Temporality is also relevant to the study of the genotypes; since gene variants are inherited and do not change after conception, they precede the onset of disease indeed. In addition the temporal pattern with which a particular variant/mutation manifests itself can be relevant. In Huntington's disease, for example, there is the phenomenon of "anticipation" (younger age of disease onset in one generation than in the previous) depending on the number of the repeated triplets in the gene (which tend to increase in the offspring). For acquired genetic alterations (e.g., somatic mutations) temporality is also important; in persons living in normal conditions the timing of occurrence of the mutation often cannot be observed directly. A collection of archived specimens may help, as can knowledge on the usual course of events gained from molecular pathology studies. For epigenetic mechanisms temporality is even more crucial, but it is beyond the purpose of this article [14,16-18].

In genomics, the possibility of observing a dose-response gradient depends on the model of genotype-phenotype relationships. Even for a diallelic system at one locus, there could be recessive, dominant or codominant models. The biologic model for the action of numerous alleles at different loci is more complex and is essentially unknown for most common diseases. Only if the genetic model is codominant can a dose-response be observed. However, a different kind of dose-response is observable if we consider the cumulative effect of multiple genes or SNPs. Both the risk of lung cancer and the levels of DNA damage can increase approximately linearly with an increasing number of "at risk" gene variants [21,28]. Gene copy number variation can lead to more complex dose-response relationships. Quantitative continuous markers used in epigenetics (promoter methylation) and transcriptomics (gene expression) may be analyzed in search of dose-response effects (linear or non-linear).

In genetics experimental evidence comes mainly from animal studies in which knock-out organisms are used in order to have a pure genetic disease model. This directly tests the effect of the absence or presence of specific genetic factors on the organism. Extrapolation of the results of these experiments to humans is challenging due to differences between humans and the knock-out organisms in both the genetic make-up and the potential types of gene-gene and gene-environment interactions. Genetic experimental studies have also long been known to reproduce disease phenotypes (e.g., in mice) that are only a partial approximation of the complex human disease; an example is the Super Oxide Dismutase-1 (SOD1) mutated mouse model for Amyotrophic Lateral Sclerosis (ALS), which has different motor characteristics than the human disease [29].

7.A2 APPENDIX 2: THE CALCULUS OF THE DECISION THEORETIC FRAMEWORK (DTF)

7.A2.1 THE CALCULUS OF DTF

Conditional independence [12] is the tool DTF uses to a) express how variables are associated and b) to understand when it is possible to make inferences about causal associations from data that are observational. It is best described as follows: consider 3 variables A, B and C. Say that $Pr(A,C|B) = Pr(A|B)Pr(C|B)$ (where $Pr(.)$ means probability of).

Then we can say that A is independent of C given B - formally: A $\perp\!\!\!\perp C|B$.

This means that if we know what B is, knowing what A is gives us no further information on C; e.g., if we want to know the genetic make up of Alfred (A), we can gain some information by looking at his brother Colin (C). If however, we can see their parents Barry and Barbara (B), then knowing about Colin gives us no further information on Alfred. This shows where the "familial" terminology used in DAGs comes from.

Conditional independence is a non-graphical (and non-causal) equivalent of the d-separation criteria used in the causal DAG approach [11]. It forms the basis for the formal treatment of DTF, and its manipulation allows us to determine under what circumstances we can equate the results of observation to those of experiment [35,44].

The original role of DAGs in the statistical literature is to encode statistical associations (described, for instance, by Chi-squared tests). Thus, in DTF the lack of directed edges in a DAG is viewed as conditional or marginal independence between variables, not a lack of a causal relationship. There are two problems with interpreting DAGs encoding such associations as causal. The first problem is that often there is more than one DAG representing the same set of conditional independences (see example below). To determine which, if any of them, is causal, we must use knowledge that is not inherent in the data or the DAG (e.g., time ordering). The second problem is that we often do not have data on all the variables that play a role (causal or otherwise) in the problem we are considering. This means that the DAGs only tell us about the relationships between the variables we have observed, making a causal interpretation dangerous.

Consider the following simple example: A and B are proteins produced in the body and C is a cancer thought to be associated to the production of A and B. It is possible to artificially increase the amount of B in the system and we would eventually like to know whether this could prevent the emergence of the cancer C. However, at this point we do not know whether A or B are produced by the presence of C or indeed whether there is any natural ordering to the appearance of the three variables. We obtain the conditional independence $A \perp\!\!\!\perp C|B$ from data on a number of individuals in a case control study investigating possible causes of C. This is encoded by all three DAGs in the Figure 2. These three DAGs only tell us one thing, namely that the cancer is not directly associated to protein A (when we only consider these three variables and the individuals in the study). They do not tell us whether treating patients with B will have a positive effect on the incidence of C or indeed how A and B are associated. Thus, trying to determine whether intake of B will act as a preventive agent (i.e., whether B causes C) based only on current knowledge and the DAGs is impossible. When we face a problem that we do not understand fully, interpreting one DAG or even one particular directed edge as causal can be difficult.

7.A2.2 RANDOMISATION AND INTERVENTIONS

One way of determining whether relationships depicted in a DAG describing observational data are causal is to relate it to an equivalent situation under intervention or randomisation. It is generally accepted that the ideal for causal inference is the randomised controlled trial because confounding is eliminated or attenuated. It is generally also accepted [36] that when we perform an external intervention, such as randomisation on a system in equilibrium, we can view the consequences as causal. Thus, intervention is a formal way of asserting cause-effect relationships.

In DTF we introduce randomisation as a variable R (Figure 3). To clarify, consider the following example. Assume that X is a binary variable that can be forced to take on a particular value or "set". It takes on two values: "active" ($X = a$), or "baseline" ($X = b$). The randomising variable R has the same settings as X as well as the observational setting $R = \Phi$ (the empty set). When $R = a$ then $X = a$ with no uncertainty (imagine forcing X to take on this value, say by administering the treatment to a compliant patient). Similarly, when $R = b$, $X = b$ with no uncertainty. Finally when $R = \Phi$, X is allowed to arise without intervention and can take on the values a and b as in an observational study. For causal inference in DTF we want to estimate (usually the expected value of) the outcome Y given that an intervention has happened. For example, if we want to know which treatment, active or baseline, is better for Y, we might look at the difference in the expected value of Y given these treatments: $E(Y \mid R = a)$- $E(Y|R = b)$. This would then be a measure of the causal effect of a vs b. In observational studies, we do not have $E(Y|R = a)$ the interventional expectation; rather, we have $E(Y \mid X = a, R = \Phi)$ the observational expectation; similarly for b. The question is, therefore, how to make an inference about the former using the latter. One assumption that is often made is that all observed confounders U are observed. However, this is often not possible and other approaches that simulate randomisation, such as the instrumental variable approach known as Mendelian randomisation [37] can be used. See Dawid [41], Didelez [42], and Geneletti [43] for formal examples.

Introducing randomisation can also help us distinguish between intermediate variables and confounders, as when X is randomised the association between X and any confounders U is severed, whilst that with intermediates is not (A and B in Figure 3). Statistically, if after randomising X the distribution of U conditional on X remains the same as before randomisation, then U is a confounder rather than a mediating variable, as this means that U is independent of X when it is randomised. This corresponds precisely to the situation described by the DAG in Figure 3A. If U depends on X then we have that U is a mediator as in Figure 3B.

As also shown in Figure 3B, interventions are represented by decision nodes (square boxes) in augmented DAGs [38], and these can be used to make some causal inferences, as DAGs explicitly represent interventions. By introducing the randomisation/intervention variables explicitly into the DAG, we can use conditional independences to determine when it is possible to estimate the causal effect (based $R = a,b$) from data that are observational (based on $R = \Phi$ and $X = a,b$). Again, as a detailed description of the formal DTF is beyond the scope of this paper, we refer the interested reader to previous work [41-44].

TABLE 1: Main identified genes involved in Parkinsonism, with their biological, clinical and pathological main features

Gene (locus)	Protein	Function	Inheritance	Pathology	Clinical phenotype
1SNCA (PARK1/4)	α-synuclein	Signal transduction, membrane vesicle trafficking, and cytoskeletal dynamics	Dominant	Diffuse Lewy bodies (prominently nigral and hippocampal neuronal loss)	Early onset progressive L-Dopa responsive Parkinsonism, cognitive decline, autonomic dysfunction and dementia
LRRK2 (PARK8)	Dardarin	Cytosolic kinase with several functions (including substrate binding, protein phosphorylation and protein-protein interactions)	Dominant	Predominantly Lewy bodies disease (rare cases with neurofibrillar tangels and/or nigral neuronal loss	Parkinsonism consistent with sporadic Parkinson's Disease. Dystonia, amyotrophy, gaze palsy and dementia occasionally develop
PRKN (PARK2)	Parkin	E3 ligase (conjugating ubiquitine to proteins to target them for degradation by the proteasome)	Recessive (rare "presudo-dominant" cases reported)	Predominantly nigral neuronal loss (compound heterozygotes with Lewy bodies or tau pathology are described)	Early onset Parkinsonism, often presenting with dystopia, with diurnal fluctuations. Typically responsive to very low doses of L-Dopa
PINK1 (PARK6)	-	Mitochondrial kinase	Recessive	Undetermined	Early onset Parkinsonism, slowly progressive and responsive to low doses of L-Dopa
DJ-1 (PARK7)	-	Oxidative stress signalling molecule on mitochondria	Recessive	Undetermined	Slowly progressive early-onset Parkinsonism occasionally with psychiatric disturbances; rare compound heterozygotes with Parkinsonism and dementia or amyotrophy are described

7.A3 APPENDIX 3: PARKINSON'S DISEASE: ENVIRONMENTAL AND GENETIC RISK FACTORS

7.A3.1 PARKINSON'S DISEASE: ENVIRONMENTAL FACTORS

Large epidemiological studies aimed at identifying risk factors for Parkinson's disease have suggested a role of 1-methyl-4-phenyl-1,2,3,6-tetrahydropyridine (MPTP) (a compound accidentally produced in the manufacture of illegal drugs), of some pesticides, of certain metals and of polychlorinated biphenyls [46]. On the other hand, tea and coffee drinking, use of non-steroidal anti-inflammatory drugs, and high blood levels of uric acid have been suggested to be protective for Parkinson's disease [46].

7.A3.2 PARKINSON'S DISEASE: SINGLE GENE DISORDERS

To date, eleven monogenic forms have been identified (with *PARK1* to *11* gene acronyms); they will be selectively discussed below (Table 1) [47]. However, monogenic forms of Parkinson's explain no more than 20% of the early-onset cases of the disease, and less than 3% of the forms with onset in the old ages, a situation that is common to many chronic diseases as breast cancer (e.g., role of BRCA1) or heart disease (e.g., Familial Hypercholesterolemia). Most forms of the disease appear to be caused or at least influenced by complex interactions between several genes, or between genes and environmental factors.

The α-synuclein, encoded by the *SNCA* gene, is a protein with several functions in signal transduction and vesicle trafficking; it is also a competitive inhibitor of an enzyme involved in the L-Dopa biosynthesis. Three known dominant mutations on the *SNCA* gene have been identified in families affected by Parkinsonism with dementia characterised pathologically by diffuse Lewy bodies, mainly composed of α-synuclein. The identification of these mutations contributes to the contention as to whether the so-called Lewy body disorders (Parkinson's disease, Parkinsonism with dementia, and dementia with Lewy bodies) represent a continuum or have to be considered as distinct diseases [47]. This is thus as well an excellent example of a situation in which researchers try to elucidate the causal relationships between a complex set of genotypes and a rich spectrum of clinical phenotypes.

The *LRRK* gene encodes for a protein involved in multiple functions; three dominant mutations are known. Pathologically, the disease is characterised by a typical Lewy body pattern consistent with the post mortem diagnosis of Parkinson's disease. However, some cases with tau-positive pathology without Lewy bodies have been observed even within the same family. The pathway leading to one or the other condition is likely to be influenced by genetic and/or environmental factors that remain to be identified [47].

There are more than 50 known variants in the *parkin* gene and their effect on the disease appears to be recessive. Subjects with homozygous mutations leading to complete loss of *parkin* expression are found to have a selective loss of dopaminergic neurons in the substantia nigra and in the locus coeruleus without Lewy bodies or neurofibrillar tangles. However, subjects with compound heterozygous mutations (a diploid genotype in which two copies of a gene carry different mutations) may present pathologically with Lewy bodies or neurofibrillar pathology. This behaviour can be due to the fact that the outcome is mutation-specific: some mutations can reduce rather than abolish the protein activity affecting substrate specificity. Otherwise, these two different outcomes can share the primary cause (as for the *LRRK* case), which is subsequently influenced by gene-gene and/or gene-environment interactions [47].

For the last two recessive mutations, *PINK-1* and *DJ-1* there is no pathological information available. The protein encoded by *PINK-1* gene is a mitochondrial kinase that seems to be involved in protecting the cell from mitochondrial dysfunction and stress-induced apoptosis [47]. The protein encoded by *DJ-1* gene also is localised on mitochondria, but it seems to belong to the chaperones family, induced by oxidative stress [48]. This protein has been demonstrated to be involved in cell protection during oxidative stress. Intriguingly, reduced *DJ-1* expression in *Drosophila melanogaster* results in susceptibility to oxidative stress and proteasome inhibition, which leads to a selective sensitivity to the environmental chemical agents paraquat and rotenone [49].

7.A4 APPENDIX 4: THE GENE-ENVIRONMENT INTERACTIONS (GEI) MODELS IN FORMAL TERMS[o]

Below is a more formal treatment of the GEI models we consider in the main text. In addition to considering the conditional independence statements we also look at the observed relative risks as these can give us information about the type of interaction we are dealing with. We assume throughout that the interaction is synergistic rather than antagonistic and also that the appropriate monotonicity conditions between risks hold.

First the assumption of no dependence between genotype and exposure is given formally DJ - 1 $\perp\!\!\!\perp$ P.

Relative risks are defined as follows:

$R_{pd}/R_{\overline{pd}}$ denotes the risk of disease of $P = p$ and DJ-1 $= d$, relative to the risk given by $P = \bar{p}$ and $DJ = 1 = \bar{d}$.

7.A4.1 MODEL I

In addition to the above assumption the Model I DAG represents the following conditional independence

■ Y $\perp\!\!\!\perp$ (DJ-1, P)| $= 0$ - this tells us that when either the variant or the exposure are not present, the disease is not associated with the mutation or the exposure.

In terms of relative risks this model implies that

$$\frac{R_{pd}}{R_{\overline{pd}}} > 1 \text{ and } \frac{R_{p\bar{d}}}{R_{\overline{pd}}} = \frac{R_{\bar{p}d}}{R_{\overline{pd}}} = 1$$

7.A4.2 MODEL II

In addition to the above assumptions we have:

• which says that P does not affect Y when $DJ = 1 = \bar{d}$.

$$\frac{R_{pd}}{R_{\bar{p}d}} > \frac{R_{p\bar{d}}}{R_{\bar{p}d}} > 1 \text{ and} \frac{R_{\bar{p}d}}{R_{\bar{p}d}} = 1$$

7.A4.3 MODEL III

The formal assumptions are the complement of those in Model II.

7.A4.4 MODEL IV

$$\frac{R_{pd}}{R_{\bar{p}d}} > 1 \text{ and } \frac{R_{p\bar{d}}}{R_{\bar{p}d}} > 1$$

There are no additional assumptions here. In this case the only way to determine which model holds is to run an experiment or an observational study to estimate the effect of the interaction. In this scenario it is essential to decide on the scale of the interaction, as this will determine whether an effect is found or not. In the case of the fruit fly, there appeared to be an increase of risk of neural damage on the log scale, indicating a multiplicative model.

REFERENCES

1. Lawlor DA, Harbord RM, Sterne JA, Timpson N, Davey SG: Mendelian randomization: using genes as instruments for making causal inferences in epidemiology. Stat Med 2008, 27:1133-1163.

2. Ioannidis JP, Boffetta P, Little J, O'Brien TR, Uitterlinden AG, Vineis P, Balding DJ, Chokkalingam A, Dolan SM, Flanders WD, Higgins JP, McCarthy MI, McDermott DH, Page GP, Rebbeck TR, Seminara D, Khoury MJ: Assessment of cumulative evidence on genetic associations: interim guidelines. Int J Epidemiol 2008, 37:120-132.

3. Porta M, ed: A Dictionary of Epidemiology. 5th edition. New York: Oxford University Press; 2008. p. 34-37, 65-66, 82-84, 100-103, 116, 129-130, 152-154, 237-238

4. Greenland S, ed: Evolution of Epidemiologic Ideas. Annotated Readings on Concepts and Methods. Chestnut Hill, MA: Epidemiology Resources; 1987.

5. Morabia A: A History of Epidemiologic Methods and Concepts. Basel: Birkhäuser / Springer; 2004.

6. Fletcher RH, Fletcher SW: Clinical Epidemiology -the Essentials. 4th edition. Philadelphia: Lippincott Williams & Wilkins; 2005.

7. Haynes RB, Sackett DL, Guyatt GH, Tugwell P: Clinical epidemiology. How to do clinical practice research. 3rd edition. Philadelphia: Lippincott, Williams & Wilkins; 2006.

8. Hill AB: The environment and disease: association or causation? Proc R Soc Med 1965, 58:295-300.

9. Vineis P, Manuguerra M, Kavvoura FK, Guarrera S, Allione A, Rosa F, Di Gregorio A, Polidoro S, Saletta F, Ioannidis JP, Matullo G: A field synopsis on low-penetrance variants in DNA repair genes and cancer susceptibility. J Natl Cancer Inst 2009, 101:24-36.

10. Maraganore DM, de Andrade M, Elbaz A, Farrer MJ, Ioannidis JP, Krüger R, Rocca WA, Schneider NK, Lesnick TG, Lincoln SJ, Hulihan MM, Aasly JO, Ashizawa T, Chartier-Harlin MC, Checkoway H, Ferrarese C, Hadjigeorgiou G, Hattori N, Kawakami H, Lambert JC, Lynch T, Mellick GD, Papapetropoulos S, Parsian A, Quattrone A, Riess O, Tan EK, Van Broeckhoven C: Genetic Epidemiology of Parkinson's Disease (GEO-PD) Consortium. Collaborative analysis of alpha-synuclein gene promoter variability and Parkinson disease. JAMA 2006, 296:661-670.

11. Ioannidis JP, Trikalinos TA, Khoury MJ: Implications of small effect sizes of individual genetic variants on the design and interpretation of genetic association studies of complex diseases. Am J Epidemiol 2006, 164:609-614.

12. Yang Q, Khoury MJ, Friedman J, Little J, Flanders WD: How many genes underlie the occurrence of common complex diseases in the population? Int J Epidemiol 2005, 34:1129-1137.

13. Ioannidis JP, Trikalinos TA: Early extreme contradictory estimates may appear in published research: the Proteus phenomenon in molecular genetics research and randomized trials. J Clin Epidemiol 2005, 58:543-549.

14. Lee DH, Jacobs DR Jr, Porta M: Hypothesis: a unifying mechanism for nutrition and chemicals as lifelong modulators of DNA hypomethylation. Environ Health Perspect 2009, 117:1799-1802.

15. Glazier AM, Nadeau JH, Aitman TJ: Finding genes that underlie complex traits. Science 2002, 298:2345-2349.

16. Jirtle RL, Skinner MK: Environmental epigenomics and disease susceptibility. Nat Rev Genet 2007, 8:253-62.

17. Feinberg AP: Phenotypic plasticity and the epigenetics of human disease. Nature 2007, 447:433-440.

18. Edwards TM, Myers JP: Environmental exposures and gene regulation in disease etiology. Environ Health Perspect 2007, 115:1264-1270.

19. Bellivier F, Henry C, Szöke A, Schürhoff F, Nosten-Bertrand M, Feingold J, Launay JM, Leboyer M, Laplanche JL: Serotonin transporter gene polymorphisms in patients with unipolar or bipolar depression. Neurosci Lett 1998, 255:143-146.

20. Kim YI: 5,10-Methylenetetrahydrofolate reductase polymorphisms and pharmacogenetics: a new role of single nucleotide polymorphisms in the folate metabolic pathway in human health and disease. Nutr Rev 2005, 63:398-407.

21. Neasham D, Gallo V, Guarrera S, Dunning A, Overvad K, Tjonneland A, Clavel-Chapelon F, Linseisen JP, Malaveille C, Ferrari P, Boeing H, Benetou V, Trichopoulou A, Palli D, Crosignani P, Tumino R, Panico S, Bueno de Mesquita HB, Peeters PH, van Gib CH, Lund E, Gonzalez CA, Martinez C, Dorronsoro M, Barricarte A, Navarro C, Quiros JR, Berglund G, Jarvholm B, Khaw KT, et al.: Double-strand break DNA repair genotype predictive of later mortality and cancer incidence in a cohort of non-smokers. DNA Repair 2008.

22. Marcus PM, Vineis P, Rothman N: NAT2 slow acetylation and bladder cancer risk: a meta-analysis of 22 case-control studies conducted in the general population. Pharmacogenetics 2000, 10:115-122.

23. Vineis P, McMichael A: Interplay between heterocyclic amines in cooked meat and metabolic phenotype in the etiology of colon cancer. Cancer Causes Control 1996, 7:479-486.

24. Vineis P, Pirastu R: Aromatic amines and cancer. Cancer Causes Control 1997, 8:346-355.

25. Ochs-Balcom HM, Wiesner G, Elston RC: A meta-analysis of the association of N-acetyltransferase 2 gene (NAT2) variants with breast cancer. Am J Epidemiol 2007, 166:246-254.

26. Borlak J, Reamon-Buettner SM: N-acetyltransferase 2 (NAT2) gene polymorphisms in colon and lung cancer patients. BMC Med Genet 2006, 7:58.

27. Postmenopausal estrogen use and heart disease N Engl J Med 1986, 315:131-136.

28. Vineis P, Anttila S, Benhamou S, Spinola M, Hirvonen A, Kiyohara C, Garte SJ, Puntoni R, Rannug A, Strange RC, Taioli E: Evidence of gene gene interactions in lung carcinogenesis in a large pooled analysis. Carcinogenesis 2007, 28:1902-1905.

29. Nicholson SJ, Witherden AS, Hafezparast M, Martin JE, Fisher EM: Mice, the motor system, and human motor neuron pathology. Mamm Genome 2000, 11:1041-1052.

30. Porta M, Álvarez-Dardet C: How is causal inference practised in the biological sciences? J Epidemiol Community Healt 2000, 54:559-560.

31. Greenland S, Pearl J, Robins JM: Causal diagrams for epidemiologic research. Epidemiology 1999, 10:37-48.

32. Hernán MA, Robins JM: Instruments for causal inference: an epidemiologist's dream? Epidemiolog 2006, 17:360-372.

33. Hernán MA, Robins JM: Causal Inference. New York: Chapman & Hall/CRC; 2010.

34. Pearl J: Causality: Models, Reasoning, and Inference. Cambridge, U.K.: Cambridge University Press; 2009.

35. Dawid AP: Conditional independence in statistical theory. With discussion. J Roy Statist Soc B 1979, 41:1-31.

36. Cartwright N: Nature's capacities and their measurement. 1989.

37. Davey SG, Ebrahim S: 'Mendelian randomization': can genetic epidemiology contribute to understanding environmental determinants of disease? Int J Epidemiol 2003, 32:1-22.

38. Dawid AP: Influence diagrams for causal modelling and inference. Intern Statist Rev 2002, 70:161-189.

39. Didelez V, Sheehan N: Mendelian randomization as an instrumental variable approach to causal inference. Stat Methods Med Res 2007, 16:309-330.

40. Chen L, Davey SG, Harbord RM, Lewis SJ: Alcohol intake and blood pressure: a systematic review implementing a Mendelian randomization approach. PLoS Med 2008, 5:e52.

41. Dawid AP: Causal inference without counterfactuals. J Am Statist Ass 2000, 95:407-448.

42. Didelez V, Sheenan N: Mendelian randomisation: why epidemiology needs a formal language for causality. In Causality and probability in the sciences. College Publications London, London; 2007. ed ?

43. Geneletti S: Identifying direct and indirect effects in a non-counterfactual framework. J Roy Stat Soc B 2007, 69:199-215.

44. Lauritzen S: Graphical models. Oxford 1996.

45. Nelson LM, Tanner CM, Van Den Eeden SK, McGuire V: Neuroepidemiology. In Oxford. Oxford University Press; 2004.

46. Kuehn BM: Scientists probe role of genes, environment in Parkinson disease. JAMA 2006, 295:1883-1885.

47. Farrer MJ: Genetics of Parkinson disease: paradigm shifts and future prospects. Nat Rev Genet 2006, 7:306-318.

48. Clements CM, McNally RS, Conti BJ, Mak TW, Ting JP: DJ-1, a cancer- and Parkinson's disease-associated protein, stabilizes the antioxidant transcriptional master regulator Nrf2. Proc Natl Acad Sci USA 2006, 103:15091-15096.

49. Meulener M, Whitworth AJ, Armstrong-Gold CE, Rizzu P, Heutink P, Wes PD, Pallanck LJ, Bonini NM: Drosophila DJ-1 mutants are selectively sensitive to environmental toxins associated with Parkinson's disease. Curr Biol 2005, 15:1572-1577.

50. van Duijn CM, Dekker MC, Bonifati V, Galjaard RJ, Houwing-Duistermaat JJ, Snijders PJ, Testers L, Breedveld GJ, Horstink M, Sandkuijl LA, van Swieten JC, Oostra BA, Heutink P: Park7, a novel locus for autosomal recessive early-onset parkinsonism, on chromosome 1p36. Am J Hum Genet 2001, 69:629-634.

51. Bonifati V, Rizzu P, van Baren MJ, Schaap O, Breedveld GJ, Krieger E, Dekker MC, Squitieri F, Ibanez P, Joosse M, van Dongen JW, Vanacore N, van Swieten JC, Brice A, Meco G, van Duijn CM, Oostra BA, Heutink P: Mutations in the DJ-1 gene associated with autosomal recessive early-onset parkinsonism. Science 2003, 299:256-259.

52. Bossy-Wetzel E, Schwarzenbacher R, Lipton SA: Molecular pathways to neurodegeneration. Nat Med 2004, 10(Suppl):S2-S9.

53. Brown TP, Rumsby PC, Capleton AC, Rushton L, Levy LS: Pesticides and Parkinson's disease-is there a link? Environ Health Perspect 2006, 114:156-164.

54. Betarbet R, Sherer TB, MacKenzie G, Garcia-Osuna M, Panov AV, Greenamyre JT: Chronic systemic pesticide exposure reproduces features of Parkinson's disease. Nat Neurosci 2000, 3:1301-1306.

55. Khoury MJ, Adams MJ Jr, Flanders WD: An epidemiologic approach to ecogenetics. Am J Hum Genet 1988, 42:89-95.
56. Ottman R: An epidemiologic approach to gene-environment interaction. Genet Epidemiol 1990, 7:177-185.
57. Davey Smith G, Lawlor DA, Harbord R, Timpson N, Day I, Ebrahim S: Clustered environments and randomized genes: a fundamental distinction between conventional and genetic epidemiology. PLoS Med 2007, 4:e352.
58. Alcaro A, Huber R, Panksepp J: Behavioral functions of the mesolimbic dopaminergic system: an affective neuroethological perspective. Brain Res Rev 2007, 56:283-321.
59. VanderWeele TJ, Robins JM: Directed acyclic graphs, sufficient causes, and the properties of conditioning on a common effect. Am J Epidemiol 2007, 166:1096-1104.
60. Quik M: Smoking, nicotine and Parkinson's disease. Trends Neurosci 2004, 27:561-568.
61. VanderWeele TJ, Robins JM: The identification of synergism in the sufficient-component-cause framework. Epidemiology 2007, 18:329-339.
62. Bonifati V, Rizzu P, Squitieri F, Krieger E, Vanacore N, van Swieten JC, Brice A, van Duijn CM, Oostra B, Meco G, Heutink P: DJ-1 (PARK7), a novel gene for autosomal recessive, early onset parkinsonism. Neurol Sci 2003, 24:159-160.
63. Hague S, Rogaeva E, Hernandez D, Gulick C, Singleton A, Hanson M, Johnson J, Weiser R, Gallardo M, Ravina B, Gwinn-Hardy K, Crawley A, St George-Hyslop PH, Lang AE, Heutink P, Bonifati V, Hardy J, Singleton A: Early-onset Parkinson's disease caused by a compound heterozygous DJ-1 mutation. Ann Neurol 2003, 54:271-274.
64. Liou HH, Tsai MC, Chen CJ, Jeng JS, Chang YC, Chen SY, Chen RC: Environmental risk factors and Parkinson's disease: a case-control study in Taiwan. Neurology 1997, 48:1583-1588.
65. Petrovitch H, Ross GW, Abbott RD, Sanderson WT, Sharp DS, Tanner CM, Masaki KH, Blanchette PL, Popper JS, Foley D, Launer L, White LR: Plantation work and risk of Parkinson disease in a population-based longitudinal study. Arch Neurol 2002, 59:1787-1792.
66. Hertzman C, Wiens M, Bowering D, Snow B, Calne D: Parkinson's disease: a case-control study of occupational and environmental risk factors. Am J Ind Med 1990, 17:349-355.
67. Semchuk KM, Love EJ, Lee RG: Parkinson's disease and exposure to agricultural work and pesticide chemicals. Neurology 1992, 42:1328-1335.
68. Firestone JA, Smith-Weller T, Franklin G, Swanson P, Longstreth WT Jr, Checkoway H: Pesticides and risk of Parkinson disease: a population-based case-control study. Arch Neurol 2005, 62:91-95.
69. Corasaniti MT, Bagetta G, Rodino P, Gratteri S, Nistico G: Neurotoxic effects induced by intracerebral and systemic injection of paraquat in rats. Hum Exp Toxicol 1992, 11:535-539.
70. Bertrand KA, Spiegelman D, Aster JC, Altshul LM, Korrick SA, Rodig SJ, Zhang SM, Kurth T, Laden F: Plasma organochlorine levels and risk of non-Hodgkin lymphoma in a cohort of men. Epidemiology 2010, 21:172-180.

71. Porta M, Pumarega J, López T, Jariod M, Marco E, Grimalt JO: Influence of tumor stage, symptoms and time of blood draw on serum concentrations of organochlorine compounds in exocrine pancreatic cancer. Cancer Causes Contro 2009, 20:1893-1906.

72. McCormack AL, Thiruchelvam M, Manning-Bog AB, Thiffault C, Langston JW, Cory-Slechta DA, Di Monte DA: Environmental risk factors and Parkinson's disease: selective degeneration of nigral dopaminergic neurons caused by the herbicide paraquat. Neurobiol Dis 2002, 10:119-127.

73. Wacholder S, Chatterjee N, Caporaso N: Intermediacy and gene-environment interaction: the example of CHRNA5-A3 region, smoking, nicotine dependence, and lung cancer. J Natl Cancer Inst 2008, 100:1488-1491.

74. Weinberg CR: Can DAGs clarify effect modification? Epidemiology 2007, 18:569-572.

75. Susser M: Causal thinking in the health sciences. New York: Oxford University Press; 1973.

76. VanderWeele TJ, Robins JM: Four types of effect modification: a classification based on directed acyclic graphs. Epidemiology 2007, 18:561-568.

GENOME WIDE ASSOCIATION STUDY TO PREDICT SEVERE ASTHMA EXACERBATIONS IN CHILDREN USING RANDOM FORESTS CLASSIFIERS

MOUSHENG XU, KELAN G. TANTISIRA, ANN WU, AUGUSTO A. LITONJUA, JEN-HWA CHU, BLANCA E. HIMES, AMY DAMASK, AND SCOTT T. WEISS

8.1 BACKGROUND

Personalized medicine, the ability to predict an individual's predisposition to disease and response to therapy with genetic and phenotypic characteristics, promises to deliver more efficient health outcomes [1-4]. As a field, personalized medicine faces multiple issues when trying to predict complex diseases such as cardiovascular diseases, cancer, and asthma. This is largely due to the fact that no single genotypic or phenotypic characteristic can explain more than a small portion of any complex disease. Instead, complex diseases are influenced by multiple genetic factors and environmental exposures. For instance, the height of a person is considered to be strongly heritable, but the top 20 single nucleotide polymorphisms (SNPs)

This chapter was originally published under the Creative Commons Attribution License. Xu M, Tantisira KG, Wu A, Litonjua AA, Chu J-H, Himes BE, Damask A and Weiss ST. Genome Wide Association Study to Predict Severe Asthma Exacerbations in Children Using Random Forests Classifiers. BMC Medical Genomics 12,90 (2011). doi:10.1186/1471-2350-12-90.

chosen by p value, explain only ~2-3% of the variability in adult height [5]. In addition to the multitude of factors influencing complex traits, the genetic and environmental factors interact with each other adding to the complexity.

To integrate multiple genetic and environmental predictors into modeling, conventional statistical methods and some data mining algorithms such as an artificial neural network (ANN) can be easily over-fit typically due to a small sample size in relation to the number of potential SNPs or predictors. Nevertheless, data mining methods are available to handle this type of data that are more resistant to over-fitting. Random Forests (RF) [6,7] are a classification algorithm that is composed of a set of random decision trees, with each tree making a decision and voting for the final prediction outcome. Being able to generate a highly accurate classifier with many (even relatively weak) predictors without over-fitting [6,7], Random Forests would appear to be an ideal approach to the integration of hundreds of SNPs plus clinical traits needed to predict complex clinical phenotypes. An added benefit of Random Forests is that the decision trees naturally handle interactions among input variables.

Asthma is a complex disease known to be influenced by both genetic and environmental factors [8-16]. 26.7 million or about 9.7% of the population in the United States have had asthma during their lifetime [17]. In the year 2000, asthma exacerbations resulted in 1,499 deaths, 1.1 million hospital days, and $2.9 billion in direct expenditures in the United States [18]. The ability to predict severe asthma exacerbations would therefore have direct prognostic significance and might form the basis for the development of novel therapeutic interventions. Severe asthma exacerbations have been associated with several clinical factors including the forced expiratory volume in one second as a percent of predicted ($FEV_1\%$), oral corticosteroid usage [9,19], age [20], and sex [21]. However, these factors by themselves are limited in their ability to successfully predict severe asthma exacerbations [21,22]. To explore the potential power of a multi-SNP model as incorporated into RF together with clinical relevant risk factors to effectively predict complex diseases, we applied this algorithm to the prediction of exacerbations in a population of childhood asthmatics participating in the Childhood Asthma Management Program (CAMP).

8.2 METHODS

8.2.1 STUDY POPULATION

CAMP was a multicenter, randomized, double-blinded clinical trial testing the safety and efficacy of inhaled budesonide vs. nedocromil vs. placebo over a mean of 4.3 years. Trial design, methodology, and primary clinical outcome have been previously published (The Childhood Asthma Management Program Research Group 1999; The > Childhood Asthma Management Program Research Group 2000). Entry criteria included asthma symptoms and/or medication use for ≥ 6 months in the previous year and airway responsiveness with a provocative concentration dose (PC_{20}) of methacholine ≤ 12.5 mg/ml. 1,041 children with mild-moderate asthma were enrolled.

At baseline, data regarding demographics; home environment characteristics; asthma symptoms, severity, and treatment; allergy history; and relevant family history were collected. Each patient's parent or guardian signed a consent statement, with each child providing assent. IRB approval was obtained for all participating CAMP centers and the data coordinating center. A 6 week run-in period which included therapy limited to as needed albuterol preceded randomization. Visits occurred at randomization, at two and four months after randomization, and every four months thereafter. During these visits, an interval asthma history was obtained, including specific questions related to health care utilization related to asthma.

The CAMP Genetics Ancillary Study was approved by each individual study center's Internal Review Board, and informed consent/assent was obtained from all participants and their parents.

8.2.2 PRIMARY OUTCOME

The occurrence of either an emergency room visit or a hospitalization for asthma symptoms at any time during the clinical trial period was used to define a severe asthma exacerbation.

8.2.3 CLINICAL COVARIATES

Age, sex, pre-bronchodilator $FEV_1\%$, and treatment group are known to be associated with asthma exacerbations and were included as clinical traits in our models. Values for each predictor were those obtained at the CAMP randomization visit. Age and pre-bronchodilator $FEV_1\%$, are coded as numeric variables; sex is coded as 1 for male, 2 for female; treatment group is coded as 1, 2, 3 for three different treatments.

8.2.4 GWAS DATA

Of the CAMP participants, 422 Caucasian parent-child trios were genotyped using the Infinium II HumanHap550v3 Genotyping BeadChip (Illumina, San Diego, CA), 164 Caucasian non-trio cohort children were subsequently genotyped using the Human660W-Quad BeadChip. 5 of the 422 trios had an excess of missing genotypes and were removed from this study, and thus 417 trio children were actually used in this study. Over 500,000 SNPs were successfully genotyped in the CAMP trios, with a reproducibility of > 99.99%. Reproducibility is based on 4 samples that were each genotyped 15 times in the experiment. Genotype quality has been validated using the Mendel option of PLINK v0.99r http://pngu.mgh. harvard.edu/purcell/plink/ [23], verifying allele calls against RefSeq to ensure correct orientation, and testing for extreme departures from Hardy Weinburg equilbrium in the parents.

8.2.5 SELECTION OF SNPS

Focusing on the trio probands as our initial test population, we used RF importance scores to rank and select SNPs in two steps. At each step, we used SNPs as predictors to predict asthma exacerbations with RF, and obtained the RF importance score of each of the SNPs. At the first step, we computed RF importance scores for all SNPs genome-wide, 4,000 at a time, in chromosomal order. At the second step, we ranked all SNPs based on their RF importance scores, selected the top 4,000 SNPs, and re-ran RF with these selected SNPs to re-rank them.

8.2.6 PREDICTION MODEL BUILDING WITH RF

The 417 Caucasian trio samples (Stage 1 samples) were genotyped before the 164 cohort samples (Stage 2 samples), and were used to build and train the RF models to predict asthma exacerbations. The R package randomForest version 4.5-25 originally written in Fortran by Leo Breiman and Adele Cutler and ported to R by Andy Liaw and Matthew Wiener http://cran.r-project.org/web/packages/randomForest/index.html was used to build RF models in this study. The RF predicted score is the percentage of trees voting for "yes." During this step and the steps described in "Selection of SNPs" above, RF parameter "ntree" (number of trees to grow) were set to be 1,500—a relatively large number to ensure stable prediction results, and all other parameters, including mtry, were set to use the default values.

8.2.7 PREDICTION PERFORMANCE CONTROLS

In order to assess the performance of the RF classifier built with the selected clinical traits and SNPs as predictors, two types of controls were used in this study. One type of control is called a permutation control, the other a random SNP control. The permutation control permuted the response variable (any severe exacerbation) among samples while retaining the association of the predictors with the samples; the random SNP control randomly selected SNPs used in the Genome-Wide Association Study (GWAS) regardless of whether they are associated with the phenotype or not, and used the equivalent number of random SNPs to build predictive models. Both controls were iterated 10 times.

8.2.8 TESTING IN AN INDEPENDENT POPULATION

After the RF models were built with the Stage 1 samples, additional samples were genotyped and used as the Stage 2 population for testing. The clinical traits and SNPs of the Stage 2 samples were used to predict the asthma exacerbations with these RF models. Because RF does not allow missing values for prediction, missing alleles were imputed by randomly selecting a genotype based on the observed genotype frequency distribution among controls.

8.2.9 ROC CURVE AND AUC COMPUTATION

Receiver Operating Characteristic curve (ROC curve) and the Area Under the ROC Curve (AUC) were computed using the R package ROCR developed by Sing et al (Sing 2005), which is downloadable from http://rocr.bioinf.mpi-sb.mpg.de/. We used the AUC as our primary indicator of predictive success [24,25]. The computation of the p-value for an AUC to be different from that would be obtained by chance is described in [24,26].

8.3 RESULTS

8.3.1 SAMPLE CHARACTERISTICS

The clinical characteristics of both our training (trios) and test (probands) are shown in Table 1. The Stage 1 samples are 417 CAMP asthmatic family-trio children genotyped and used in this study. 127 (30%) of them experienced at least one severe asthma exacerbations during the four year follow-up period as indicated by an emergency room visit or hospitalization (Table 1). Children with severe exacerbations were more likely to be male, have lower pre-bronchodilator FEV_1%, and be untreated with drugs. The Stage 2 samples are 164 cohort children, who are independent of the Stage 1 samples. A similar percentage of the Stage 2 children experienced exacerbations in the follow-up period when compared with Stage 1 samples. Two of the four clinical traits (gender and treatment group) in the study are different in the Stage 2 samples from the Stage 1 samples. The clinical traits are used as covariates for the outcome prediction.

TABLE 1: Sample Characteristics (All Subjects Are Caucasian)

	Training Population N = 417		Testing Population N = 164	
	Exac.	Non-exac.	Exac.	Non-exac.
Subjects	127 (30%)	290 (70%)	50 (30%)	114 (70%)
Age (mean ± s.d.)	8.41 ± 2.07	8.89 ± 2.07	8.54 ± 2.28	9.45 ± 2.19
Male	69%	61%	46%	53%
$FEV_1\%$ (mean ± s.d.)	92.9 ± 15.7	93.5 ± 13.2	95.4 ± 17.1	95.4 ± 13.5
Treatment				
Budesonide	20%	31%	36%	32%
Nedocromil	28%	29%	30%	32%
Placebo	52%	39%	34%	36%

8.3.2 THE IMPORTANCE SCORE LANDSCAPE OF SNPS GENOME-WIDE

RF importance score measures the relative contribution of a predictor to the prediction. The importance score of each of the SNPs is plotted in Figure 1 in chromosomal order. The demarcation separates the top 4k SNPs with the highest importance scores from the rest. This plot is similar to the "Manhattan plot" seen in GWAS analysis except the y-axis is the RF importance score instead of the -log(p).

8.3.3 PREDICTION OF SEVERE ASTHMA EXACERBATIONS

Using clinical traits age, sex, pre-bronchodilator FEV1%, and treatment group, plus different numbers of SNPs selected based on RF importance score (see Methods) as predictors, RF predicted severe asthma exacerbations with varying degrees of success. With just the 4 clinical attributes as predictors, the predictive model had an externally replicated AUC of about

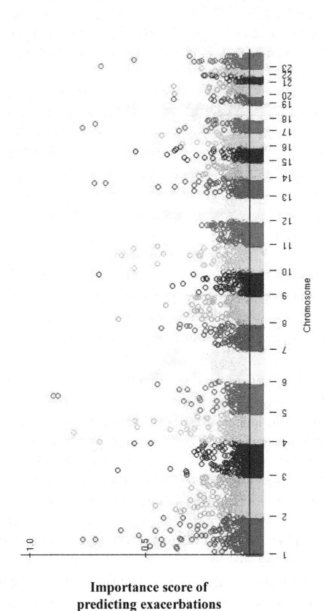

FIGURE 1: The "manhattan plot" of RF importance scores of all the 550k SNPs. X-axis: the SNPs in chromosomal order; Y-axis: the RF importance scores. The black demarcation separates the top 4k SNPs from the rest.

0.56 (Figure 2). Since, an AUC of 0.5 indicates prediction equivalent to chance, clinical predictors alone had weak predictability. The addition of the 10 SNPs with the highest RF importance score for exacerbations increased the AUC to 0.57. The addition of SNPs continued to increase the predictability of asthma exacerbations, with an independently replicated AUC of 0.62, 0.66, and 0.66 for 40, 160 and 320 SNPs, respectively. The ROC curves for prediction using 160 SNPs in the training and independent populations are shown in Figure 3. The p-value for the independent replication AUC 0.66 to be different from 0.5 by random guess is 0.000266. Starting at 160 SNPs the AUC reached 0.66 and began to plateau with additional SNPs. The top 160 SNPs together with the closest genes are listed in Additional File 1, Table S1.

8.3.4 MODEL VALIDATION

To evaluate the RF models, we performed permutation and random SNP controls and used an independent replication population (Figure 2). Permutation control: after permuting exacerbations labels among samples, RF models were built and tested for predictability in terms of AUC. For all RF models built with permuted data, the AUC scores were about 0.5, suggesting the true predictability of RF models built with original data. Random SNP control: random SNPs showed AUC scores slightly higher than 0.5 (data not shown). The evidence for weak predictability in the Random SNP control models likely comes from the clinical traits used in the models rather than the random SNPs. These results indicate that the RF selected SNPs contain information about exacerbation, while the random SNPs do not.

8.4 DISCUSSION

One of the biggest challenges of complex trait prediction is the lack of statistical power that is the direct result of small effects of many causal factors and relatively small sample sizes. These problems are exacerbated when consideration is given to the potential for interaction among the

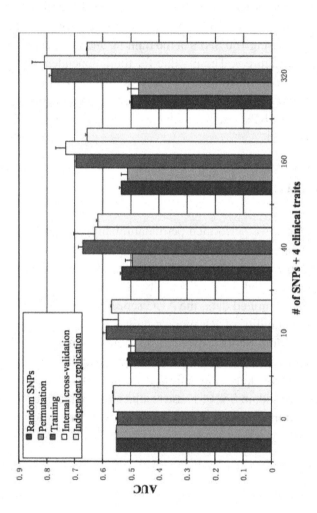

FIGURE 2: Comparison of performance of predicting severe asthma exacerbation with different methods. Y-axis: AUC; X-axis: the number of SNPs used in a model. "Random SNPs": SNPs are chosen randomly from all SNPs and used as input variables to predict asthma exacerbations, and this process has been iterated 10 times [see Methods for details]; "Permuted": asthma exacerbation is permuted across samples while clinical traits and SNPs are kept with the samples, and this process has been iterated 10 times [see Methods for details]; "Training": the AUC of the model trained and built with all the Stage 1 samples predicting on the same samples; "Internal cross-validation": the AUC of the model built with 90% of the randomly selected Stage 1 samples predicting on the rest (10%) of the Stage 1 samples; "Independent replication": the AUC of the model built with all the Stage 1 samples predicting on all the Stage 2 samples.

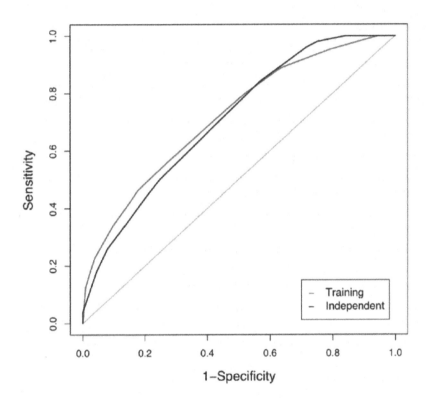

FIGURE 3: ROC curves using clinical attributes plus 160 SNPs as predictors. The red curve is obtained for the training of the Stage 1 samples, the blue curve is for the testing of the Stage 2 samples, the grey diagonal line is a theoretical curve representing random guess. Both the red and the blue curves are higher than the grey line, indicating better than random prediction; and they are similar to each other, suggesting the true predictability of the RF model. The p-value for the independent testing AUC to be different from 0.5 is 0.000266.

causal factors to interact with one another. We have shown that RF modeling can produce accurate results using hundreds of SNPs obtained from a relatively small study (131 cases, 291 controls). With only 417 subjects, using 160 SNPs, we are able to generate a good predictive model for childhood asthma exacerbations, with a > 0.66 AUC and about 0.66 sensitivity and 0.6 specificity (Figures 2, 3). Depending on the portion of the ROC curve that is used, this can equate to a positive predictive value (PPV) of 0.81 and a negative predictive value (NPV) of 0.74 with proportion of exacerbators = 0.3 as shown in Table 1 and choosing a scoring threshold corresponding to sensitivity = 0.2 and specificity = 0.95, allowing for reasonable prediction of asthma exacerbations. The permutation control, random SNP control, and independent replication results all support the validity and robustness of the random forest predictive model. The ROC curve obtained for the model training using the Stage 2 (independent replication) samples is very similar to that obtained for the Stage 1 (training) samples (Figure 3), and the p-value for the independent replication AUC is < 0.05, indicating reproducibility of the predictive accuracy in the model using 160 SNPs.

The 160 SNPs are in or near to 140 genes (Additional File 1, Table S1). Among the top 160 SNPs, one SNP (rs10496476) is located within the intron of gene DPP10, which has been shown to be associated with asthma in multiple populations, based on a recent review [27]. All other genes are not on the list of replicated asthma genes reported by [27], suggesting most SNPs and genes identified by our RF method are novel. A couple of factors may contribute to the discovery of new SNPs and genes: 1) RF evaluates individual SNPs in the context of interactions. This is different from conventional statistical methods such as logistic regression, applied in GWAS which searches SNPs one by one without consideration of SNP-SNP interactions; 2) asthma exacerbations are related to but different phenotypes from asthma diagnosis.

Our study highlights an innovative way of integrating a large number of individually weak predictors to effectively build a reasonable predictive model for asthma exacerbations. Given that complex trait studies so far have used only up to a dozen predictors (i.e. an order of magnitude fewer than what we use here) with limited consideration of interaction and have generated relatively poor predictability, our approach of employing RF with hundreds of predictors with a relatively small sample size gives hope for additional improvement in complex trait prediction using a variety of machine learning approaches. Talmud, et al, studied 20 SNPs derived from genome-wide association studies of type 2 diabetes susceptibility in a population of 5,535 subjects followed for 10 years [28]. They noted that clinical factors outperformed genetic markers in the prediction of incident diabetes and that the addition of the SNPs produced minimal improvement in risk estimation based only on clinical variables. In contrast to this study, which focused on the additive effects of 20 SNPs, our RF model simultaneously accounts for both additive and interactive effects using 160 SNPs to more effectively predict asthma exacerbations compared with clinical factors alone.

Most complex traits such as adult height, cardiovascular diseases, cancer, diabetes, autism, and asthma etc. are likely to be encoded by a large number of both genetic and environmental factors [5,29-32]. Asthma exacerbations, as shown in this study, is associated with at least several hundred genetic markers and environmental factors. The top 10 SNPs has AUC score 0.57, showing marginal predictability. But with 160 SNPs, the AUC of the RF model approached 0.66. Our study suggests that in order to get good prediction of a complex trait, methods capable of integrating hundreds of predictors, such as machine learning approaches, like random forests, will be valuable.

Asthma exacerbations have historically been difficult to predict. Several clinical models have been designed to try to enhance the ability to predict exacerbations [21,33-36]. Most studies [21,33,36] attempted to isolate predictive clinical variables individually without accounting for interaction using odds ratio or regression analysis. The results of these studies are reported as odds ratios or as p-values for individual factors, and cannot be directly compared with ours using AUC.

There have been several publications that have evaluated the use of a clinical classification tree in the development of a prognostic model for asthma exacerbations [34]. One study evaluated six clinical variables including prior year hospitalization, the classification tree method was able to achieve—without independent replication—94% sensitivity and 68% specificity, better than logistic regression (87% sensitivity and 48% specificity) or an additive risk model (46% sensitivity and 93% specificity), suggesting the value of accounting for interactions among predictive variables. A recent study [35] reported 66.8% sensitivity and 85.8% specificity (with no independent validation testing) on childhood asthma exacerbations (defined as rescue oral corticosteroid use, an unscheduled visit to a physician or emergency room, or hospitalization) prediction with daytime cough, daytime wheeze, and β2-agonist use at night 1 day before the exacerbations as predictors. However, none of the clinical models developed to date have been independently validated. In our model, we successfully used both internal (e.g. permutation) controls as well as external replication in an independent subset of subjects to demonstrate predictive power of our model. While the independent subset of subjects were derived from the same source population, there were some differences in baseline characteristics between the two samples (Table 1), further supporting the generalizability of our model. RF also uses a classification tree, but with a difference—it uses many classification trees (1500 trees in our models), not just one, and it can handle a greater number of input variables without over-fitting.

A critical issue for complex disease prediction is the difficulty of extending the predictive power of a model obtained from one population to an independent population. None of the studies mentioned in the proceeding paragraph has tested their models in independent populations. One important factor that makes researchers hesitate to do so is the concerns of small sample sizes and the heterogeneity of asthma exacerbations. We applied the RF models built with the Stage 1 samples to predict the independent Stage 2 samples (Figure 2). Overall, the independent test samples paralleled the predictive accuracy of the Stage 1 (training) samples with increasing numbers of SNPs until 160 SNPs. At 160, the replicating AUC reached its maximum and flattens out thereafter. As such, we cite the 160 SNP model as our best performing model. The independent replication AUCs are obviously higher than 0.5, indicating true predictability of the RF models. However, they are lower than the training and internal cross-validation AUCs for 160 and 320 SNPs, suggesting certain degree of over-fitting may still exist.

As discussed above, clinical traits alone did not produce desirable predictability for asthma exacerbation. We did, however, exclude one predictor that is a strong predictor of severe exacerbations—prior exacerbations

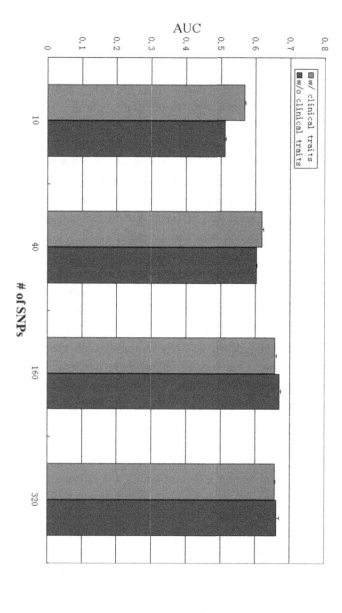

FIGURE 4: Performance comparison of predicting severe asthma exacerbation with or without clinical traits. Y-axis: AUC; X-axis: the number of SNPs used for prediction. Blue: SNPs plus clinical traits; Red: SNPs alone.

[37]. The rationale for excluding this predictor was that we were interested in developing a predictive model based upon determinants of exacerbations; these determinants would by their nature include both prior and current exacerbations. Moreover, since we sought to determine genetic predictors of exacerbations, the inclusion of prior exacerbations would mitigate the strength of the genetic association in our analyses.

One of the reasons that clinical predictors may not have provided the same strength of prediction as our genetic models is that many of the clinical traits themselves are genetically determined. Indeed, our results (Figure 4) have shown that without clinical traits, SNPs alone can predict as well as with the clinical traits, suggesting asthma exacerbations are at least partly caused by genetic factors. For instance, among our clinical predictors, sex is genetically determined; age itself is not genetic, but it may be associated with age of onset due to the patient recruitment process, and age of onset in turn can be genetic [38,39]; and pre-bronchodilator FEV1% is influenced by genetics, especially in children.

There were several potential limitations to our study. We have already discussed the limitation due to a limited sample size. One potential problem is that with more than 160 SNPs, the training AUC keeps increasing (Figure 2), but the replicating AUC does not. This suggests that the chance of getting false positive SNPs increases with the number of SNPs used for prediction. One way to reduce false positive SNPs is to increase the sample size, which is costly.

8.5 CONCLUSIONS

In conclusion, we have demonstrated that reasonable prediction of asthma exacerbations can be achieved through the use of hundreds of SNPs in a random forests model. This model can increase our understanding of the biologic mechanisms behind why only certain individuals with asthma are at risk for exacerbations, as well as the basis for the epistatic (gene-gene) interactions underlying asthma severity, providing insight into novel preventative and therapeutic strategies.

REFERENCES

1. Bodmer W, Bonilla C: Common and rare variants in multifactorial susceptibility to common diseases. Nat Genet 2008, 40(6):695-701.
2. Haga SB, Khoury MJ, Burke W: Genomic profiling to promote a healthy lifestyle: not ready for prime time. Nat Genet 2003, 34(4):347-350.
3. Katsanis SH, Javitt G, Hudson K: Public health. A case study of personalized medicine. Science 2008, 320(5872):53-54.
4. Tate SK, Goldstein DB: Will tomorrow's medicines work for everyone? Nat Genet 2004, 36(11 Suppl):S34-42.
5. Weedon MN, Lango H, Lindgren CM, Wallace C, Evans DM, Mangino M, Freathy RM, Perry JR, Stevens S, Hall AS, Samani NJ, Shields B, Prokopenko I, Farrall M, Dominiczak A, Diabetes Genetics Initiative, Wellcome Trust Case Control Consortium, Johnson T, Bergmann S, Beckmann JS, Vollenweider P, Waterworth DM, Mooser V, Palmer CN, Morris AD, Ouwehand WH, Cambridge GEM Consortium, Zhao JH, Li S, Loos RJ, et al.: Genome-wide association analysis identifies 20 loci that influence adult height. Nat Genet 2008, 40(5):575-583.
6. Breiman L: Random Forests. Machine Learning 2001, 45:5-32.
7. Banfield RE, Hall LO, Bowyer KW, Kegelmeyer WP: A comparison of decision tree ensemble creation techniques.
8. IEEE Trans Pattern Anal Mach Intell 2007, 29(1):173-180.
9. Berce V, Repnik K, Potocnik U: Association of CCR5-delta32 mutation with reduced risk of nonatopic asthma in Slovenian children. J Asthma 2008, 45(9):780-784.
10. Fuhlbrigge AL, Weiss ST, Kuntz KM, Paltiel AD: Forced expiratory volume in 1 second percentage improves the classification of severity among children with asthma. Pediatrics 2006, 118(2):e347-355.
11. Hersh CP, Raby BA, Soto-Quiros ME, Murphy AJ, Avila L, Lasky-Su J, Sylvia JS, Klanderman BJ, Lange C, Weiss ST, Celedón JC: Comprehensive testing of positionally cloned asthma genes in two populations. Am J Respir Crit Care Med 2007, 176(9):849-857.
12. Moffatt MF: Genes in asthma: new genes and new ways. Curr Opin Allergy Clin Immunol 2008, 8(5):411-417.
13. Movahedi M, Mahdaviani SA, Rezaei N, Moradi B, Dorkhosh S, Amirzargar AA: IL-10, TGF-beta, IL-2, IL-12, and IFN-gamma cytokine gene polymorphisms in asthma. J Asthma 2008, 45(9):790-794.
14. Ho SM: Environmental epigenetics of asthma: an update. J Allergy Clin Immunol 2010, 126(3):453-465.
15. Gelfand EW: Pediatric asthma: a different disease. Proc Am Thorac Soc 2009, 6(3):278-282.
16. Eder W, Ege MJ, von Mutius E: The asthma epidemic. N Engl J Med 2006, 355(21):2226-2235.
17. Cookson W: The alliance of genes and environment in asthma and allergy. Nature 1999, 402(6760 Suppl):B5-11.

18. Mannino DM, Homa DM, Akinbami LJ, Moorman JE, Gwynn C, Redd SC: Surveillance for asthma-United States, 1980-1999. MMWR Surveill Summ 2002, 51(1):1-13.

19. Krishnan V, Diette GB, Rand CS, Bilderback AL, Merriman B, Hansel NN, Krishnan JA: Mortality in patients hospitalized for asthma exacerbations in the United States. Am J Respir Crit Care Med 2006, 174(6):633-638.

20. Razi CH, Turktas I, Bakirtas A: Comparison of single 2000-microg dose treatment vs. sequential repeated-dose 500-microg treatments with nebulized budesonide in acute asthma exacerbations. Ann Allergy Asthma Immunol 2008, 100(4):370-376.

21. Walsh-Kelly CM, Kelly KJ, Drendel AL, Grabowski L, Kuhn EM: Emergency department revisits for pediatric acute asthma exacerbations: association of factors identified in an emergency department asthma tracking system. Pediatr Emerg Care 2008, 24(8):505-510.

22. Arnold DH, Gebretsadik T, Minton PA, Higgins S, Hartert TV: Assessment of severity measures for acute asthma outcomes: a first step in developing an asthma clinical prediction rule. Am J Emerg Med 2008, 26(4):473-479.

23. Kunkov S, Pinedo V, Silver EJ, Crain EF: Predicting the need for hospitalization in acute childhood asthma using end-tidal capnography. Pediatr Emerg Care 2005, 21(9):574-577.

24. Purcell S, Neale B, Todd-Brown K, Thomas L, Ferreira MA, Bender D, Maller J, Sklar P, de Bakker PI, Daly MJ, Sham PC: PLINK: a tool set for whole-genome association and population-based linkage analyses. Am J Hum Genet 2007, 81(3):559-575.

25. Lasko TA, Bhagwat JG, Zou KH, Ohno-Machado L: The use of receiver operating characteristic curves in biomedical informatics. J Biomed Inform 2005, 38(5):404-415.

26. Swets JA: Signal detection theory and ROC analysis in psychology and diagnostics: Collected papers. 1995.

27. DeLong ER, DeLong DM, Clarke-Pearson DL: Comparing the areas under two or more correlated receiver operating characteristic curves: a nonparametric approach. Biometrics 1988, 44(3):837-845.

28. Weiss ST, Raby BA, Rogers A: Asthma genetics and genomics 2009. Curr Opin Genet Dev 2009, 19(3):279-282.

29. Talmud PJ, Hingorani AD, Cooper JA, Marmot MG, Brunner EJ, Kumari M, Kivimaki M, Humphries SE: Utility of genetic and non-genetic risk factors in prediction of type 2 diabetes: Whitehall II prospective cohort study. BMJ 2010, 340:b4838.

30. Altshuler D, Daly MJ, Lander ES: Genetic mapping in human disease. Science 2008, 322(5903):881-888.

31. Gail MH: Discriminatory accuracy from single-nucleotide polymorphisms in models to predict breast cancer risk. J Natl Cancer Inst 2008, 100(14):1037-1041.

32. Gail MH, Brinton LA, Byar DP, Corle DK, Green SB, Schairer C, Mulvihill JJ: Projecting individualized probabilities of developing breast cancer for white females who are being examined annually. J Natl Cancer Inst 1989, 81(24):1879-1886.

33. Rosner B, Colditz GA, Iglehart JD, Hankinson SE: Risk prediction models with incomplete data with application to prediction of estrogen receptor-positive breast cancer: prospective data from the Nurses' Health Study. Breast Cancer Res 2008, 10(4):R55.

34. Alvarez GG, Schulzer M, Jung D, Fitzgerald JM: A systematic review of risk factors associated with near-fatal and fatal asthma. Can Respir J 2005, 12(5):265-270.
35. Li D, German D, Lulla S, Thomas RG, Wilson SR: Prospective study of hospitalization for asthma. A preliminary risk factor model. Am J Respir Crit Care Med 1995, 151(3 Pt 1):647-655.
36. Swern AS, Tozzi CA, Knorr B, Bisgaard H: Predicting an asthma exacerbation in children 2 to 5 years of age. Ann Allergy Asthma Immunol 2008, 101(6):626-630.
37. Wasilewski Y, Clark NM, Evans D, Levison MJ, Levin B, Mellins RB: Factors associated with emergency department visits by children with asthma: implications for health education. Am J Public Health 1996, 86(10):1410-1415.
38. Miller MK, Lee JH, Miller DP, Wenzel SE: Recent asthma exacerbations: a key predictor of future exacerbations. Respir Med 2007, 101(3):481-489.
39. Bouzigon E, Corda E, Aschard H, Dizier MH, Boland A, Bousquet J, Chateigner N, Gormand F, Just J, Le Moual N, Scheinmann P, Siroux V, Vervloet D, Zelenika D, Pin I, Kauffmann F, Lathrop M, Demenais F: Effect of 17q21 variants and smoking exposure in early-onset asthma. N Engl J Med 2008, 359(19):1985-1994.
40. Liang PH, Shyur SD, Huang LH, Wen DC, Chiang YC, Lin MT, Yang HC: Risk factors and characteristics of early-onset asthma in Taiwanese children. J Microbiol Immunol Infect 2006, 39(5):414-421.

There is a supplemental file that is not available in this version of the article. To view this additional information, please use the citation information cited on the first page of this chapter.

POTENTIAL UTILITY OF NATURAL PRODUCTS AS REGULATORS OF BREAST CANCER-ASSOCIATED AROMATASE PROMOTERS

SHABANA I. KHAN, JIANPING ZHAO, IKHLAS A. KHAN, LARRY A. WALKER, AND ASOK K. DASMAHAPATRA

9.1 BACKGROUND

Aromatase is a member of the cytochrome P450 enzyme family and a product of the *CYP 19A1* gene [1]. This membrane-bound protein (aromatase) is the rate limiting enzyme in the conversion of androstenedione to estrone (E1) and of testosterone to estradiol (E2) (Figure 1). Aromatase consists of two components: the hemoprotein aromatase cytochrome P450 encoded by the *CYP19A1* gene and expressed only in steroidogenic cells, and the flavoprotein NADPH-cytochrome P450 reductase, expressed ubiquitously in many cell types [2-4]. The enzyme (aromatase) is localized in the endoplasmic reticulum of a cell, and catalyzes three hydroxylation reactions that convert androstenedione to E1 and testosterone to E2 [5,6]. The enzyme activity is increased by alcohol, age, obesity, insulin and

This chapter was originally published under the Creative Commons Attribution License. Khan SI, Zhao J, Khan IA, Walker LA and Dasmahapatra AK. Potential Utility of Natural Products as Regulators of Breast Cancer-Associated Aromatase Promoters. Reproductive Biology and Endocrinology *9,91 (2011). doi:10.1186/1477-7827-9-91.*

gonadotropins [7]. The *CYP19A1* gene is highly expressed in the human placenta and in the granulosa cells of the ovarian follicles. However, many nonglandular tissues including liver, muscle, brain, bone, cartilage, blood vessels, breast (both normal and carcinogenic) and adipose tissues have lower level of *CYP 19A1* expression under the control of tissue-specific promoters [8]. Inhibition of aromatase enzyme activity has been shown to reduce estrogen production throughout the body and aromatase inhibitors (AIs) are being used clinically to retard the development and progression of hormone-responsive breast cancer [6,7].

9.2 THE AROMATASE GENE AND TISSUE-SPECIFIC PROMOTER EXPRESSION

Human aromatase is a 58 kDa protein which was first purified from placental microsomes in 1980s [9]. Only recently has the crystal structure of human placental aromatase been described [5]. Aromatase is encoded by a single copy of the *CYP19A1* gene which is ~123 kb long, located on the short arm of the chromosome 15 (15q21), and is transcribed from the telomere to the centromere [2,10-12]. The coding region spans 30 kb and includes nine translated exons (II-X) with two alternative polyadenylation sites [2]. The ATG translation initiation site is located on the exon II. There are a number of alternative non-coding first exons (I.1, I.2, I.3, I.4, I.5, I.6, I.7, and PII) which are expressed in tissue-specific manner, lie upstream to the coding region and are spliced to a common acceptor sites in exon 2 [13-15] (Figure 2). The distal promoter I.1 which drives transcription in placenta is located approximately 89 kb upstream of exon II. The proximal promoter found immediately upstream of exon II is PII which is expressed in the gonad. In between these two promoters, several other first exons and promoters have been identified, such as 2a in the placental minor, I.3 in the adipose tissue specific promoter, I.4 in the promoters in skin fibroblast and preadipocytes, I.5 in fetal, I.6 in bone, I.f in brain, and I.7 in endothelial cells [2,14,16-18]. As various tissues utilize their own promoters and associated enhancers and suppressors, the tissue-specific regulation of estrogen synthesis is very complex. Due to the use of alternative promoters, aromatase transcripts in various expression sites contain unique

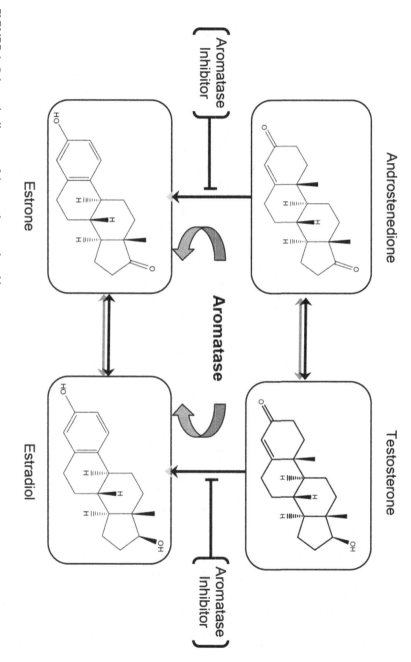

FIGURE 1: Schematic diagram of the reaction catalyzed by aromatase enzyme.

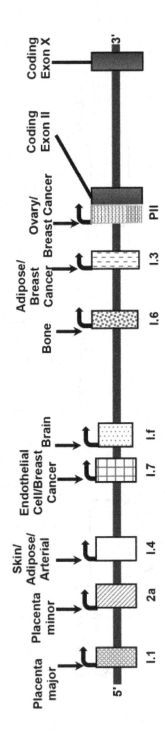

FIGURE 2: Partial structure of human CYP19 gene. Human aromatase gene is located on chromosome 15 and transcribes from telomere towards centromere. The aromatase gene is ~ 123 kb long contains nine coding exons (II-X) and two alternative polyadenylation sites. Partially tissue specific promoters direct aromatase gene transcription.

5'-untranslated first exons, which are spliced onto the coding exon II at the common 3'-splice site upstream of the ATG translation start codon [14]. Although expression of the aromatase gene is under the control of distinct tissue-specific promoters, the coding region of aromatase transcripts and the resulting protein is identical in all expression sites [9,14] and [19].

In healthy breast tissue, expression of *CYP 19* is under the control of promoter I.4 with synergistic actions of class I cytokines such as IL-6, IL-11, tumor necrosis factor-α (TNF-α) and glucocorticoids [9,20-22]. In tumorous tissue aromatase expression is switched to promoters I.3 and II which are transactivated by protein kinase A (PKA) and cAMP-dependent signaling pathways [8,23]. Depending on the microenvironment the promoter switching in the malignant breast tissue results in the enhancement of aromatase gene transcription, protein expression, and the enzymatic activity compared to the normal breast tissue. Moreover, this promoter switching is the primary reason for the increased estrogen production in adipose stromal cells surrounding the breast cancer [18,24,25]. Promoter I.7 is also considered to be a novel breast cancer associated aromatase promoter situated midway between promoter I.4 and promoter I.3/II [14,22]. Promoters I.3 and II lie 215 bp apart from each other and are coordinately regulated by prostaglandin E2 (PGE2) via a cAMP-PKA-dependent pathway, and not by cytokines as seen in normal breast tissue [8]. Signaling effects/transcriptional regulators that mediate PGE2 action include the activator pathways p38/CREB-ATF and JNK/jun and the inhibitory factor breast cancer 1 (BRCA1) in breast adipose fibroblasts [14,22].

9.3 BREAST CANCER AND AROMATASE

Breast cancer is an important public health problem worldwide. In the United States, breast cancer represents the most common neoplasm and second most frequent cause of cancer death in women [26]. Estrogens have been implicated in the etiology of breast cancer and have been added to the list of known human carcinogens [27,28]. Estrogens are suggested to cause breast cancer by stimulating cell growth and proliferation through receptor-mediated processes and via their genotoxic metabolites [29,30]; therefore, inhibition of estrogen production/effect is nowadays a common practice for breast cancer treatment [9]. The general strategies to inhibit estrogen action are to block estrogen receptor (ER) binding to its specific ligand or to disrupt estrogen production by altering the aromatase gene expression or enzyme activities [15]. ER antagonists can block estrogenic actions; however, estrogen production can be inhibited by aromatase inhibitors (AI).

It is very important to know that the E2 production site in women changes with the increase of age [6]. In the pre-menopausal period the ovaries are the major source of aromatase and its substrate, androstenedione and thus E2. In humans, androstenedione is produced by the theca folliculi cells, and is converted to E1 and subsequently to E2 in the granulosa cells by aromatase. Therefore, during the reproductive years, E2 mainly works as an endocrine factor acting on estrogen-sensitive tissues. In the post-menopausal period the ovaries lose the expression of aromatase; however, they are still able to produce androstenedione. At this stage adrenal glands are the major producer of androgens, which are converted to estrogens in peripheral tissues such as liver, fat, muscle, skin, bone, and mammary tissue [6,31-33]. In post-menopausal women E2 synthesized in extragonadal sites acts locally at these peripheral sites as intracrine, autocrine, paracrine or juxtacrine factors, and acts directly in the cells that synthesize estrogen or on the neighboring cells [34,35]. Moreover, in post-menopausal breast cancer patients, the concentration of E2 in breast tissue is ~20-fold greater than in plasma, suggesting that intratumoral estrogen synthesis, its retention, and cellular uptake plays important role in the progression of ER+ breast cancer [6,36]. Although the exact localization of aromatase in human breast tumor is still controversial [37,38], in majority of the breast cancer cases aromatase activity and aromatase mRNA levels show higher levels than those observed in non-malignant mammary tissues [39]; this supports the concept that in-situ production of E2 by aromatase plays a major role in breast cancer progression [40].

Considering the importance of E2 in hormone receptor positive breast cancer, many therapeutic approaches have been developed to deprive E2 signaling [7,9,15]. Two main chemical approaches have been successfully utilized [15]. The traditional method of E2 inhibition is to interfere with E2 interaction with its receptors (ERα and ERβ) using selective estrogen receptor modulators (SERMs) such as tamoxifen and raloxifene [41,42].

Another approach is to reduce E2 signaling by using AIs to decrease E2 synthesis [43]. While SERMs are effective both in pre-and post-menopausal women, AIs are not appropriate to use for pre-menopausal women, because in pre-menopausal women, AIs, by lowering the E2 levels, stimulate the secretion of gonadotropins from the pituitary gland. Subsequently, the gonadotropins stimulate the ovaries to produce estrogens which can counteract AIs effect and possibly causing ovarian cysts [44]. Moreover, due to indiscriminate reduction of aromatase activity in all expression sites of the body, AIs can induce many side effects such as bone loss, hepatic steatosis and abnormal lipid metabolism [14,45-49]. Therefore it is desirable to design selective aromatase modulators that target the over-expression of this enzyme (aromatase) in breast epithelial cells and surrounding fibroblasts, while other sites of estrogen production remained unaltered [50,51]. With this regard, selective inhibition of aromatase promoter I.3/II activities may be a fruitful approach to inhibit estrogen production in breast tumor while allowing aromatase expression via alternative promoters in other regions of the body like brain and bone.

9.4 INHIBITORY AGENTS OF AROMATASE PROMOTER I.3/II

There are several potential synthetic agents available for inactivation of aromatase promoter I.3/II. Studies in human breast adipose fibroblasts revealed that sodium butyrate, peroxisome proliferator activated receptor γ (PPAR γ) agonists, retinoid X-receptor (RXR) agonists, and inhibitors of p38 and JNK are capable of inhibiting aromatase promoter I.3/II activity. The action of these agents has been summarized in a recent review by Chen et al [14]. However, these synthetic products are also known to induce side effects. Troglitazone, rosiglitazone and pioglitazone are PPARγ agonists (FDA approved rosiglitazone and pioglitazone for the treatment of type 2 diabetes). These drugs caused edema, reduced hemoglobin and hematocrit levels, increased plasma LDL-and HDL cholesterol and increased body weight [52-55]. The RXR agonist LG101305 (the FDA approved drug is bexarotene) induced hypertriglyceridemia, hypercholesterolemia, hypothyroidism and leucopenia. Sodium butyrate induced bradycardia [55-57] while p38 inhibitor SB202190 is toxic to liver and the JNK inhibitor AS601245 have no reported side effects compared to others [58-60].

9.5 NATURAL PRODUCTS TARGETING AROMATASE GENE PROMOTERS

With the clinical success of several synthetic AIs in the treatment of postmenopausal ER-positive breast cancer, researchers have also been focused onto the potential of natural products as AIs [61]. These compounds (natural products) are mostly obtained from terrestrial and marine organisms and are still in the forefront of drug discovery. Moreover, the rich structural diversity and complexity of these compounds prompted the researchers to synthesize them in the laboratory for therapeutic applications. Many chemopreventive drugs used today are derived from the natural products [62-68]. In addition, many natural products that have been used traditionally for nutritional or medicinal purposes as botanical dietary supplements (BDS) may also afford as AIs with reduced side effects [61,69,70]. Because many natural products are associated with low toxicity, they are potentially excellent candidates for use as chemopreventive agents [71-73]. Epidemiological evidence suggests that women living in Asia, where diets have traditionally included soybean products, report fewer postmenopausal symptoms and experience fewer breast cancers than women in Western countries [74-77]. More specifically, Asian women have a 3-fold lower breast cancer risk than women in the United States, independent of body weight [78]. Furthermore, serum concentrations of E2 are 40% lower in Asian women compared with their Caucasian counterparts [79]. Thus, environmental and dietary factors may explain at least some of the discrepancy in breast cancer risk between Asian and western populations [74,75]. Despite the known AIs, there is still a need of searching for new AIs from natural products for future drug development [68].

Among the natural products tested as AIs, phytoestrogens, such as flavones and isoflavones are able to bind ER and induce estrogen action [77]. The binding characteristics and the structural requirements necessary for the inhibition of human aromatase by flavones and isoflavones were obtained by using computer modeling and confirmed by site-

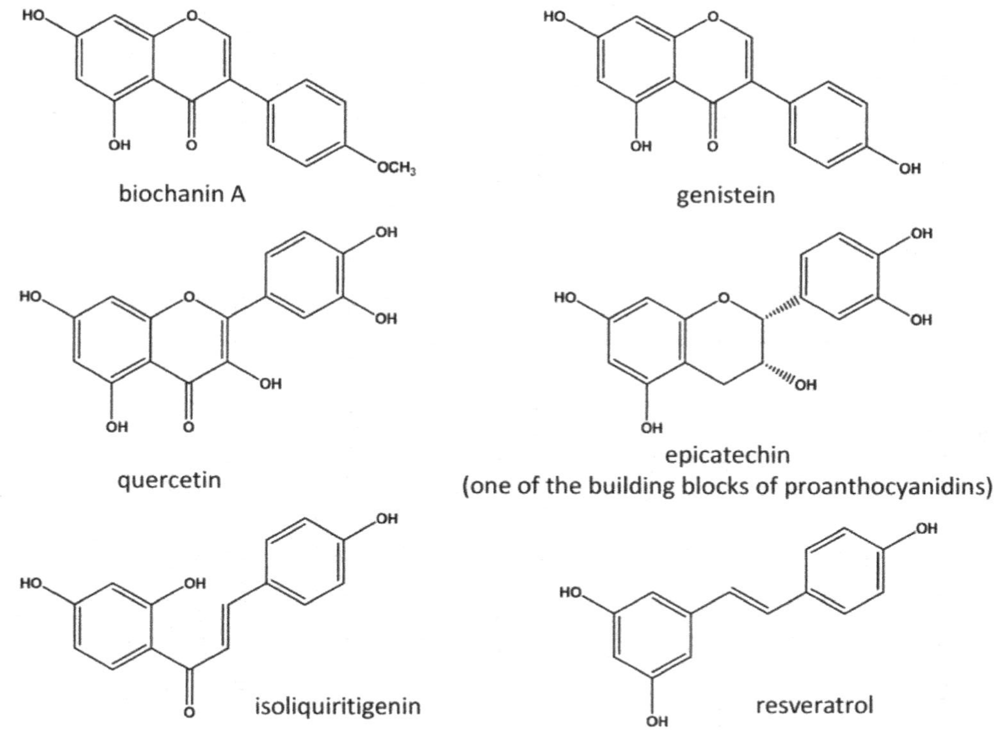

FIGURE 3: The chemical structures of biochanin A, genistein, quercetin, epicatechin, isoliquiritigenin, and resveratrol.

directed mutagenesis [80-82]. It was found that these compounds bind to the active site of aromatase in an orientation in which their rings A and C mimic rings D and C of the androgen substrate, respectively [80]. Until now ~ 300 natural products, most of them are phytoestrogens, have been evaluated for their ability to inhibit aromatase using noncellular (mostly using human microsome as a source of aromatase enzyme), cell-based, and in vivo aromatase inhibition assays [61,83-85]; however, only a few studies (biochanin A from red clover, genistein from soybean, quercetin, isoliquiritigenin from licorice, resveratrol from grape peel and extracts of grape seeds, Figure 3) have been reported for their effect on aromatase promoter I.4, I.3/II activity [86-91]. The exact mechanisms how these plant products adapted to inhibit aromatase gene expression or enzyme activity is not fully understood.

Biochanin A (5, 7-dihydroxy-4'-methoxyisoflavone) is an isoflavone extracted from red clover (*Trifolium pretense*) by Pope et al. [92]. The first evidence that red clover has estrogenic activity were reported by Bennets et al. [93] after observing breeding problems of sheep grazing on red clover pastures which have been attributed to the isoflavone and coumestrol content of red clover. Serious fertility disturbances indicating estrogenic stimulation of cattle fed with red clover silage were reported [94-96]. Although biochanin A was moderately active in inhibiting microsomal aromatase activity (IC_{50}: 5-10 µM) but was strongly active when tested in JEG-3 cells (human placental choriocarcinoma cell line). However, it did not inhibit aromatase activity in granulosa-luteal cells, and human preadipocyte cells and was also inactive in trout ovarian aromatase assay [61]. Interestingly, in MCF-7 cells (ER-positive breast cancer cells) biochanin A exhibited a dual action. It inhibited aromatase activity at low concentrations, but was estrogenic at high concentrations [97]. Furthermore, in SK-BR3 cells (ER-negative breast cancer cells) biochanin A was reported to inhibit aromatase enzyme activity and reduce mRNA expression. By using a luciferase reporter gene assay it was demonstrated that this phytochemical (biochanin A) was able to suppress the activation of breast-specific promoter I.3/II [88]. However, it is not known whether this inhibition is mediated through a PGE-2 or cAMP dependent PKA mechanisms. When genistein (a major metabolite of biochanin A) was tested in the same model, it was also found to suppress promoter I.3/II activation and showed an inhibition of aromatase enzyme activity [88]. Therefore, the inhibitory effect of biochanin A on aromatase promoter activation was suggested by the authors to be due to its metabolic conversion to genistein rather than its direct effect [88].

Genistein is a major phytoestrogen isolated from soybean, a potential nutraceutical, geared for women suffering from perimenopausal symptoms [98-101]. Genistein is also found in a number of other plants such as fava beans, lupin, kudzu, and psoralea [102]. Genistein is believed to be a chemopreventive agent against various types of cancers, including prostate, cervix, brain, breast, esophagus and colon [103]. Genistein was shown to increase aromatase activity in human adrenocortical carcinoma (H295R) cells and in isolated rat ovarian follicles [104,105]. Dietary genistein, which produced circulating concentrations consistent with human exposures, did not act as an aromatase inhibitor; rather, dietary intake of genistein negated the inhibitory effect of an aromatase inhibitor letrozole (a 3rd generation aromatase inhibitor), by stimulating the growth of aromatase-expressing estrogen-dependent breast tumors [106]. This study raises concerns about the consumption of genistein-containing products by postmenopausal women with advanced breast cancer who may be treated with letrozole. Genistein suppressed promoter I.3/II transactivity in SK-BR-3 cells (an ER-negative breast cancer cell line), however, in HepG2 cells, genistein was found to induce promoter-specific aromatase mRNA expression with significant increases in promoters I.3 and II [89]. In addition, the phosphorylated forms of PKCα, p38, MEK and ERK1/2 kinases were also induced in HepG2 cells by genistein [89]. There are also some reports of a weak inhibition of aromatase enzyme activity by genistein as well [80,107] and a decrease in the transcription of *Cyp19* mRNA in human granulosa luteal cells [108].

Quercetin is one of the most abundant flavonols found in plants. Quercetin was found to inhibit human aromatase activity in placental microsomes [109]. When tested in cellular systems utilizing adrenocortical carcinoma cells, preadipocyte cells, or in co-culture experiments, it exhibited either a mild or no effect [86,110,111]. In the primary culture of human granulosa-luteal cells quercetin was able to reduce aromatase mRNA expression in a dose-dependent manner after an exposure period of 48 h [108]. In another study, H295R human adrenocortical carcinoma cells were exposed to quercetin for 24 h and an increase in aromatase enzyme activity was observed at lower concentration, while a decrease in the enzyme activity was observed at higher concentrations [105]. Quercetin increased p II and I.3-specific aromatase transcripts about 2.6-and 2-fold in H295R cells after 24 h exposure probably by enhancing intracellular cAMP levels [105].

Isoliquiritigenin, a flavonoid from licorice (*Glycyrrhiza glabra*), was found to be an inhibitor of aromatase enzyme activity in vitro [90]. Moreover, this compound was able to block MCF-7aro cells(MCF-7 cells stably transfected with CYP19) growth and when added in diet inhibited significantly the xenograft growth in ovariectomized athymic mice transplanted with MCF-7aro cells [90]. Isoliquiritigenin also inhibited aromatase mRNA expression and suppressed the activity of CYP19 promoters I.3 and II [90] in MCF-7 cells. Furthermore, binding of C/EBP to PII promoter of CYP19 was suppressed by isoliquiritigenin [90]. This study indicated that isoliquirititigenin has the potential to be used as a tissue-specific aromatase inhibitor in breast cancer.

The aromatase inhibitory activity of grapes and grape seed extracts (GSE) has been studied by many investigators [61,83,91]. The active chemicals found in grapes and red wine are procyanidin dimers that are also present in high concentrations in grape seeds [87]. GSE is composed of about 74-78% of proanthocyanidins and <6% of free flavanol monomers such as catechin, epicatechin, and their gallic acid esters [87]. Through the suppression of the expression of CREB-1 and glucocorticoid receptor (GR), grape seed extracts (GSE) has been found to decrease the expression of aromatase in MCF-7 and SK-BR-3 cells by suppressing the activity of promoters I.3/II, and I.4 in a dose-dependent manner [87]. The GSE (IH636) is in phase I clinical trials for the prevention of breast cancer in postmenopausal women who have an increased risk of breast cancer development [61].

The grape peel contains resveratrol, a polyphenolic compound which has structural similarity with estrogen [91]. This nonflavonoid phytoestrogen inhibited aromatase activity in MCF-7aro cells. In SK-BR-3 cells resveratrol significantly reduced aromatase mRNA and protein expression in a dose-dependent manner [91]. Moreover, this compound was able to repress the transactivation of CYP19 promoters I.3 and II in SK-BR-3 cells [91], which indicate that resveratrol could be able to reduce localized estrogen production in breast cancer cells.

9.6 FUTURE DIRECTIONS

The expected direct outcome of aromatase inhibition is the maintenance of low levels of estrogen in the breast and surrounding adipose tissue. Understanding the molecular mechanism by which aromatase promoters I.4 and I.3/II are regulated is clinically significant and useful for developing new drugs. Although only a few plant products have been documented to mediate their effects through aromatase promoters, there are many more potent natural products (such as white button mushroom (*Agaricus bisporus*) which is in phase I trials [83]) which could be potential candidates for future study. Moreover, accumulating evidence suggests that beside transcription factors and co-regulators there are many other factors such as cyclooxygenases (COX) which are involved in tissue-specific aromatase promoter regulation [112,113]. Selective COX inhibitors from natural products can be used to suppress *CYP19A1* gene expression. Studies also indicate that *CYP 19A1* regulations are also under epigenetic control, including DNA methylation, and histone modification, which can add a new layer of complexity in the regulation of the aromatase gene [114]. DNA methylation generally occurs in gene promoters where the CpG rich dinucleotides are located. However, DNA methylation of CpG-poor promoter regions has also been shown as a mechanism of mediating tissue-specific gene transcription through the inhibition of transcription factor binding [115,116]. Aromatase promoter I.3/II has six CpG dinucleotides subjected to methylation of cytosines and can be considered as CpG-poor promoter. However, in human skin fibroblasts hypermethylation of almost all six CpG sites resulted in markedly reduced aromatase promoter I.3/II activity, whereas hypomethylation of only two of the six sites led to increased promoter activity associated with an increase in cAMP [14]. In contrast to these studies, in breast adipose fibroblasts (BAF) promoter I.4 and I.3/II derived mRNA were not dependent on the CpG methylation status within respective aromatase promoters [114]. Further, DNA methylation is catalyzed by DNA methyl transferases (DNMTs). Inhibition of DNA methylation by 5-aza-2'-deoxycytidine, which is also a specific DNMT inhibitor, increased *CYP19* mRNA expression in BAFs and breast cell lines [114]. These studies indicate that disruption in epigenetic regulation may give rise to increase in aromatase levels in the breast [114]. There are many synthetic chemicals that are undergoing clinical trials to be used as epigenetic drugs (epidrugs) for breast cancer treatment [117]. The major problems of these drugs are the unwanted side effects. Many natural products have the potential to be used as better epidrugs than synthetic epidrugs. One of the best examples is (-) - epigallocatechin-3-gallate from green tea which is used as demethylating agents for breast cancer patients [118-120]. Therefore extensive investigations in natural products seem promising or necessary.

9.7 CONCLUSIONS

Aromatase is a well-established molecular target and the AIs are proving to be an effective new class of agent for the chemoprevention of breast cancer. Regulation of aromatase expression in human tissues is a complex phenomenon, involving alternative promoter sites that provide tissue specific control. The promoters I.3 and II are the major promoters directing aromatase expression in breast cancer. The drugs that can selectively inhibit aromatase expression may be useful to obviate side effects induced by the nonselective AIs. Although many synthetic chemicals are used to inhibit tissue-specific inactivation of aromatase promoters I.3 and II, in the literature only a few natural products (we have included six of them) have been reported with such activities. More studies on natural products are necessary to find an appropriate tissue-specific AI.

REFERENCES

1. Simpson ER: Aromatase: biologic relevance of tissue specific expression. Semin Reprod Med 2004, 22:11-23.
2. Means GD, Mahendroo MS, Corbin CJ, Mathis JM, Powell FE, Mendelson CR, Simpson ER: Structural analysis of the gene encoding human aromatase cyto-

chrome P-450, the enzyme responsible for estrogen biosynthesis. J Biol Chem 1989, 264:19385-19391.

3. Zhao Y, Agarwal VR, Mendelson CR, Simpson ER: Transcriptional regulation of CYP 19 gene (aromatase) expression in adipose stromal cells in primary culture. J Steroid Biochem Mol Biol 1997, 61:203-210.

4. Simpson ER, Clyne C, Rubin G, Boon WC, Robertson K, Britt K, Speed C, Jones M: Aromatase-a brief overview. Annu Rev Physiol 2002, 64:93-127.

5. Ghosh D, Griswold J, Erman M, Pangborn W: Structural basis for androgen specificity and oestrogen synthesis in human aromatase. Nature 2009, 457(7226):219-223.

6. Milani M, Jha G, Potter DA: Anastrozole use in early stage breast cancer of postmenopausal women. Clin Med Ther 2009, 1:141-156.

7. Smith IE, Dowsett M: Aromatase inhibitors in breast cancer. N Engl J Med 2003, 348(24):2431-2442.

8. Simpson ER: Sources of estrogen and their importance. J Steroid Biochem Mol Biol 2003, 86(3-5):225-230.

9. Czajka-Oraniec I, Simpson ER: Aromatase research and its clinical significance. Endokrynol Pol 2010, 61:126-134.

10. Harada N, Yamada K, Saito K, Kibe N, Dohmae S, Takagi Y: Structural characterization of the human estrogen synthetase (aromatase) gene. Biochem Biophys Res Commun 1990, 166:365-372.

11. Nelson DR, Koymans L, Kamataki T, Stegeman JJ, Feyereisen R, Waxman DJ, Waterman MR, Gotoh O, Coon MJ, Estabrook RW, Gunsalus IC, Nebert DW: P450 superfamily: update on new sequences, gene mapping, accession numbers and nomenclature. Pharmacogenetics 1996, 6:1-42.

12. Bulun SE, Lin Z, Imir G, Amin S, Demura M, Yilmaz B, Martin R, Utsunomiya H, Thung S, Gurates B, Tamura M, Langoi D, Deb S: Regulation of aromatase expression in estrogen-responsive breast and uterine disease: from bench to treatment. Pharmacol Rev 2005, 57:359-383.

13. Bulun SE, Simpson ER: Aromatase expression in women's cancer. Adv Exp Med Biol 2008, 630:112-132.

14. Chen D, Reierstad S, Lu M, Lin Z, Ishikawa H, Bulun SE: Regulation of breast cancer-associated aromatase promoters. Cancer Lett 2009, (273):15-27.

15. Jiao J, Xiang H, Liao Q: Recent advancement in nonsteroidal aromatase inhibitors for treatment of estrogen-dependent breast cancer. Curr Med Chem 2010, 17:3476-3487.

16. Mahendroo MS, Means GD, Mendelson CR, Simpson ER: Tissue-specific expression of human P-450AROM. The promoter responsible for expression in adipose tissue is different from that utilized in placenta. J Biol Chem 1991, 266:11276-11281.

17. Simpson ER, Michael MD, Agarwal VR, Hinshelwood MM, Bulun SE, Zhao Y: Expression of the CYP19 (aromatase) gene: an unsual case of alternative promoter usage. FASEB J 1997, 11:29-36.

18. Sebastian S, Takayama K, Shozu M, Bulun SE: Cloning and characterization of a novel endothelial promoter of the human CYP19 (aromatase P450) gene that is up-regulated in breast cancer tissue. Mol Endocrinol 2002, 16:2243-2254.

19. Bulun SE, Takayama K, Suzuki T, Sasano H, Yilmaz B, Sebastian S: Organization of the human aromatase p450 (CYP19) gene. Semin Reprod Med 2004, (22):5-9.

20. Zhao Y, Mendelson CR, Simpson ER: Characterization of the sequences of human CYP19 (aromatase) gene that mediate regulation by glucocorticoids in adipose stromal cells and fetal hepatocytes. Mol Endocrinol 1995, 9:340-349.

21. Zhao Y, Nichols JE, Bulun SE, Mendelson CR, Simpson ER: Aromatase p450 gene expression in human adipose tissue. Role of Jak/STAT pathway in regulation of the adipose-specific promoter. J Biol chem 1995, 270:16449-16457.

22. Bulun SE, Lin Z, Zhao H, Lu M, Amin S, Reierstad S, Chen D: Regulation of aromatase expression in breast cancer tissue. Ann NY Acad Sci 2009, 1155:121-131.

23. Zhou J, Gurates B, Yang S, Sebastian S, Bulun SE: Malignant breast epithelial cells stimulate aromatase expression via promoter II in human adipose fibroblasts: an epithelial-stromal interaction in breast tumors mediated by CCAAT/enhancer binding protein beta. Cancer Res 2001, 61:2328-2334.

24. Utsumi T, Harada N, Maruta M, Takagi Y: Presence of alternatively spliced transcripts of aromatase gene in human breast cancer. J Clin Endocrinol Metab 1996, 81:2344-2349.

25. Agarwal VR, Bulun SE, Leitch M, Rohrich R, Simpson ER: Use of alternative promoters to express the aromatase cytochrome P450 (CYP19) gene in breast adipose tissues of cancer-free and breast cancer patients. J Clin Endocrinol Metab 1996, 81:3843-3849.

26. American Cancer Society: Cancer statistics. [http://www.cancer.org/Research/CancerFactsFigures/CancerFactsFigures/index] 2006.

27. IARC (International Agency of Research on Cancer): Overall evaluation of Carcinogenicity: An updating of IARC Monographs Volumes 1 to 42. IARC Monogr Eval Carcinog Risks Hum Suppl 1987, 7:272-310.

28. IARC (International Agency for Research on Cancer): Hormonal concentration and postmenopausal hormone therapy. IARC Monogr Eval Carcinog Risks Hum 1999, 72:474-530.

29. Cavalieri E, chakravarti D, Guttenplan J, Hart E, Ingle J, Jankowiak R, Muti P, Rogan E, Russo J, Santen R, Sutter T: Catechol estrogen quinones as initiators of breast and other human cancers: implications for biomarkers of susceptibility and cancer prevention. Biochim Biophys Acta 2006, 1766:63-78.

30. Yager JD, Davidson NE: Estrogen carcinogenesis in breast cancer. N Engl J Med 2006, 354:270-282.

31. Longcope C, Pratt JH, Schneider SH, Fineberg SE: Aromatization of androgens by muscle and adipose tissue in vivo. J Clin Endocrinol Metab 1978, 46:146-152.

32. Sasano H, Uzuki M, Sawai T, Nagura H, Matsunaga G, Kashimoto O, Harada N: Aromatase in human bone tissue. J Bone Miner Res 1997, 12:1416-1423.

33. Subramanian A, Salhab M, Mokbel K: Oestrogen producing enzymes and mammary carcinogenesis: a review. Breast Cancer Res Treat 2008, 111:191-202.

34. Harada N, Sasano H, Murakami H, Ohkuma T, Nagura H, Takagi Y: Localized expression of aromatase in human vascular tissues. Cir Res 1999, 84:1285-1291.

35. Simpson ER, Davis SR: Minireview: aromatase and the regulation of estrogen biosynthesis-some new perspectives. Endocrinology 2001, 142:4589-4594.

36. Castagnetta LA, Lo Casto M, Granata OM, Polito L, Calabro M, Lo Bue A, Bellavia V, Carruba G: Estrogen content and metabolism in human breast tumor tissues and cells. Ann NY Acad Sci 1996, 784:314-324.

37. Miki Y, Suzuki T, Sasano H: Controversies of aromatase localization in human breast cancer-stromal versus parenchymal cells. J Steroid Biochem Mol Biol 1990, 37:1055-1059.

38. Suzuki T, Miki Y, Akahira J-I, Moriya T, Ohuchi N, Sasano H: Aromatase in human breast carcinoma as a key regulator of intratumoral sex steroid concentrations. Endocrine J 2008, 55:455-463.

39. Miller WR, Anderson TJ, Jack WJ: Relationship between tumor aromatase acitivity, tumor characteristics and response to therapy. J steroid Biochem Mol Biol 1990, 37:1055-1059.

40. Suzuki T, Moriya T, Ishida T, Ohuchi N, Sasano H: Intracrine mechanism of estrogen synthesis in breast cancer. Biomed Pharmacother 2003, 57:460-462.

41. Nadji M, Gomez-Fernandez C, Ganjei-Azar P, Morales AR: Immunohistochemistry of estrogen and projesteron receptors reconsidered: experience with 5,993 breast cancers. Am J Clin pathol 2005, 123:21-27.

42. Wang T, You Q, Huang FS, Xiang H: Recent advances in selective estrogen receptor modulators for breast cancer. Mini Rev Med Chem 2009, 9:1191-1201.

43. Brueggemeier RW, Hackett JC, Diaz-Cruz ES: Aromatase inhibitors in the treatment of breast cancer. Endocr Rev 2005, 26:331-345.

44. Nabholtz JM: Long-term safety of aromatase inhibitors in the treatment of breast cancer. Ther Clin Risk Manag 2008, 4:189-204.

45. Edwards BJ, Raisch DW, Shankaran V, McKoy JM, Gradishar W, Bunta AD, Samaras AT, Boyle SN, Bennett CL, West DP, Guise TA: Cancer therapy associated bone loss: implications for hip fractures in mid-life women with breast cancer. Clin cancer Res 2011, 17:560-568.

46. Mazziotti G, Canalis E, Giustina A: Drug-induced osteoporosis: mechanisms and clinical implications. Am J Med 2010, 123:877-884.

47. Murata Y, Ogawa Y, Saibara T, Nishioka A, Fujiwara Y, Fukumoto M, Inomata T, Enzan H, Onishi S, Yoshida S: Unrecognized hepatic steatosis and non-alcoholic steatohepatitis in adjuvant tamoxifen for breast cancer patients. Oncol Rep 2000, 7:1299-1304.

48. Pinto HC, Baptista A, Camilo ME, de Costa EB, Valente A, de Moura MC: Tamoxifen-associated steatohepatitis report of three cases. J Hepatol 1995, 23:95-97.

49. Oien KA, Moffat D, Curry GW, Dickson J, Habeshaw T, Mills PR, MacSween RN: Cirrhosis with steatohepatitis after adjuvant tamoxifen. Lancet 1999, 353:36-37.

50. Simpson E, Davis S: Why do the clinical sequelae of estrogen deficiency affect women more than men? J Clin Endocrinol Metab 1998, 83:2214.

51. Simpson E, Rubin G, Clyne C, Robertson K, Donnell L, Jones M, Davis S: The role of local estrogen biosynthesis in the males and females. Trends Endocrinol Metab 2000, 11:184-188.

52. Safi R, Kovacic A, Gaillard S, Mutara ER, Simpson ER, McDonnell DP, Clyne CD: Coactivation of liver receptor homologue-1 by peroxisome proliferator-activated receptor gamma coactivator-1 aplha on aromatase promoter II and its inhibition by activated retinoid × receptor suggest a novel target for breast-specific antiestrogen therapy. Cancer Res 2005, 65:11762-11770.

53. Rubin GL, Duong JH, Clyne CD, Speed CJ, Murata Y, Gong C, Simpson ER: Ligands of the peroxisomal proliferator-activated receptor gamma and the retinoid ×

receptor inhibit aromatase cytochrome P450 (CYP19) expression mediated by pro-moter II in human breast adipose. Endocrinology 2002, 143:, 2863-2871.

54. Lebovitz HE: Differentiating members of the thiazolidinedione class: a focus on safety. Diabetes Metab Res Rev 2002, 18(suppl 2):S23-S29.

55. Sharma R, Sharma R, Verma U, Bhat NK: Novel drugs targeting retinoic acid recep-tors. JK Science 2005, 7:1-2.

56. Deb S, Zhou J, Amin SA, Imir AG, Yimaz MB, Lin Z, Bulun SE: A novel role of sodium butyrate in the regulation of cancer-associated aromatase promoters I.3 and II by disrupting transcriptional complex in breast adipose fibroblasts. J Biol Chem 2006, 281:2585-2597.

57. Weidle UH, Grossmann A: Inhibition of histone deacetylases: a new strategy to tar-get epigenetic modifications of anticancer treatment. Anticancer Res 2000, 20:1471-1485.

58. Chen D, Reierstad S, Lin Z, Lu M, Brooks C, Li N, Innes J, Bulun SE: Prostaglandin E (2) induces breast cancer related aromatase promoters via activation of p38 and c-jun NH(2)-terminal kinase in adipose fibroblast. Cancer Res 2007, 67:8914-8922.

59. Gore SD, Carducci MA: Modifying histones to tame cancer: clinical development of sodium phenylbutyrate and other histone deacetylase inhibitors. Expert Opin In-vestig drugs 2006, 15:721-727.

60. Braddock M, Murray C: 10th anniversary inflammation and immune diseases Drug Discovery and Development Summit. 20-21 March 2006, New Brunswick, USA. Expert Opin Investig Drugs 2006, 15:721-727.

61. Balunas MJ, Su B, Brueggemeier RW, Kinghorn AD: Natural products as aromatase inhibitors. Anticancer Agents Med Chem 2008, 8:646-682.

62. Daly JW: Marine toxins and nonmarine toxins: convergence or symbiotic organ-isms. J Nat Prod 2004, 67:1211-1215.

63. Cardy J, Walsh C: Lessons from natural molecules. Nature 2004, 432:829-837.

64. Butler MS: Natural products to drugs: natural product-derived compounds in clinical trials. Nat Prod Rep 2008, 25:475-516.

65. Newman DJ, Cragg GM: Microbial antitumor drugs: natural products of microbial origin as anticancer agents. Curr Opin Investig Drugs 2009, 10:1280-1296.

66. Mayer AM, Glaser KB, Cuevas C, Jacobs RS, Kem W, Little RD, McIntosh JM, Newman DJ, Potts BC, Shuster DE: The odyssey of marine pharmaceuticals: a cur-rent pipeline perspective. Trends Pharmacol Sci 2010, 31:255-265.

67. Cragg GM, Grothaus PG, Newman DJ: Impact of natural products on developing new anti-cancer agents. Chem Rev 2009, 109:3012-3042.

68. Eisenberg DM, Harris ES, Littlefield BA, Cao S, Craycroft JA, Scholten R, Bayliss P, Fu Y, Wang W, Qiao Y, Zhao Z, Chen H, Liu Y, Kaptchuk T, Hahn WC, Wang X, Roberts T, Shamu CE, Clardy J: Developing a library of authenticated Traditional Chinese medicinal (TCM) plants for systematic biological evaluation-rationale, methods and preliminary results from a Sino-American collaboration. Fitoterapia 2011, 82:17-33.

69. Basly JP, Lavier MC: Dietary phytoestrogens: potential selective estrogen enzyme modulators? Planta Med 2005, 71:287-294.

70. Edmunds KM, Holloway AC, Crankshaw DJ, Agarwal SK, Foster WG: The effects of dietary phytoestrogens on aromatase activity in human endometrial stromal cells. Reprod Nutr Dev 2005, 45:709-720.

71. Whitehead SA, Lacey M: Phytoestrogens inhibit aromatase but not 17β-hydroxysteroid dehydrogenase (HSD) type 1 in human granulosa-luteal cells: evidence for FSH induction of 17β-HSD. Human Repro 2003, 18:487-494.

72. Rice S, Whitehead SA: Phytoestrogens and breast cancer-promoters or protectors? Endocrine-Related Cancer 2006, 13:995-1015.

73. Bal Z, Gust R: Breast cancer, estrogen receptor and ligands. Arch Pharm Chem Life Sci 2009, 342:133-149.

74. Adlercreutz H: Epidemiology of phytoestrogens. Bailliers Clin Endocrinol Metab 1998, 12:605-623.

75. Nichenametla SN, Taruscio TG, Barney DL, Exon JH: A review of the effects of mechanisms of polyphenolics in cancer. Crit Rev Food Sci Nutr 2006, 46:161-183.

76. Usui T: Pharmaceutical prospects of phytoestrogens. Endocrine J 2006, 53:7-20.

77. Mense SM, Hei TK, Ganju RK, Bhat HK: Phytoestrogens and breast cancer prevention: possible mechanisms of action. Environ Health Persp 2008, 166:426-433.

78. Ursin G, Bernstein L, Pike MG: Breast cancer. Cancer Surv 1994, 19-20:241-264.

79. Peeters PH, Keinan-Boker L, van der Schouw YT, Grobbee DE: Phytoestrogens and breast cancer risk. Review of the epidemiological evidence. Breast cancer Res Treat 2003, 77:171-183.

80. Kao YC, Zhou C, Sherman M, Laughton CA, Chen S: A site-directed mutagenesis study Molecular basis of the inhibition of human aromatase (estrogen synthetase) by flavone and isoflavone phytoestrogens. Environ Health Perspect 1998, 106:85-92.

81. Chen S, Zhang F, Sherman MA, Kijima I, Cho M, Yuan YC, Toma Y, Osawa Y, Zhou D, Eng ET: Structure-function studies of aromatase and its inhibitors: a progress report. J Steroid Biochem Mol Biol 2003, 86:231-237.

82. Paoletta S, Steventon GB, Wildeboer D, Ehrman TM, Hylands PJ, Barlow DJ: Screening of herbal constituents for aromatase inhibitory activity. Bioorganic Med Chem 2008, 16:8466-8470.

83. Adam S, Chen S: Phytochemicals for breast cancer prevention by targeting aromatase. Front Biosci 2009, 14:3846-3863.

84. Zhao J, Dasmahapatra AK, Khan SI, Khan IA: Anti-aromatase activity of the constituents from damiana (Turnera diffusa). J Ethnopharmacol 2008, 120:387-393.

85. Balunas MC, Kinghorn AD: Natural compounds with aromatase inhibitory activity: an update. Planta Med 2010, 76:1087-1093.

86. Sanderson JT, Hordijk J, Denison MS, Springsteel MF, Nantz MH, van den Berg M: Induction and inhibition of aromatase (CYP19) activity by natural and synthetic flavonoid compounds in H295R human adrenocortical carcinoma cells. Toxicol Sci 2004, 82:70-79.

87. Kijima I, Phung S, Hur G, Kwok SL, Chen S: Grape seed extract is an aromatase inhibitor and a suppressor of aromatase expression. Cancer Res 2006, (66):5960-5967.

88. Wang Y, Gho WM, Chan FL, Chen S, Leung LK: The red clover (trifolium pretense) isoflavone biochenin A inhibits aromatase activity and expression. Brit J Nutr 2008, 99:303-310.

89. Ye L, Chan MY, Leung LK: The soy isoflavone genistein induces estrogen synthesis in the extragonadal pathway. Mol Cell Endocrinol 2009, (302):73-80.

90. Ye L, Gho WM, Chan FL, Chen S, Leung LK: Dietary administration of the licorice flavonoid isoliquiritigenin deters the growth of MCF-7 cells overespressing aromatase. Int J can 2009, 124:1028-1036.

91. Wang Y, Lee KW, Chan FL, Chen S, Leung LK: The red wine polyphenol reseveratrol displays bilevel inhibition on aromatase in breast cancer cells. Toxicol Sci 2006, 92:71-77.

92. Pope GS, Elcoate PV, Simpson SA, Andrews DG: Isolation of an oestrogenic isoflavone (biochanin A) from red clover. Chem Indus 1953, :1092.

93. Bennets HW, Underwood EJ, Shier FL: A specific breeding problem of sheep on subterranean clover pastures in western Australia. Aust Vet J 1946, 22:2-12.

94. Linder HR: Occurrence of anabolic agents in plants and their importance. Environ Qual saf Suppl 1976, 5:151-158.

95. Kallela K, Heinonen K, saloniemi H: Plant oestrogens; the cause of decresed fertility in cows. A case report. Nord Vet Med 1984, 36:124-129.

96. Saloniemi H, Wahala K, Nykanen-Kurki P, Kallela K, Saastamoinen I: Phytoestrogen content and estrogenic effect of legume fodder. Proc Soc Exp Biol Med 1995, 208:13-17.

97. Almstrup K, Fernandez MF, Petersen JH, Olea N, Skakkebaek NE, Leffers H: Dual effects of phytoestrogens results in u-shaped dose-response curves. Environ Health perspect 2002, 110:743-748.

98. Franke AA, Custer LJ: High-performance liquid chromatographic assay of isoflavonoids and coumestrol from human urine. J chromatogram B Biomed Appl 1994, 662:47-60.

99. Mazur W, Fotsis T, Wahala K, Ojala S, Salakka A, Adlercreutz H: Isotope dilution gas chromatographic-mass spectrometric method for the determination of isoflavonoids, coumestrol, and lignans in food samples. Anal Biochem 1996, 233:169-180.

100. Nestel PJ, Yamashita T, sasahara T, Pomeroy S, Dart A, Komesaroff P, Owen A, Abbey M: Soy isoflavones improve systemic arterial compliance but not plasma lipids in menopausal and perimenopausal women. Arterioscler thromb Vasc Biol 1997, 17:3392-3398.

101. Manonai J, Songchitsomboon S, Chanda K, Hong JH, Komindr S: The effect of a soy-rich diet on urogenital atrophy: a randomized, cross-over trial. Maturitas 2006, 54:135-140.

102. Meeran SM, Ahmad A, Tollefsbol TO: Epigenetic targets of bioactive dietary components for cancer prevention and therapy. Clin Epigenetics 2010, 1:101-116.

103. Barnes S: Effect of genistein on in vitro and in vivo model of cancer. J nutr 1995, 125:777s-783s.

104. Myllymaki S, Haavisto T, Vainio M, Toppari J, Paranko J: In vitro effects of diethylstilbestrol, genistein, 4-tert-butylphenol, and 4-tert-octylphenol on steroidogenic activity of isolated mature rat ovarian follicles. Toxicol Appl Pharmacol 2005, 204:69-80.

105. Sanderson JT, Hordijk J, Denison MS, Springsteel MF, Nantz MH, van der Berg M: Induction and inhibition of aromatase (CYP19) activity by natural and synthetic

flavonoid compounds in H295R human adrenocortical carcinoma cells. Toxicol Sci 2004, 82:70-79.

106. Ju YH, Doerge DR, Woodling KA, Hartman JA, Kwak J, Helferich WG: Dietary genistein negates the inhibitory effect of latrozole on the growth of aromatase-expressing estrogen-dependent human breast cancer cells (MCF-7Ca) in vivo. Carcinogenesis 2008, 29:2162-2168.

107. Pelissero C, Lenczowski MJ, Chinzi D, Davail-Cuisset B, Sumpter JP, Fostier A: Eflavonoids on aromatase activity, an in vitro study. J steroid Biochem Mol boil 1996, 57:215-223.

108. Rice S, Mason HD, Whitehead SA: Phytoestrogens and their low dose combinations inhibit mRNA expression and activity of aromatase in human granulosa-luteal cells. J Steroid Biochem Mol Biol 2006, 101:216-225.

109. Kellis JT, Vickery LE: Inhibition of human estrogen synthase (aromatase) by flavones. Science 1984, 225:1032-1034.

110. Wang C, Makela T, hase T, Kurzer MS: Lignans and flavonoids inhibit aromatase enzyme in human preadipocytes. J steroid Biochem Mol Biol 1994, 50:205-212.

111. van Meeuwen JA, Korthagen PC, de Jong PC, Piersma AH, van den Berg M: (Anti) estrogenic effects of phytochemicals on human primary mammary fibroblasts, MCF-7 cells and their co-culture. Toxicol appl Pharmacol 2007, 221:372-383.

112. Prosperi JR, Robertson FM: Cyclooxygenase-2 directly regulates gene expression of P450 Cyp19 aromatase promoter regions pII, p1.3, and pI.7 and estradiol production in human breast tumor cells. Prostaglandins Other Lipid Mediat 2006, 81:55-70.

113. Brueggemeier RW, Su B, Darby MV, Sugimoto Y: Selective regulation of aromatase expression for drug discovery. J Steroid Biochem Mol Biol 2010, 118:207-210.

114. Knower KC, To SQ, Simpson ER, Clyne CD: Epigenetic mechanisms resulting CYP19 transcription in human breast adipose fibroblasts. Mol Cell Endocrinol 2010, 321:123-130.

115. Fujii G, nakamura Y, Tsukamoto D, Ito M, Shiba T, Takamatsu N: CpG methylation at the USF-binding site is important for the liver-specific transcription of the chipmunk HP-27 gene. Biochem J 2006, 395:203-209.

116. Jones B, Chen J: Inhibition of INF-gamma transcription by site-specific methylation during T helper cell development. EMBO J 2006, 25:2443-2452.

117. Miyamoto K, Ushijima T: Diagnostic and therapeutic applications of epigenetics. Jap J Clin Oncol 2005, 35:293-301.

118. Fang MZ, Wang Y, Ai N, Hou Z, Sun Y, Lu H, Welsh W, Yang CS: Tea polyphenol (-)-epigallocatechin-3-gallate inhibits DNA methyltransferase and reactivates methylation-silenced genes in cancer cell lines. Cancer Res 2003, 63:7563-7570.

119. Moyers SB, Kumar NB: Green tea polyphenols and cancer chemoprevention: multiple mechanisms and endpoints for phase II trials. Nutr Rev 2004, 62:204-211.

120. Krik H, Cefalu WT, Ribnicky D, Liu Z, Eilertsen KJ: Botanicals as epigenetic modulators for mechanisms contributing to development of metabolic syndrome. Metab Clinic Exp 2008, 57(suppl 1):S16-S23.

CHAPTER 10

THERAPEUTIC POTENTIAL OF CLADRIBINE IN COMBINATION WITH STAT3 INHIBITOR AGAINST MULTIPLE MYELOMA

JIAN MA, SHUILIANG WANG, MING ZHAO, XIN-SHENG DENG, CHOON-KEE LEE, XIAO-DAN YU, AND BOLIN LIU

10.1 BACKGROUND

Multiple myeloma (MM) is a plasma cell malignancy characterized by specific genetic and epigenetic changes. Although many advances have been achieved in recent studies, MM remains an incurable disease and novel treatment strategies or agents are urgently needed [1,2]. A number of purine nucleoside analogs are rationally designed anticancer drugs that exert cytotoxicity via inhibition of DNA and RNA synthesis, and are currently used in the treatment of hematologic malignancies [3,4]. Cladribine (also known as 2-chlorodeoxyadenosine, 2-CDA) is an adenosine deaminase-resistant 2-deoxypurine nucleoside analog which requires phosphorylation by deoxycytidine kinase. Since this enzyme is mainly expressed in lymphocytes, cladribine is primarily active in lymphoid tissues [5]. Cladribine exerts remarkable activity in hairy cell leukemia (HCL), a chronic B-cell lymphoproliferative disorder, producing prolonged complete remissions in most patients [6,7]. Although cladribine is particularly cytotoxic to malignant B-cells and T-cells, and is widely used in HCL [8-10], it has not been approved to treat other lymphoid malignancies. Increasing evidences suggest that cladribine administered in combination with recently approved novel agents may be a valuable and safe treatment for patients with chronic lymphocutic leukemia (CLL) [11,12] and other lymphoid disorders, such as lymphoplasmacytic lymphoma, marginal zone lymphoma, and mantle cell lymphoma [13].

Although cladribine has been used for patients with low grade lymphoma and Waldenstrom's macroglobulinemia [14], it has only been studied in a limited manner in patients with MM, without much success [15]. Several studies have suggested that since "cladribine has a narrow spectrum of activity within the B-cell progeny" it may yet prove to be useful in subsets of patients with MM [16], because the self-renewing population of MM, arises at early B-cell precursors [17]. In vitro, the inhibitory effects of cladribine on MM cell lines are conflicting. While some studies observe completely negative results [18,19], others showing that cladribine has a marked heterogeneous effect on different MM cell lines [5] and clearly inhibits proliferation of RPMI8226 cells at high concentrations [20]. The precise molecular mechanisms by which MM cells show different responsiveness to cladribine remain unclear. It has been reported that cladribine induces accumulation of DNA strand breaks, and subsequently activates the tumor suppressor p53 in lymphocytes [21]. While mutation or deletion of *p53* is rarely detected in untreated MM [22,23], it is not known whether *p53* status in MM cell lines may influence their sensitivity to cladribine. Recent studies also suggest that frequent activation of STAT3 signaling provides survival advantage for MM cells [24-26], and STAT3 may serve as a novel target for the treatment of hematological tumors, including MM [27]. To date, there is no report indicating whether cladribine may modulate STAT3 activity in MM cells. Here, we studied cladribine's activity against different MM cell lines with either wild type (WT) or mutant *p53*, investigated its inhibitory effects on STAT3, and explored the therapeutic potential of cladribine in combination with a specific STAT3 inhibitor.

10.2 METHODS

10.2.1 REAGENTS AND ANTIBODIES

Cladribine or 2-chlorodeoxyadenosine (2-CDA) was purchased from Sigma-Aldrich Corp. (St. Louis, MO). STAT3 inhibitor VI (S3I-201) was obtained from EMD Chemicals, Inc. (Gibbstown, NJ). Antibodies for western blot analysis were from following sources: caspase-8 mouse mAb (1C12), caspase-9 polyclonal antibody, caspase-3 rabbit mAb (8G10), Poly (ADP-ribose) polymerase (PARP) rabbit mAb, phospho-STAT3 rabbit mAb and STAT3 (Cell Signaling Technology, Inc., Beverly, MA); b-actin mouse mAb (clone AC-75) (Sigma). All other reagents were purchased from Sigma unless otherwise specified.

10.2.2 CELLS AND CELL CULTURE

Human MM cell line U266 was kindly provided by Dr. Lisheng Wang (Institute of Radiology, Academy of Military Medical Sciences, Beijing, China). Human MM cell line RPMI8226 was purchased from the American Type Culture Collection (ATCC, Manassas, VA). Human MM cell line MM1.S was kindly provided by Dr. Steven Rosen (Department of Medicine, Robert H. Lurie Comprehensive Cancer Center, Northwestern University, Chicago, IL). All cell lines were maintained in RPMI1640 cell culture medium supplemented with 10% fetal bovine serum (FBS) at a 37°C humidified atmosphere containing 95% air and 5% CO_2 and were split twice a week.

10.2.3 CELL PROLIFERATION ASSAYS

The CellTiter96™ AQ non-radioactive cell proliferation kit (Promega Corp., Madison, WI) was used to determine cell viability as we previously described [28]. In brief, cells were plated onto 96-well plates with either 0.1 ml complete medium (5% FBS) as control, or 0.1 ml of the same medium containing a series of doses of cladribine, and incubated for 72 hrs. After reading all wells at 490 nm with a micro-plate reader, the percentages of surviving cells from each group relative to controls, defined as 100% survival, were determined by reduction of MTS (3-(4,5-dimethylthiazol-2-yl)-5-(3-carboxymethoxy   phenyl)-2-(4-sulfophenyl)-2H-tetrazolium, inner salt).

10.2.4 FLOW CYTOMETRIC ANALYSIS OF CELL CYCLE AND APOPTOSIS

Flow cytometric analyses were performed as described previously [28] to define the cell cycle distribution and apoptosis for treated and untreated cells. For cell cycle analysis, cells grown in 100-mm culture dishes were harvested and fixed with 70% ethanol. Cells were then stained for total DNA content with a solution containing 50 µg/ml propidium iodide and 100 µg/ml RNase A in PBS for 30 min at 37°C. Cell cycle distribution was analyzed with a FACScan flow cytometer (BD Biosciences, San Jose, CA). For apoptosis analysis, harvested cells were stained with Annexin V-FITC and propidium iodide according to the manufacturer's instruction and then subjected to the same analyzer.

10.2.5 QUANTIFICATION OF APOPTOSIS

An apoptosis ELISA kit (Roche Diagnostics) was used to quantitatively measure cytoplasmic histone-associated DNA fragments (mononucleosomes and oligonucleosomes) as previously reported [28].

10.2.6 WESTERN BLOT ANALYSIS

Protein expression levels were determined by western blot analysis as previously described [28]. Briefly, cells were lysed in a buffer containing 50 mM Tris, pH 7.4, 50 mM NaCl, 0.5% NP-40, 50 mM NaF, 1 mM Na_3VO_4, 1 mM phenylmethylsulfonyl fluoride, 25 μg/ml leupeptin, and 25 μg/ml aprotinin. The protein concentrations of the total cell lysates were determination by the Coomassie Plus protein assay reagent (Pierce Chemical Co., Rockford, IL). Equal amounts of cell lysates were boiled in Laemmli SDS-sample buffer, resolved by SDS-PAGE, transferred to nitrocellulose membrane (Bio-Rad Laboratories, Hercules, CA), and probed with specific antibodies as described in the figure legends. After the blots were incubated with horseradish peroxidase-labeled secondary antibody (Jackson ImmunoResearch Laboratories, Inc., West Grove, PA), the signals were detected using the enhanced chemiluminescence reagents (Amersham Life Science, Piscataway, NJ).

10.2.7 STATISTICAL ANALYSIS

Statistical analyses of the experimental data were performed using a two-sided Student's t test. Significance was set at a $P < 0.05$.

10.3 RESULTS

10.3.1 CLADRIBINE INHIBITS CELL PROLIFERATION/ SURVIVAL OF MM CELLS IN VITRO

To explore whether cladribine might be a potential therapeutic agent against MM, we investigated its anti-proliferative/anti-survival effects on three MM cell lines: U266, RPMI8226 with mutant *p53*; and MM1.S which retains and expresses WT *p53* [23]. Although the three MM cell lines exhibited different sensitivities, cladribine was able to inhibit proliferation/survival of all cells in a dose-dependent manner (Figure 1). While U266 was the least sensitive cell line, MM1.S was the most sensitive one to cladribine. The IC_{50}s of cladribine for U266, RPMI8226, MM1.S cells were approximately 2.43, 0.75, and 0.18 μmol/L, respectively. To determine

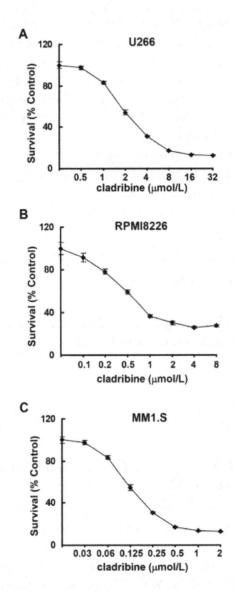

FIGURE 1: Cladribine inhibits proliferation/survival of MM cells. Human MM cells (1 × 10^4 cells/well) were plated onto 96-well plates with complete culture medium (RPMI1640, 10% FBS). After 24 hrs, the medium was replaced with fresh medium (0.5% FBS) or same medium containing indicated concentrations of cladribine for another 72 hrs. The percentages of surviving cells as compared to controls, defined as 100% survival, were determined by reduction of MTS. Data shows the representative of three independent experiments. Bars, SD. A, U266; B, RPMI8226; C, MM1.S

the molecular mechanisms by which cladribine inhibited proliferation/survival of MM cells, we first investigated the effects of cladribine on cell cycle progression. Both U266 and RPMI8226 cells with mutant p53 were treated with cladribine at the same concentration (2 μmol/L). U266 cells were collected at different time points (24, 48, or 72 hrs), and then analyzed with flow cytometry. Treatment with cladribine gradually increased the percentage of cells in the G1 phase of the cell cycle and reduced the percentage of cells in S phase (Figure 2A). Similar results were obtained in RPMI8226 cells with the treatment of cladribine for 24 hrs (Figure 2B). Cladribine appeared to increase G2-M phase in U266 cells upon 24 hr-treatment, it had no significant effect on G2-M phase either in U266 cells with 48 or 72 hr-treatment or in RPMI8226 cells (Figure 2A & 2B). It remains unclear why cladribine affected G2-M phase in U266 cells only by 24 hr-treatment. MM1.S cells were treated with cladribine at a much lower concentration (0.5 μmol/L) for 24 hrs. Cladribine induced a minor increase in G1 phase, decreased the percentage cells in S phase, and had no effect on G2-M phase in MM1.S cells (Figure 2C). Although our cell proliferation assays indicated that the IC50 of cladribine was much lower for MM1.S cells than the IC_{50}s for U266 and RPMI8226 cells (Figure 1), it appeared G1 arrest-induced by cladribine in MM1.S cells was not as profound as that we observed in the other two cell lines (Figure 2). It is likely that the potent anti-proliferative/anti-survival effects of cladribine on MM1.S cells may be mainly due to its strong capability to induce apoptosis as we discovered in the following studies (Figures 3 & 4). Collectively, our data suggest that induction of cell cycle G1 arrest contributes to cladribine-mediated growth inhibition in MM cells.

10.3.2 CLADRIBINE INDUCES APOPTOSIS IN MM CELLS

We next studied whether cladribine might also induce apoptosis in these MM cells, using two different methods. U266 cells were double-stained with Annexin V and propidium iodide, and then analyzed by a FACScan flow cytometer. These studies showed that cladribine induced apoptosis in U266 cells in a dose-dependent manner. The percentages of apoptotic cells evidenced by Annexin V-positive staining were 5%, 15%, 21%, and

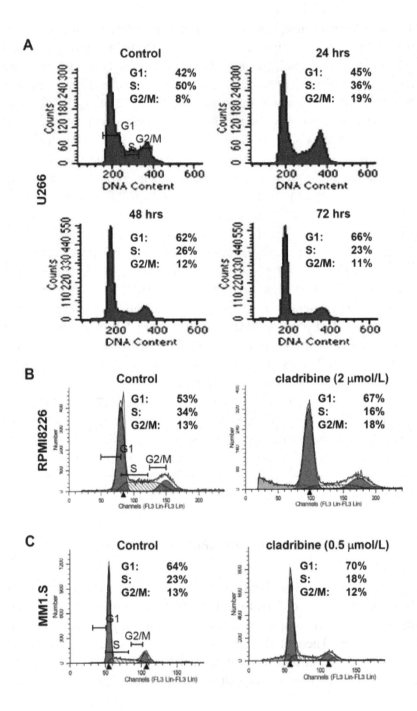

FIGURE 2: Cladribine induces cell cycle G1 arrest in MM cells. A, U266 cells were cultured with RPMI1640 (0.5% FBS) in the absence or presence of cladribine (2 µmol/L) for 24, 48, or 72 hrs. Cells were harvested and subjected to flow cytometry analysis of cell cycle distribution. Data shows the representative of three independent experiments. B & C, RPMI8226 (B) and MM1.S (C) cells cultured with RPMI1640 (0.5% FBS) in the absence or presence of cladribine for 24 hrs were harvested and subjected to flow cytometry analysis of cell cycle distribution. Data shows the representative of three independent experiments.

33% when U266 cells were untreated or treated with 2, 5, 10 µmol/L of cladribine, respectively (Figure 3A). When an ELISA methodology was used to quantify apoptosis in RPMI8226 and MM1.S treated with cladribine, a dose-dependent increase in apoptosis was seen in both RPMI8226 and MM1.S cells (Figure 3B & 3C). Consistent with the cell proliferation data (Figure 1), MM1.S was more sensitive to cladribine than RPMI8226 cells. To explore whether cladribine induced apoptosis through caspase-dependent mechanism, we carried out western blot assays to examine activation of caspases and PARP cleavage. In U266 cells, we were able to observe caspase-3 and caspase-8 activation and PARP cleavage only with cladribine at a higher concentration (10 µmol/L), however, it had no significant effect on caspase-9 activation (Figure 4A). Similar results were obtained in RPMI8226 cells treated with 1 µmol/L of cladribine for 48 hrs (Figure 4B). In contrast, treatment with cladribine at 0.2 µmol/L dramatically induced activation of caspase-3, -8, and -9 and PARP cleavage in a time-dependent manner in MM1.S (Figure 4C). Consistent with previous data derived from the apoptotic-ELISA (Figure 3B & 3C), the lowest concentration of cladribine induced strongest activation of caspases and PARP cleavage in MM1.S cells (Figure 4). Taken together, our studies indicate that caspase-dependent apoptosis contributes to cladribine-mediated anti-proliferation/anti-survival effects on MM cells. Among the three MM cell lines tested, MM1.S is the most sensitive one to cladribine-induced apoptosis.

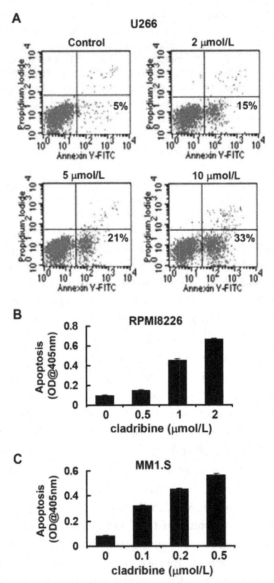

FIGURE 3: Cladribine induces apoptosis in MM cells. A, U266 cells were cultured with RPMI1640 (0.5% FBS) in the absence or presence of indicated concentrations of cladribine for 24 hrs. Cells were harvested and double-stained with Annexin V/PI, and then subjected to FACScan. The percentages of Annexin V-positive staining cells, indicative of apoptosis, were shown. B & C, RPMI8226 and MM1.S cells were cultured with RPMI1640 (0.5% FBS) in the absence or presence of indicated concentrations of cladribine for 24 hrs. Cells were collected and subjected to a specific apoptotic-ELISA. Bars, SD.

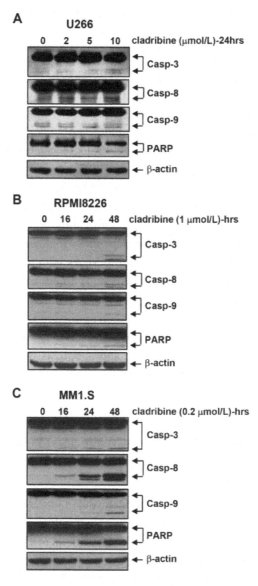

FIGURE 4: Cladribine induces activation of caspase-3, -8, -9 and PARP cleavage in MM cells. A, U266 cells were untreated or treated with indicated concentrations of cladribine for 24 hrs. B & C, RPMI8226 or MM1.S cells were untreated or treated with cladribine (1 μmol/L or 0.2 μmol/L, respectively) for 16, 24, or 48 hrs. Cells were collected and subjected to western blot analyses with specific antibodies directed against caspase-3 (Casp-3), caspase-8 (Casp-8), caspase-9 (Casp-9), PARP, or β-actin.

10.3.3 CLADRIBINE INACTIVATES STAT3 SIGNALING IN MM CELLS

It has been reported that constitutive activation of STAT3 is common in many human and murine cancer cells, and leads to cellular transformation [29,30]. Since aberrant activation of STAT3 plays a critical role in the development of human cancers, including MM [27], numerous studies have tried to identify novel anticancer strategies/agents targeting STAT3 [27,31]. To test whether cladribine's inhibitory activity against MM cells is due to STAT3 inactivation, we performed western blot analysis to determine the phosphorylation status of STAT3 in cladrabine-treated MM cells. In all three MM cell lines, cladribine significantly decreased the phospho-STAT3 (P-STAT3) levels in a dose-dependent manner, but had no effect on the total STAT3 protein levels (Figure 5). As with our cell proliferation (Figure 1) and apoptosis data (Figures 3 & 4), treatment with low doses of cladribine (0.2 μmol/L) was as effective in reducing P-STAT3 in MM1.S cells (Figure 5C) as high doses were when applied to U266 (2 μmol/L) and RPMA8226 (1 μmol/L) cells (Figure 5A & 5B). These data suggest that cladribine-induced growth inhibition and apoptosis in MM cells may be associated with its inactivation of STAT3.

10.3.4 COMBINATIONS OF CLADRIBINE AND S3I-201, A SPECIFIC STAT3 INHIBITOR, SIGNIFICANTLY PROMOTE MM CELLS UNDERGOING APOPTOSIS

Since STAT3 activation is important in the development of human cancers, including MM [27], and cladribine was able to inhibit STAT3 in MM cells (Figure 5), we hypothesized that the combinations of cladribine and a specific STAT3 inhibitor might exhibit super activity in inducing apoptosis in MM cells. S3I-201, which selectively inhibits STAT3 DNA-binding activity [32], was chosen to test this hypothesis. It has been shown that treatment with 30 μmol/L of S3I-201 for 48 hrs induces significant apoptosis in human breast cancer cell line MDA-MB-435, which harbors constitutive active STAT3 [32]. S3I-201 with 5 μmol/L was used in the following assays, as this concentration alone did not induce apoptosis in all the three

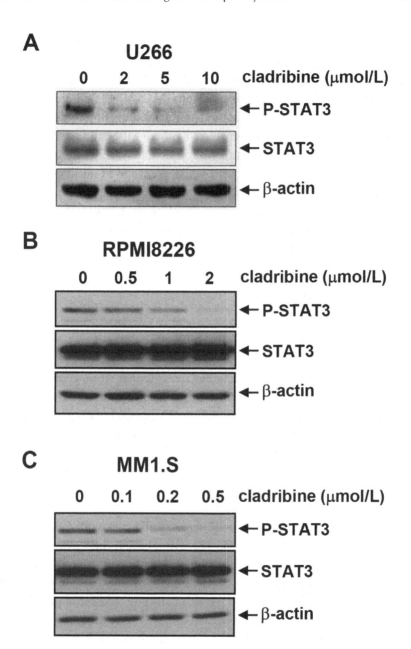

FIGURE 5: Cladribine inactivates STAT3 in MM cells in a dose-dependent manner. U266 (A), RPMI8226 (B), and MM1.S (C) cells untreated or treated with indicated concentrations of cladribine for 24 hrs collected and subjected to western blot analyses with specific antibodies directed against P-STAT3, STAT3, or β-actin.

MM cell lines (Figure 6). In contrast, different concentrations of cladribine were used in the combinational studies: 2 μmol/L for U266 cells, 1 μmol/L for RPMI8226 cells, and 0.2 μmol/L for MM1.S cells, because treatment with cladribine at this concentration for 24 hrs did decrease P-STAT3 levels (Figure 5), but had no significant induction of caspase activation and PARP cleavage for each of the three MM cell lines (Figure 4). As expected, the combinations of cladribine and S3I-201 induced strong activation of caspase-3 and -8, and PARP cleavage in all three MM cell lines (Figure 6A). Furthermore, apoptotic-ELISA demonstrated that their combinations, as compared to either agent alone, significantly promoted MM cells undergoing apoptosis (Figure 6B, P < 0.002, P < 0.0007, P < 0.002 for U266, RPMI8226, MM1.S, respectively).

10.4 DISCUSSION

Although cladribine inhibited cell proliferation and induced apoptosis in all three MM cell lines tested, we used a wide range of concentrations of cladribine. Pharmacokinetic studies indicate that when given as a 2-hr bolus at a dose of 0.14 mg/kg, the mean peak plasma concentration of cladribine reaches 198 nmol/L and falls to 22.5 nmol/L within 6-hr [33,34]. The MM1.S cell line was the only one showing significant growth inhibition and apoptosis-induced by cladribine within this concentration range (Figures 1C, 3C, & 4C). While our studies are consistent with a previous report indicating that cladribine has a heterogeneous effect on different MM cell lines [5], they suggest that cladribine may be useful to treat a subset of MM patients whose cells share similarities with MM1.S cells, which retain and express WT p53 [23]. In addition, like other clinically important nucleoside analogs, cladribine's effectiveness may be critically determined by the expression levels of deoxycytidine kinase (DCK), as this kinase is required to phosphorylate cladribine, and subsequently convert the inactive pro-drug into its active form [21]. We are currently testing whether cladribine may activate the tumor suppressor p53 in MM1.S cells, and whether or not this line expresses higher levels of DCK than U266 and RPMI8226 cells. Since cladribine at the clinically relevant concentrations dramatically reduced the levels of P-STAT3 in MM1.S cells (Figure 5C),

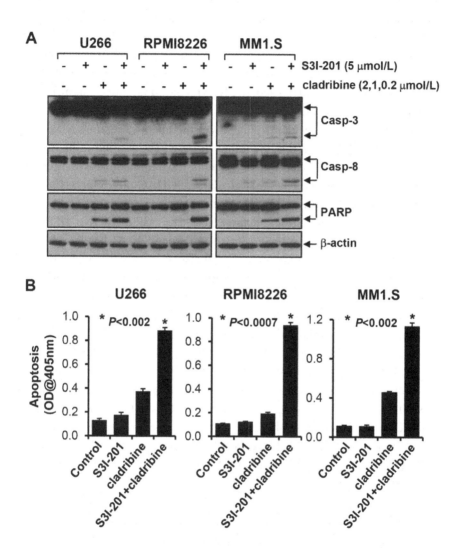

FIGURE 6: The combinations of cladribine and S3I-201 significantly induce apoptosis in MM cells. MM cells were untreated or treated with either S3I-201 (5 μmol/L), or cladribine (2 μmol/L for U266, 1 μmol/L for RPMI8226, 0.2 μmol/L for MM1.S) alone, or the combinations of S3I-201 and cladribine for 24 hrs. A, Cells were collected and subjected to western blot analyses with specific antibodies directed against caspase-3 (Casp-3), caspase-8 (Casp-8), PARP, or β-actin. B, Cells were collected and subjected to a specific apoptotic-ELISA. Bars, SD. P values vs single agent.

this might serve as an *in vitro* screen for identifying potential cladribine candidates. These findings also suggest that cladribine-resistance may be attributed, in part, to a hyperactive STAT3 signaling pathway, which frequently occurs in MM [24-26]. In this report, we have focused our studies on modulation of STAT3 activity. Our data showed that the combinations of caldribine and S3I-201, a specific STAT3 inhibitor, indeed significantly induced apoptosis in all three MM cell lines (Figure 6).

Recent advances in identifying novel therapeutics against MM have provided new hope for this incurable disease. The inhibitors of histone deacetylase (HDAC) are promising agents for treatment of MM [35,36]. Our recent studies indicate that a class I HDAC inhibitor (HDACi), SNDX-275 exhibits strong anti-MM activities via enhanced DNA damage response and induction of apoptosis [28]. Although two HDACis, LBH589 and AR-42, have been shown to reduce STAT3 levels in human lung cancer cells and malignant mast cell disease, respectively [37,38], the effects of SNDX-275 on STAT3 activation and/or expression in MM cells remain unknown. It is not clear if SNDX-275 could reverse the cladribine resistant phenotype. It would be interesting and in clinical relevance to test the combinational activities of cladribine and SNDX-275 in MM.

It has been reported that the insulin-like growth factor-1 (IGF-1) and interleukin-6 (IL-6) are two major MM growth factors promoting cell proliferation and survival, and play a critical role in MM development [39,40]. Strategies targeting IGF-1 receptor (IGF-1R)—blocking antibodies and small molecule inhibitors—show very encouraging preclinical results against MM cells [41], and both strategies are now in clinical trials [42]. IGF-1 and IL-6 binds their specific receptors and subsequently result in activation of several signal transduction pathways [35], including the JAK/STAT3, PI-3K/Akt, Ras/MAPK, NF-κB and β-catenin pathway. The PI-3K/Akt signaling is a well-known cell survival pathway, and its activation often leads to resistance to therapeutic agents in cancer treatment [43,44]. Currently, it is unclear whether the autocrine or paracrine IGF-1/IGF-1R loop in MM and through which downstream signaling pathways may also contribute to cladribine-resistance as we observed in U266 and RPMI8226 cells.

10.5 CONCLUSIONS

Cladribine-induced growth inhibition and apoptosis in MM cells correlated with its ability to inactivate STAT3. Cladribine in combination with S3I-201, a specific STAT3 inhibitor, resulted in significant apoptosis in all three MM cell lines as compared to either agent alone. Although cladribine as a single agent seems active in MM cells with WT p53, our studies suggest that the combinational regimens consisting of cladribine and STAT3 inhibitors may be more promising for MM patients.

REFERENCES

1. Kyle RA, Rajkumar SV: Multiple myeloma. N Engl J Med 2004, 351:1860-1873.
2. Naumann F, Weingart O, Kruse E, Schulz H, Bohlius J, Hulsewede H, Engert A: Fifth biannual report of the cochrane haematologic malignancies group--focus on multiple myeloma. J Natl Cancer Inst 2006, 98:E2-E.
3. Robak T, Korycka A, Kasznicki M, Wrzesien-Kus A, Smolewski P: Purine nucleoside analogues for the treatment of hematological malignancies: pharmacology and clinical applications. Curr Cancer Drug Targets 2005, 5(6):421-444.
4. Robak T, Lech-Maranda E, Korycka A, Robak E: Purine nucleoside analogs as immunosuppressive and antineoplastic agents: mechanism of action and clinical activity. Curr Med Chem 2006, 13:3165-3189.
5. Hjertner O, Borset M, Waage A: Comparison of the effects of 2-chlorodeoxyadenosine and melphalan on myeloma cell lines. Leuk Res 1996, 20:155-160.
6. Gidron A, Tallman MS: 2-CdA in the treatment of hairy cell leukemia: a review of long-term follow-up. Leuk Lymphoma 2006, 47(11):2301-2307.
7. Huynh E, Sigal D, Saven A: Cladribine in the treatment of hairy cell leukemia: initial and subsequent results. Leuk Lymphoma 2009, 50(Suppl 1):12-17.
8. Chadha P, Rademaker AW, Mendiratta P, Kim B, Evanchuk DM, Hakimian D, Peterson LC, Tallman MS: Treatment of hairy cell leukemia with 2-chlorodeoxyadenosine (2-CdA): long-term follow-up of the Northwestern University experience. Blood 2005, 106:241-246.
9. Cheson BD, Sorensen JM, Vena DA, Montello MJ, Barrett JA, Damasio E, Tallman M, Annino L, Connors J, Coiffier B, Lauria F: Treatment of hairy cell leukemia with 2-chlorodeoxyadenosine via the Group C protocol mechanism of the National Cancer Institute: a report of 979 patients. J Clin Oncol 1998, 16:3007-3015.
10. Jehn U, Bartl R, Dietzfelbinger H, Haferlach T, Heinemann V: An update: 12-year follow-up of patients with hairy cell leukemia following treatment with 2-chlorodeoxyadenosine. Leukemia 2004, 18:1476-1481.

11. Bertazzoni P, Rabascio C, Gigli F, Calabrese L, Radice D, Calleri A, Gregato G, Negri M, Liptrott SJ, Bassi S, Nassi L, Sammassimo S, Laszlo D, Preda L, Pruneri G, Orlando L, Martinelli G: Rituximab and subcutaneous cladribine in chronic lymphocytic leukemia for newly diagnosed and relapsed patients. Leuk Lymphoma 2010, 51:1485-1493.

12. Leupin N, Schuller JC, Solenthaler M, Heim D, Rovo A, Beretta K, Gregor M, Bargetzi MJ, Brauchli P, Himmelmann A, Hanselmann S, Zenhäusern R: Efficacy of rituximab and cladribine in patients with chronic lymphocytic leukemia and feasibility of stem cell mobilization: a prospective multicenter phase II trial (protocol SAKK 34/02). Leuk Lymphoma 2010, 51:613-619.

13. Sigal DS, Miller HJ, Schram ED, Saven A: Beyond hairy cell: the activity of cladribine in other hematologic malignancies. Blood 2010, 116:2884-2896.

14. Dimopoulos MA, Kantarjian H, Estey E, O'Brien S, Delasalle K, Keating MJ, Freireich EJ, Alexanian R: Treatment of Waldenstrom macroglobulinemia with 2-chlorodeoxyadenosine. Ann Intern Med 1993, 118:195-198.

15. Dimopoulos MA, Kantarjian HM, Estey EH, Alexanian R: 2-Chlorodeoxyadenosine in the treatment of multiple myeloma. Blood 1992, 80:1626.

16. Niesvizky R, Siegel D, Michaeli J: 2-Chlorodeoxyadenosine for multiple myeloma. Blood 1993, 81:868-869.

17. Niesvizky R, Siegel D, Michaeli J: Biology and treatment of multiple myeloma. Blood Rev 1993, 7:24-33.

18. Krett NL, Ayres M, Nabhan C, Ma C, Nowak B, Nawrocki S, Rosen ST, Gandhi V: In vitro assessment of nucleoside analogs in multiple myeloma. Cancer Chemother Pharmacol 2004, 54:113-121.

19. Nagourney RA, Evans SS, Messenger JC, Su YZ, Weisenthal LM: 2 chlorodeoxyadenosine activity and cross resistance patterns in primary cultures of human hematologic neoplasms. Br J Cancer 1993, 67:10-14.

20. Bagley RG, Roth S, Kurtzberg LS, Rouleau C, Yao M, Crawford J, Krumbholz R, Lovett D, Schmid S, Teicher BA: Bone marrow CFU-GM and human tumor xenograft efficacy of three antitumor nucleoside analogs. Int J Oncol 2009, 34:1329-1340.

21. Johnston JB: Mechanism of Action of Pentostatin and Cladribine in Hairy Cell Leukemia. Leuk Lymphoma 2011.

22. Chesi M, Bergsagel PL: Epigenetics and microRNAs combine to modulate the MDM2/p53 axis in myeloma. Cancer Cell 2010, 18:299-300.

23. Pichiorri F, Suh SS, Rocci A, De Luca L, Taccioli C, Santhanam R, Zhou W, Benson DM Jr, Hofmainster C, Alder H, et al.: Downregulation of p53-inducible microRNAs 192, 194, and 215 impairs the p53/MDM2 autoregulatory loop in multiple myeloma development. Cancer Cell 2010, 18:367-381.

24. Burger R, Bakker F, Guenther A, Baum W, Schmidt-Arras D, Hideshima T, Tai YT, Shringarpure R, Catley L, Senaldi G, Gramatzki M, Anderson KC: Functional significance of novel neurotrophin-1/B cell-stimulating factor-3 (cardiotrophin-like cytokine) for human myeloma cell growth and survival. Br J Haematol 2003, 123:869-878.

25. Catlett-Falcone R, Landowski TH, Oshiro MM, Turkson J, Levitzki A, Savino R, Ciliberto G, Moscinski L, Fernandez-Luna JL, Nunez G, Dalton WS, Jove R: Con-

stitutive activation of Stat3 signaling confers resistance to apoptosis in human U266 myeloma cells. Immunity 1999, 10:105-115.

26. Hodge DR, Xiao W, Wang LH, Li D, Farrar WL: Activating mutations in STAT3 and STAT5 differentially affect cellular proliferation and apoptotic resistance in multiple myeloma cells. Cancer Biol Ther 2004, 3:188-194.

27. Al Zaid Siddiquee K, Turkson J: STAT3 as a target for inducing apoptosis in solid and hematological tumors. Cell Res 2008, 18:254-267.

28. Lee CK, Wang S, Huang X, Ryder J, Liu B: HDAC inhibition synergistically enhances alkylator-induced DNA damage responses and apoptosis in multiple myeloma cells. Cancer Lett 2010, 296:233-240.

29. Bromberg JF, Wrzeszczynska MH, Devgan G, Zhao Y, Pestell RG, Albanese C, Darnell JE Jr: Stat3 as an oncogene. Cell 1999, 98:295-303.

30. Yu H, Jove R: The STATs of cancer--new molecular targets come of age. Nat Rev Cancer 2004, 4:97-105.

31. Yue P, Turkson J: Targeting STAT3 in cancer: how successful are we? Expert Opin Investig Drugs 2009, 18:45-56.

32. Siddiquee K, Zhang S, Guida WC, Blaskovich MA, Greedy B, Lawrence HR, Yip ML, Jove R, McLaughlin MM, Lawrence NJ, et al.: Selective chemical probe inhibitor of Stat3, identified through structure-based virtual screening, induces antitumor activity. Proc Natl Acad Sci USA 2007, 104:7391-7396.

33. Liliemark J, Juliusson G: On the pharmacokinetics of 2-chloro-2'-deoxyadenosine in humans. Cancer Res 1991, 51:5570-5572.

34. Sonderegger T, Betticher DC, Cerny T, Lauterburg BH: Pharmacokinetics of 2-chloro-2'-deoxyadenosine administered subcutaneously or by continuous intravenous infusion. Cancer Chemother Pharmacol 2000, 46:40-42.

35. Hideshima T, Mitsiades C, Tonon G, Richardson PG, Anderson KC: Understanding multiple myeloma pathogenesis in the bone marrow to identify new therapeutic targets. Nat Rev Cancer 2007, 7:585-598.

36. Podar K, Chauhan D, Anderson KC: Bone marrow microenvironment and the identification of new targets for myeloma therapy. Leukemia 2009, 23:10-24.

37. Edwards A, Li J, Atadja P, Bhalla K, Haura EB: Effect of the histone deacetylase inhibitor LBH589 against epidermal growth factor receptor-dependent human lung cancer cells. Mol Cancer Ther 2007, 6:2515-2524.

38. Lin TY, Fenger J, Murahari S, Bear MD, Kulp SK, Wang D, Chen CS, Kisseberth WC, London CA: AR-42, a novel HDAC inhibitor, exhibits biologic activity against malignant mast cell lines via down-regulation of constitutively activated Kit. Blood 2010, 115:4217-4225.

39. Mitsiades CS, Mitsiades N, Munshi NC, Anderson KC: Focus on multiple myeloma. Cancer Cell 2004, 6:439-444.

40. Sprynski AC, Hose D, Caillot L, Reme T, Shaughnessy JD Jr, Barlogie B, Seckinger A, Moreaux J, Hundemer M, Jourdan M, Meissner T, Jauch A, Mahtouk K, Kassambara A, Bertsch U, Rossi JF, Goldschmidt H, Klein B: The role of IGF-1 as a major growth factor for myeloma cell lines and the prognostic relevance of the expression of its receptor. Blood 2009, 113:4614-4626.

41. Mitsiades CS, Mitsiades NS, McMullan CJ, Poulaki V, Shringarpure R, Akiyama M, Hideshima T, Chauhan D, Joseph M, Libermann TA, García-Echeverría C, Pearson

MA, Hofmann F, Anderson KC, Kung AL: Inhibition of the insulin-like growth factor receptor-1 tyrosine kinase activity as a therapeutic strategy for multiple myeloma, other hematologic malignancies, and solid tumors. Cancer Cell 2004, 5:221-230.

42. Menu E, van Valckenborgh E, van Camp B, Vanderkerken K: The role of the insulin-like growth factor 1 receptor axis in multiple myeloma. Arch Physiol Biochem 2009, 115:49-57.

43. Knuefermann C, Lu Y, Liu B, Jin W, Liang K, Wu L, Schmidt M, Mills GB, Mendelsohn J, Fan Z: HER2/PI-3K/Akt activation leads to a multidrug resistance in human breast adenocarcinoma cells. Oncogene 2003, 22:3205-3212.

44. Wang S, Huang X, Lee CK, Liu B: Elevated expression of erbB3 confers paclitaxel resistance in erbB2-overexpressing breast cancer cells via upregulation of Survivin. Oncogene 2010, 29:4225-4236.

CHAPTER 11

EPIGENETIC UNDERSTANDING OF GENE-ENVIRONMENT INTERACTIONS IN PSYCHIATRIC DISORDERS: A NEW CONCEPT OF CLINICAL GENETICS

TAKEO KUBOTA, KUNIO MIYAKE, AND TAKAE HIRASAWA

11.1 BACKGROUND

Until recently, in clinical genetics, epigenetics was a minor field, of which two unusual genetic phenomena (genomic imprinting and X-chromosome inactivation (XCI)) were the main aspects under investigation. Based on the findings related to these phenomena, epigenetic disorders were considered to be very rare. However, as epigenetics has become more popular, it has developed into a huge research field that extends beyond genetics, encompassing not only biology and medicine, but also nutrition, education, health and social sciences. It now appears that epigenetics bridges the two major disease-causing factors (environmental and genetic) in medicine. Therefore, it is time to review epigenetics in the light of recent findings.

This chapter was originally published under the Creative Commons Attribution License. Kubota T, Miyake K, Takae Hirasawa T. Epigenetic Understanding of Gene-Environment Interactions in Psychiatric Disorders: A New Concept of Clinical Genetics. Clinical Epigenetics **4**,1 (2012). doi:10.1186/1868-7083-4-1.

In this review, we explain the epigenetic mechanisms that cause congenital disorders, show examples of environmental factors that can alter the epigenetic status, and discuss recent topics in epigenetics, such as the possibility of its inheritance and the use of epigenetic strategies for the treatment of diseases.

11.1.1 EPIGENETICS: A FIELD THAT BRIDGES GENETIC AND ENVIRONMENTAL FACTORS

It has long been thought that environmental and genetic factors are involved in the pathogenesis of common diseases such as cancer, diabetes, and psychiatric disorders [1-5]. For instance, environmental factors, such as drugs, viral infection, toxins and vaccines were proposed to be associated with the recent increase in the frequency of autism [6-9].

In the meantime, a number of genes related to autism have been identified, which are mutated in a subset of autistic children. Most of these genes encode synaptic proteins, including synaptic scaffolding proteins, receptors, transporters, and cell-adhesion molecules [10,11]. A recent comprehensive study confirmed that there were differences between autistic and control brains in the expression levels of genes encoding synaptic proteins and proteins related to inflammation [12]. Based on these findings, autism is now considered as a 'synaptogenesis disorder' [13,14],, and designated 'synaptic autism' [15] (Figure 1, left).

It was recently reported that short-term mental stress caused by maternal separation during the neonatal period alters the epigenetic status of the glucocorticoid receptor (Gr) promoter in the rat hippocampus, which leads to changes in gene expression. This altered epigenetic status and abnormal gene expression persisted throughout life, and resulted in abnormal behavior [16]. This finding led us to posit a new paradigm in which epigenetics links genetics to environmental science [16]. Since then, similar observations have been reported [17,18], and epigenetics is now considered to be an intrinsic mechanism that bridges the gap between environmental and genetic factors (Figure 1, right).

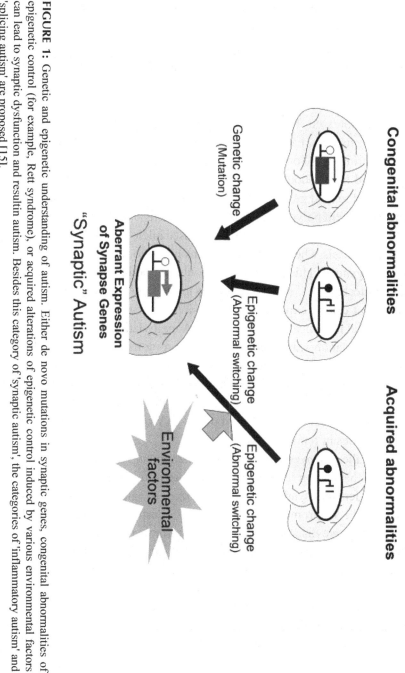

FIGURE 1: Genetic and epigenetic understanding of autism. Either de novo mutations in synaptic genes, congenital abnormalities of epigenetic control (for example, Rett syndrome), or acquired alterations of epigenetic control induced by various environmental factors can lead to synaptic dysfunction and resultin autism. Besides this category of 'synaptic autism', the categories of 'inflammatory autism' and 'splicing autism' are proposed [15].

11.1.2 THE FIRST EPIGENETIC PHENOMENA TO BE ASSOCIATED WITH DISORDERS

Genomic imprinting and XCI were the first two epigenetic phenomena discovered in mammals. Genomic imprinting is a unique genetic phenomenon in which only one of two parental alleles is expressed, while the other allele is suppressed. These genes are called 'imprinted genes'; the term 'imprinting' refers to a parent-of-origin specific epigenetic mark for suppression. Imprinting is considered to be a reversible mechanism, because the suppressed allele should be reactivated during gametogenesis when it is transmitted to next generation. For instance, the gene for small nuclear ribonucleoprotein polypeptide N (*SNRPN*) is only expressed by the paternal allele [19,20], but the maternally suppressed allele should be active during spermatogenesis when the allele is transmitted to the next generation via the male gamete. This phenomenon could not be interpreted by the usual genetic mechanisms, such as a change in the DNA sequence (that is, mutation), but can be explained by reversible epigenetic mechanisms based on chemical modifications, such as DNA methylation. In fact, differential DNA methylation was discovered in the promoter region of SNRPN between the paternal and maternal alleles [19].

XCI is another epigenetic phenomenon, which occurs only in females, because it compensates for the difference in the number of X chromosomes between females (XX) and males (XY), by silencing one of the X chromosomes in females [21].

Since the discovery of these two phenomena, abnormalities in these processes have been identified in a number of disorders, including Beckwith-Wiedemann syndrome (characterized by gigantism at birth [22]) Prader-Willi syndrome (characterized by obesity and features of obsessive-compulsive disorder), Angelman syndrome, (characterized by intractable epilepsy [19,20]), and XCI disorders such as ring Turner syndrome (which occurs when both the X and small ring X chromosomes are active, and is characterized by severe developmental delay that starts at birth [21]). Complete failure of XCI results in embryonic abortion [23,24]. These findings imply that proper epigenetic gene regulation is essential for normal development (Figure 1, middle).

11.1.3 MECP2: A MOLECULE THAT BRIDGES EPIGENETICS AND NEUROSCIENCE

Two of the first disorders identified in an epigenetic molecule were ICF (immunodeficiency-centromeric instability-facial anomalies) syndrome [25] and Rett syndrome (RS). The latter is characterized by epilepsy, ataxia and autistic features [26,27]. Because it is an X-linked dominant disease (it is embryonic lethal in males, thus patients are all female), the X chromosome was analyzed to identify the causative gene. At first, it was thought that the gene encoded a synaptic protein. However, the identified gene, the methyl-CpG binding protein 2 (*MECP2*) gene, encodes a transcriptional repressor [26] that is rarely seen, thus this unexpected result introduced a new paradigm, 'epigenetics,' and highlighted the importance of epigenetics in the brain.

Once the gene was identified, the next step in RS research was to understand the pathogenesis of this disorder in relation to the function of MeCP2. Because MeCP2 is a transcriptional repressor, it was expected that the brains of patients with RS would have abnormal upregulation of neuronal genes[28], and in fact, several dysregulated neuronal genes have been identified [29-31]. Because RS has an autistic feature that is caused by epigenetic failure, it was speculated that autism can be caused not only by mutations of synaptic molecules (as described in the introduction) but also by the aberrant expression of these molecules; this has been confirmed, as a synaptic function has been proven for protocadherins, which depends on their targeting by MeCP2 [32].

The MeCP2 protein also stabilizes genomic DNA by suppressing L1 retrotransposition (a genetic phenomenon in which an L1 sequence is inserted into various genomic regions when the L1 sequence is hypomethylated) [33]. The DNA sequence is different in each neuron because L1 retrotransposition occurs somatically in neurons [34], and MeCP2 deficiency accelerates this retrotransposition, suggesting that there is greater variation in DNA sequences and in expression pattern in the brains of patients with RS than in the brains of controls [33], as retrotransposition-driven L1 insertions can affect expression of adjacent genes [35]. Therefore, although no differences have been found in the genome sequences of monozygotic twins with disease discordance for multiple sclerosis [36], some differences may be detected in the sequences of monozygotic twins with RS.

RS is a congenital disease, in which the neurological features do not start at birth, but are first detected in late infancy or childhood (1-3 years of age). This is because the patients are heterozygous females, thus on average, 50% of their cells are normal cells, in which the X chromosome carrying the normal allele expresses *MECP2* under random XCI. In addition, MeCP2 does not encode a protein related to neurogenesis, but to neuronal maturation [37]. Therefore, it is possible that RS might be treatable if the level of MeCP2 could be supplemented to take it to the normal level during the maturation stage after birth. Indeed, this hypothesis was recently proven in the mouse model described below [38].

Mecp2 knockout mice mimic the neurological symptoms seen in patients with RS, including seizures, ataxic gait, and hind-limb clasping [39]. A new *Mecp2* 'knock-in' mouse model was created based on a first-generation *Mecp2*-knockout mouse, created by insertion of an 'exogenous' *Mecp2* gene [38]. To produce this phenotype, the exogenous *Mecp2* is initially silenced by an inserted stop codon, but it can be reactivated by treatment with tamoxifen (an estrogen analog), which causes the Cre-estrogen receptor fusion protein to translocate from the cytoplasm, where it is inactive, to the nucleus, where the Cre recombinase acts to recombine the two loxP sites that flank the inserted stop codon. Therefore, these mice exhibit neurological symptoms shortly after birth; however, after treatment with tamoxifen, the symptoms became much milder and the mice survived longer than the first-generation *Mecp2* knockout mice. These results indicate that the developmental absence of MeCP2 does not irreversibly damage neurons and that the subsequent neurological defects are not irrevocable. Furthermore, the results indicate that neurodevelopmental disorders caused by mutations in epigenetic molecules or epigenetic gene dysregulation are potentially treatable after birth. However, this strategy cannot immediately be applied to humans, because it is not possible to generate a *MECP2* knock-in human before birth. Thus, we need to identify chemicals that activate the expression of *MECP2* in patients with RS (Figure 2).

In addition to experiments using chemicals as described above, recent experiments have shown that appropriate environmental conditions (for

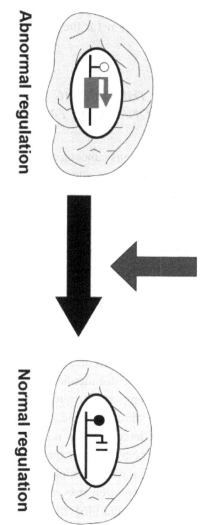

FIGURE 2: Epigenetic switching with various epimutable factors. A number of factors are known to exert epimutable effects. These factors alter the expression status by changing the epigenetic switches.

example, providing toys that stimulate the brain) could ameliorate the neurological features of Mecp2 knockout mice by altering gene expression and synaptogenesis in the brain [40-43]. These results suggest that it is important to provide a stimulating educational environment for patients with RS, as this can potentially alter the epigenetic status. Thus, epigenetics may provide useful scientific information for the assessment of specific educational conditions.

11.1.4 EPIGENETICS: KEY TO THE GENETIC UNDERSTANDING OF ENVIRONMENTAL FACTORS

Epigenetic alterations are seen in various cancers, and are currently used clinically as diagnostic markers [44]. These alterations occur in response to internal or external environmental cues [45], and occur over a long time period during carcinogenesis. However, mental stress (for example, decreased pup licking and grooming, and arched-back nursing) induced in rat mothers had effects on their offspring, with alterations in the DNA methylation and histone acetylation status of the glucocorticoid receptor (*Gr*) promoter seen in the hippocampus of the pups during the first week of life [16]. This was the first indication that epigenetic changes can be induced by environmental stimuli over a short period. Since then, other environmental factors, including consumption of folic acid [46] and royal jelly (confirmed in honeybees, but not yet in mammals) [47], malnutrition during the fetal period [48], use of drugs for mental disorders [49-53], and neuronal stimulation [54], have been reported to alter the epigenetic status.

These factors do not affect the whole genome, but target specific genomic regions in certain tissues. Dietary protein restriction during pregnancy in rats results in DNA hypomethylation at the promoters of the *Gr* and peroxisomal proliferator-activated receptor alpha (*Ppara*) genes in the offspring's liver; folic acid supplementation prevented this hypomethylation even during the post-weaning period [46]. In a mouse model of depression induced by chronic social defeat stress [49], chronic administration of imipramine, a commonly used antidepressant, induced long-lasting histone H3 acetylation at the P3 and P4 promoters and H3-K4 dimethylation at the P3 promoter of the brain-derived neurotrophic factor (*Bdnf*) gene, with increased expression in the hippocampus. An antiepileptic drug, valproic acid (VPA), which is an inhibitor of histone deacetylases (HDACs), blocked seizure-induced aberrant neurogenesis by normalizing the expression of the HDAC-dependent glutamate receptor 2 gene (*GluR2*) in the rat hippocampus, which protected the animals from seizure-induced cognitive impairment [50]. In a study on mice in which the *Reln* promoter was hypermethylated by pretreatment with L-methionine, clozapine and sulpiride (atypical antipsychotics for schizophrenia and bipolar disorder) decreased DNA methylation at the reelin (*Reln*) promoter and the N-terminus of the 67 kDa glutamic acid decarboxylase (*Gad67*) promoter in the frontal cortex and striatum [51]. This demethylation effect of clozapine and sulpiride was enhanced in combination with VPA, and the effect was specific to the brain, as it was not observed in the liver [51]. This demethylation effect of VPA at the *Reln* and *Gad67* promoters in the frontal cortex of mice was further confirmed by a different research group [52]; however, the precise mechanism underlying this demethylation process in the brain still remains to be elucidated. Lithium, another drug used to treat bipolar disorder, was found to have an epigenetic effect in a study on induced pluripotent stem cells (iPSCs). In this study, iPSC generation was enhanced with lithium treatment, which resulted in the downregulation of lysine-specific histone demethylase (LSD)1, an H3K4-specific histone demethylase, and a consequent increase in the endogenous expression of *Nanog*, an essential factor for induction of iPSCs [53].

These findings suggest that neurodevelopmental disorders such as autism can be caused not only by congenital genetic and epigenetic defects, but also by epigenetic dysregulation in the brain induced by various environmental factors (Figure 1, right). All of these findings were obtained through animal experiments, but there are also greater differences in epigenomic patterns between older monozygotic twins than between younger twins [55], suggesting that the epigenome is also affected by environmental factors in humans.

11.1.5 EPIGENETICS: A CONCEPT FOR THE TRANSGENERATIONAL INHERITANCE OF ACQUIRED CHARACTERISTICS

It has long been believed that acquired characteristics are not inherited by the next generation, a belief based on Darwinian theory. However, Lamarck suggested that genetic changes can be influenced and directed by environmental factors, and DNA methylation is now thought to underlie this theory.

Epigenetic markers allow the transmission of gene activity states from one cell to its daughter cells; however, until recently, epigenetic marks were thought to be completely erased and then re-established in each generation. However, there have been several reports indicating that this erasure is incomplete at some loci in the genome of several model organisms, and that an epigenetic marker acquired in one generation can be inherited by the next generation. This phenomenon is now called 'transgenerational epigenetic inheritance' [56,57], and is an explanation of lamarckism, the idea of the heritability of acquired characteristics.

The transgenerational epigenetic inheritance of metastable epialleles was first demonstrated in a mouse strain, in which the methylation status of the Axin (Fu) allele, which is linked to the shape of the tail in the mature sperm, reflects the methylation status in the somatic tissue. In this strain, this allele did not undergo epigenetic reprogramming during gametogenesis [58]. This observation was recently confirmed in a different species, namely yeast, in which an aberrant epigenetic marker that was acquired in one generation after heat-shock treatment was inherited by the next generation [59]. Furthermore, it was recently reported that mental stress (separation from the mother) not only changes the DNA methylation status in the brain of separated pups, but also changes it in the sperm of the males, and the changed status is transmitted to the next generation. In the next generation, the changed status is visible in the brain of offspring, and also produces alterations in the corticotropin releasing factor receptor 2 (*Crfr2*) gene expression and in the animal's behavior [60,61]. Although further evidence is needed, these findings imply that a susceptibility to mental disorders that is inherited by succeeding generations depends not only upon specific genomic changes (mutations in genes) but also upon specific epigenomic changes that are initially induced by environmental factors. Future studies are necessary to identify therapeutic strategies that take advantage of the reversibility of stress-induced epigenetic modifications. These studies could also help us to identify appropriate environments for maintaining a healthy physical and mental condition [62,63].

11.1.6 FUTURE PERSPECTIVES

The clinical application of epigenomic information has improved in recent years. Its first application was a single gene-based DNA methylation assay to diagnose two imprinted disorders (Prader-Willi and Angelman syndromes) by taking advantage of the differential methylation present in a CpG region within an imprinted gene [20]. Recently, a microarray-based epigenomic assay has been developed as a second-generation test, which covers CpG sites in an entire region of a single chromosome [64]. More recently, a high-density BeadChip-based epigenomic assay has been developed as a third-generation test, and now covers 450,000 CpG sites distributed throughout the human genome. Using this method, a methylated site that was specific to heavy smokers was discovered within a gene that is possibly associated with cardiovascular complications [65].

Another important application of epigenetics relates to folic acid, which is a nutrient that provides methyl residues and is essential for the maintenance of DNA methylation. Folic acid is used to prevent neural tube defects such as spina bifida, and it is known that folic acid supplements can alter DNA methylation status [66,67]. Folic acid supplements can have a positive effect on several features of autism in children, although the underlying mechanism is not completely understood [68-70]. Folic acid is expected to exert a global effect on the genome; however, if we can identify genes in which the epigenome is changed in particular disorders (for example, the *SNRPN* gene in Prader-Willi syndrome during gametogenesis [19,20] and the coagulation factor II (thrombin) receptor-like 3 (*F2RL3*) gene in heavy smokers [65]), it might be possible to selectively restore the specific epigenomic status of the causative gene region. One method is to use pyrrole-imidazole (PI) polyamides, which are small chemicals that recognize and attach to the minor groove of DNA, and can be designed to target any DNA sequences. PI polyamide can be attached to inhibitors of DNA methylation or histone deacetylases [71], and it was recently reported that such a construct was delivered to a target gene and altered its expression [72].

As discussed above, acquired characteristics can be inherited by the next generation as an epigenetic marker, as suggested by Lamarck. Recent research on animals has shown that behavioral characteristics can be inherited [60]. Thus, if gene-specific epigenomic therapy using PI polyamides could be delivered to the affected genes (for example,, Crfr2 [61]), it might correct the altered epigenomic status, gene expression and behavior of the subject, and thus might prevent inheritance of the abnormal epigenetic status by future generations.

Recent sequencing technology has led to a precise understanding of the sequence structure of the human genome, and revealed the presence of copy-number variations (CNVs), which are associated with susceptibility to common diseases [73,74]. The presence of CNVs is currently a more favored genetic concept than epigenetics in some psychiatric disorders, such as autism [75]. However, the advantage of studying epigenetics over CNVs is that if we can understand the epigenetic basis of the inheritance of acquired characteristics, it might be possible to develop a new therapeutic strategy using the intrinsic reversibility of epigenetics and also to develop a new method of prevention can be developed for the following generation. Therefore, further understanding of interactions between genes and environment with respect to epigenetics is important, and will provide a new concept of clinical genetics.

11.2 CONCLUSIONS

The failure of epigenetic gene regulation is known to cause various rare congenital disorders. However, this dysregulation also causes common diseases that are induced by environmental factors, as the epigenetic status is affected and changed by various environmental factors. Furthermore, the changed epigenetic status in the genome can be transmitted to the succeeding generations. Therefore, a precise understanding of the interactions between genes and environment in the light of epigenetics is necessary, and will form a new concept of clinical genetics.

REFERENCES

1. Feinberg AP, Irizarry RA, Fradin D, Aryee MJ, Murakami P, Aspelund T, Eiriks-dottir G, Harris TB, Launer L, Gudnason V, Fallin MD: Personalized epigenomic signatures that are stable over time and covary with body mass index. Sci Transl Med 2010, 2:49ra67.
2. Flintoft L: Complex disease: epigenomics gets personal. Nat Rev Genet 2010, 11:746-747.
3. Pollin TI: Epigenetics and diabetes risk: not just for imprinting anymore? Diabetes 2011, 60:1859-1860.
4. Stitzel ML, Sethupathy P, Pearson DS, Chines PS, Song L, Erdos MR, Welch R, Parker SC, Boyle AP, Scott LJ, NISC Comparative Sequencing Program, Margulies EH, Boehnke M, Furey TS, Crawford GE, Collins FS: Global epigenomic analysis of primary human pancreatic islets provides insights into type 2 diabetes susceptibility loci. Cell Metab 2010, 12:443-455.
5. Nolan CJ, Damm P, Prentki M: Type 2 diabetes across generations: from pathophysiology to prevention and management. Lancet 2011, 378:169-181.
6. London EA: The environment as an etiologic factor in autism: a new direction for research. Environ Health Perspect 2000, 108(Suppl 3):401-404.
7. Goldman LR, Koduru S: Chemicals in the environment and developmental toxicity to children: a public health and policy perspective. Environ Health Perspect 2000, 108(Suppl 3):443-448.
8. Finegold SM: Desulfovibrio species are potentially important in regressive autism. Med Hypotheses 2011, 77:270-274.
9. Taylor B, Miller E, Farrington CP, Petropoulos MC, Favot-Mayaud I, Li J, Waight PA: Autism and measles, mumps, and rubella vaccine: no epidemiological evidence for a causal association. Lancet 1999, 353:2026-2029.
10. Persico AM, Bourgeron T: Searching for ways out of the autism maze: genetic, epigenetic and environmental clues. Trends Neurosci 2006, 29:349-358.
11. Herbert MR: SHANK3, the synapse, and autism. N Engl J Med 2011, 365:173-175.
12. Voineagu I, Wang X, Johnston P, Lowe JK, Tian Y, Horvath S, Mill J, Cantor RM, Blencowe BJ, Geschwind DH: Transcriptomic analysis of autistic brain reveals convergent molecular pathology. Nature 2011, 474:380-384.
13. Zoghbi HY: Postnatal neurodevelopmental disorders: meeting at the synapse? Science 2003, 302:826-830.
14. Bourgeron T: A synaptic trek to autism. Curr Opin Neurobiol 2009, 19:23123-124.
15. Korade Z, Mirnics K: Gene expression: the autism disconnect. Nature 2011, 474:294-295.

16. Weaver IC, Cervoni N, Champagne FA, D'Alessio AC, Sharma S, Seckl JR, Dymov S, Szyf M, Meaney MJ: Epigenetic programming by maternal behavior. Nat Neurosci 2004, 9:847-854.

17. Szyf M: The early life social environment and DNA methylation; DNA methylation mediating the long-term impact of social environments early in life. Epigenetics 2011, 6:971-978.

18. Murgatroyd C, Spengler D: Epigenetics of early child development. Front Psychiatry 2011, 2:16.

19. Glenn CC, Porter KA, Jong MT, Nicholls RD, Driscoll DJ: Functional imprinting and epigenetic modification of the human SNRPN gene. Hum Mol Genet 1993, 2:2001-2005.

20. Kubota T, Das S, Christian SL, Baylin SB, Herman JG, Ledbetter DH: Methylation-specific PCR simplifies imprinting analysis. Nat Genet 1997, 16:16-17.

21. Kubota T, Wakui K, Nakamura T, Ohashi H, Watanabe Y, Yoshino M, Kida T, Okamoto N, Matsumura M, Muroya K, Ogata T, Goto Y, Fukushima Y: Proportion of the cells with functional X disomy is associated with the severity of mental retardation in mosaic ring X Turner syndrome females. Cytogenet Genome Res 2002, 99:276-284.

22. Kubota T, Saitoh S, Matsumoto T, Narahara K, Fukushima Y, Jinno Y, Niikawa N: Excess functional copy of allele at chromosomal region 11p15 may cause Wiedemann-Beckwith (EMG) syndrome. Am J Med Genet 1994, 49:378-383.

23. Xue F, Tian XC, Du F, Kubota C, Taneja M, Dinnyes A, Dai Y, Levine H, Pereira LV, Yang X: Aberrant patterns of X chromosome inactivation in bovine clones. Nat Genet 2002, 31:216-220.

24. Nolen LD, Gao S, Han Z, Mann MR, Gie Chung Y, Otte AP, Bartolomei MS, Latham KE: X chromosome reactivation and regulation in cloned embryos. Dev Biol 2005, 279:525-540.

25. Okano M, Bell DW, Haber DA, Li E: DNA methyltransferases Dnmt3a and Dnmt3b are essential for de novo methylation and mammalian development. Cell 1999, 99:247-257.

26. Amir RE, Van den Veyver IB, Wan M, Tran CQ, Francke U, Zoghbi HY: Rett syndrome is caused by mutations in X-linked MECP2, encoding methyl-CpG-binding protein 2. Nat Genet 1999, 23:185-188.

27. Chunshu Y, Endoh K, Soutome M, Kawamura R, Kubota T: A patient with classic Rett syndrome with a novel mutation in MECP2 exon 1.

28. Clin Genet 2006, 70:530-531.

29. Chahrour M, Jung SY, Shaw C, Zhou X, Wong ST, Qin J, Zoghbi HY: MeCP2, a key contributor to neurological disease, activates and represses transcription.

30. Science 2008, 320:1224-1229.

31. Chen WG, Chang Q, Lin Y, Meissner A, West AE, Griffith EC, Jaenisch R, Greenberg ME: Derepression of BDNF transcription involves calcium-dependent phosphorylation of MeCP2. Science 2003, 302:885-889.

32. Martinowich K, Hattori D, Wu H, Fouse S, He F, Hu Y, Fan G, Sun YE: DNA methylation-related chromatin remodeling in activity-dependent BDNF gene regulation. Science 2003, 302:890-893.

33. Itoh M, Ide S, Takashima S, Kudo S, Nomura Y, Segawa M, Kubota T, Mori H, Tanaka S, Horie H, Tanabe Y, Goto Y: Methyl CpG-binding protein 2 (a mutation of which causes Rett syndrome) directly regulates insulin-like growth factor binding protein 3 in mouse and human brains. J Neuropathol Exp Neurol 2007, 66:117-123.

34. Miyake K, Hirasawa T, Soutome M, Itoh M, Goto Y, Endoh K, Takahashi K, Kudo S, Nakagawa T, Yokoi S, Taira T, Inazawa J, Kubota T: The protocadherins, PCDHB1 and PCDH7, are regulated by MeCP2 in neuronal cells and brain tissues: implication for pathogenesis of Rett syndrome. BMC Neurosci 2011, 12:81.

35. Muotri AR, Marchetto MC, Coufal NG, Oefner R, Yeo G, Nakashima K, Gage FH: L1 retrotransposition in neurons is modulated by MeCP2. Nature 2010, 468:443-446.

36. Coufal NG, Garcia-Perez JL, Peng GE, Yeo GW, Mu Y, Lovci MT, Morell M, O'Shea KS, Moran JV, Gage FH: L1 retrotransposition in human neural progenitor cells. Nature 2009, 460:1127-1131.

37. Muotri AR, Chu VT, Marchetto MC, Deng W, Moran JV, Gage FH: Somatic mosaicism in neuronal precursor cells mediated by L1 retrotransposition. Nature 2005, 435:903-910.

38. Baranzini SE, Mudge J, van Velkinburgh JC, Khankhanian P, Khrebtukova I, Miller NA, Zhang L, Farmer AD, Bell CJ, Kim RW, May GD, Woodward JE, Caillier SJ, McElroy JP, Gomez R, Pando MJ, Clendenen LE, Ganusova EE, Schilkey FD, Ramaraj T, Khan OA, Huntley JJ, Luo S, Kwok PY, Wu TD, Schroth GP, Oksenberg JR, Hauser SL, Kingsmore SF: Genome, epigenome and RNA sequences of monozygotic twins discordant for multiple sclerosis. Nature 2010, 464:1351-1356.

39. Shahbazian MD, Antalffy B, Armstrong DL, Zoghbi HY: Insight into Rett syndrome: MeCP2 levels display tissue- and cell-specific differences and correlate with neuronal maturation. Hum Mol Genet 2002, 11:115-124.

40. Guy J, Gan J, Selfridge J, Cobb S, Bird A: Reversal of neurological defects in a mouse model of Rett syndrome. Science 2007, 315:1143-1147.

41. Guy J, Herndrich B, Hormes M Martinc JE, Bird A: A mouse Mecp2-null mutation causes neurological symptoms that mimic Rett syndrome. Nat Genet 2001, 27:322-326.

42. Kondo M, Gray LJ, Pelka GJ, Christodoulou J, Tam PP, Hannan AJ: Environmental enrichment ameliorates a motor coordination deficit in a mouse model of Rett syndrome--Mecp2 gene dosage effects and BDNF expression. Eur J Neurosci 2008, 27:3342-3350.

43. Nag N, Moriuchi JM, Peitzman CG, Ward BC, Kolodny NH, Berger-Sweeney JE: Environmental enrichment alters locomotor behaviour and ventricular volume in Mecp2 1lox mice. Behav Brain Res 2009, 196:44-48.

44. Kerr B, Silva PA, Walz K, Young JI: Unconventional transcriptional response to environmental enrichment in a mouse model of Rett syndrome. PLoS One 2010, 5:e11534.

45. Lonetti G, Angelucci A, Morando L, Boggio EM, Giustetto M, Pizzorusso T: Early environmental enrichment moderates the behavioral and synaptic phenotype of MeCP2 null mice. Biol Psychiatry 2010, 67:657-665.

46. Ushijima T: Detection and interpretation of altered methylation patterns in cancer cells. Nat Rev Cancer 2005, 5:223-231.

47. Feinberg AP: Phenotypic plasticity and the epigenetics of human disease. Nature 2007, 447:433-440.

48. Lillycrop KA, Phillips ES, Jackson AA, Hanson MA, Burdge GC: Dietary protein restriction of pregnant rats induces and folic acid supplementation prevents epigenetic modification of hepatic gene expression in the offspring. J Nutr 2005, 135:1382-1386.

49. Kucharski R, Maleszka J, Foret S, Maleszka R: Nutritional control of reproductive status in haneybees via DNA methylation. Science 2008, 319:1827-1830.

50. Lillycrop KA, Slater-Jefferies JL, Hanson MA, Godfrey KM, Jackson AA, Burdge GC: Induction of altered epigenetic regulation of the hepatic glucocorticoid receptor in the offspring of rats fed a protein-restricted diet during pregnancy suggests that reduced DNA methyltransferase-1 expression is involved in impaired DNA methylation and changes in histone modifications. Br J Nutr 2007, 97:1064-1073.

51. Tsankova NM, Berton O, Renthal W, Kumar A, Neve RL, Nestler EJ: Sustained hippocampal chromatin regulation in a mouse model of depression and antidepressant action. Nat Neurosci 2006, 9:519-525.

52. Jessberger S, Nakashima K, Clemenson GD Jr, Mejia E, Mathews E, Ure K, Ogawa S, Sinton CM, Gage FH, Hsieh J: Epigenetic modulation of seizure-induced neurogenesis and cognitive decline. J Neurosci 2007, 27:5967-5975.

53. Dong E, Nelson M, Grayson DR, Costa E, Guidotti A: Clozapine and sulpiride but not haloperidol or olanzapine activate brain DNA demethylation. Proc Natl Acad Sci USA 2008, 105:13614-13619.

54. Dong E, Chen Y, Gavin DP, Grayson DR, Guidotti A: Valproate induces DNA demethylation in nuclear extracts from adult mouse brain. Epigenetics 2010, 5:730-735.

55. Wang Q, Xu X, Li J, Liu J, Gu H, Zhang R, Chenv J, Kuang Y, Fei J, Jiang C, Wang P, Pei D, Ding S, Xie X: Lithium, an anti-psychotic drug, greatly enhances the generation of induced pluripotent stem cells. Cell Res 2011. doi: 10.1038/cr.2011.108

56. Ma DK, Jang MH, Guo JU, Kitabatake Y, Chang ML, Pow-Anpongkul N, Flavell RA, Lu B, Ming GL, Song H: Neuronal activity-induced Gadd45b promotes epigenetic DNA demethylation and adult neurogenesis. Science 2009, 323:1074-1077.

57. Fraga MF, Ballestar E, Paz MF, Ropero S, Setien F, Ballestar ML, Heine-Suñer D, Cigudosa JC, Urioste M, Benitez J, Boix-Chornet M, Sanchez-Aguilera A, Ling C, Carlsson E, Poulsen P, Vaag A, Stephan Z, Spector TD, Wu YZ, Plass C, Esteller M: Epigenetic differences arise during the lifetime of monozygotic twins. Proc Natl Acad Sci USA 2005, 102:10604-10609.

58. Horsthemke B: Heritable germline epimutations in humans. Nat Genet 2007 39:573-574.

59. Daxinger L, Whitelaw E: Transgenerational epigenetic inheritance: more questions than answers. Genome Res 2010, 20:1623-1628.

60. Rakyan VK, Chong S, Champ ME, Cuthbert PC, Morgan HD, Luu KV, Whitelaw E: Transgenerational inheritance of epigenetic states at the murine Axin(Fu) allele occurs after maternal and paternal transmission. Proc Natl Acad Sci USA 2003, 100:2538-2543.

61. Seong KH, Li D, Shimizu H, Nakamura R, Ishii S: Inheritance of stress-induced, ATF-2-dependent epigenetic change. Cell 2011, 145:1049-1061.

62. Franklin TB, Russig H, Weiss IC, Gräff J, Linder N, Michalon A, Vizi S, Mansuy IM: Epigenetic transmission of the impact of early stress across generations. Biol Psychiatry 2010, 68:408-415.

63. Weiss IC, Franklin TB, Vizi S, Mansuy IM: Inheritable effect of unpredictable maternal separation on behavioral responses in mice. Front Behav Neurosci 2011, 5:3.

64. Thayer ZM, Kuzawa CW: Biological memories of past environments: epigenetic pathways to health disparities. Epigenetics 2011, 6:798-803.

65. Arai JA, Feig LA: Long-lasting and transgenerational effects of an environmental enrichment on memory formation. Brain Res Bull 2011, 85:30-35.

66. Sakazume S, Ohashi H, Sasaki Y, Harada N, Nakanishi K, Sato H, Emi M, Endoh K, Sohma R, Kido Y, Nagai T, Kubota T: Spread of X-chromosome inactivation into chromosome 15 is associated with Prader-Willi syndrome phenotype in a boy with a t(X;15)(p21.1;q11.2) translocation. Hum Genet 2011.

67. Breitling LP, Yang R, Korn B, Burwinkel B, Brenner H: Tobacco-smoking-related differential DNA methylation: 27K discovery and replication. Am J Hum Genet 2011, 88:450-457.

68. Burdge GC, Lillycrop KA, Phillips ES, Slater-Jefferies JL, Jackson AA, Hanson MA: Folic acid supplementation during the juvenile-pubertal period in rats modifies the phenotype and epigenotype induced by prenatal nutrition. J Nutr 2009, 139:1054-1060.

69. Junaid MA, Kuizon S, Cardona J, Azher T, Murakami N, Pullarkat RK, Brown WT: Folic acid supplementation dysregulates gene expression in lymphoblastoid cells - Implications in nutrition. Biochem Biophys Res Commun 2011, 412:688-692.

70. Rimland B: Controversies in the treatment of autistic children: vitamin and drug therapy. J Child Neurol 1988, 3(Suppl):S68-72.

71. James SJ, Cutler P, Melnyk S, Jernigan S, Janak L, Gaylor DW, Neubrander JA: Metabolic biomarkers of increased oxidative stress and impaired methylation capacity in children with autism. Am J Clin Nutr 2004, 20:1611-1617.

72. Moretti P, Sahoo T, Hyland K, Bottiglieri T, Peters S, del Gaudio D, Roa B, Curry S, Zhu H, Finnell RH, Neul JL, Ramaekers VT, Blau N, Bacino CA, Miller G, Scaglia F: Cerebral folate deficiency with developmental delay, autism, and response to folinic acid. Neurology 2005, 64:1088-1090.

73. Ohtsuki A, Kimura MT, Minoshima M, Suzuki T, Ikeda M, Bando T, Nagase H, Shinohara K, Sugiyama H: Synthesis and properties of PI polyamide-SAHA conjugate. Tetrahedron Lett 2009, 50:7288-7292.

74. Matsuda H, Fukuda N, Ueno T, Katakawa M, Wang X, Watanabe T, Matsui S, Aoyama T, Saito K, Bando T, Matsumoto Y, Nagase H, Matsumoto K, Sugiyama H: Transcriptional inhibition of progressive renal disease by gene silencing pyrrole-imidazole polyamide targeting of the transforming growth factor-β1 promoter. Kidney Int 2011, 79:46-56.

75. Sebat J, Lakshmi B, Malhotra D, Troge J, Lese-Martin C, Walsh T, Yamrom B, Yoon S, Krasnitz A, Kendall J, Leotta A, Pai D, Zhang R, Lee YH, Hicks J, Spence SJ, Lee AT, Puura K, Lehtimäki T, Ledbetter D, Gregersen PK, Bregman J, Sutcliffe JS, Jobanputra V, Chung W, Warburton D, King MC, Skuse D, Geschwind DH, Gilliam TC, Ye K, Wigler M: Strong association of de novo copy number mutations with autism. Science 2007, 316:445-449.

76. Glessner JT, Wang K, Cai G, Korvatska O, Kim CE, Wood S, Zhang H, Estes A, Brune CW, Bradfield JP, Imielinski M, Frackelton EC, Reichert J, Crawford EL, Munson J, Sleiman PM, Chiavacci R, Annaiah K, Thomas K, Hou C, Glaberson W, Flory J, Otieno F, Garris M, Soorya L, Klei L, Piven J, Meyer KJ, Anagnostou E, Sakurai T, Game RM, Rudd DS, Zurawiecki D, McDougle CJ, Davis LK, Miller J, Posey DJ, Michaels S, Kolevzon A, Silverman JM, Bernier R, Levy SE, Schultz RT, Dawson G, Owley T, McMahon WM, Wassink TH, Sweeney JA, Nurnberger JI, Coon H, Sutcliffe JS, Minshew NJ, Grant SF, Bucan M, Cook EH, Buxbaum JD, Devlin B, Schellenberg GD, Hakonarson H: Autism genome-wide copy number variation reveals ubiquitin and neuronal genes. Nature 2009, 459:569-573.
77. Eapen V: Genetic basis of autism: is there a way forward? Curr Opin Psychiatry 2011, 24:226-236.

CHAPTER 12

AN IMPRINTED RHEUMATOID ARTHRITIS METHYLOME SIGNATURE REFLECTS PATHOGENIC PHENOTYPE

JOHN W. WHITAKER, ROBERT SHOEMAKER, DAVID L. BOYLE, JOSH HILLMAN, DAVID ANDERSON, WEI WANG, AND GARY S. FIRESTEIN

12.1 BACKGROUND

RA is a chronic inflammatory disease marked by synovial hyperplasia and invasion into cartilage and bone. This process is mediated, in part, by cytokines like IL-1, IL-6, and TNF that activate a broad array of cell signaling mechanisms and leads to the release of destructive enzymes [1]. Fibroblast-like synoviocytes (FLS), which form the inner lining of the synovium, play an active role in joint destruction by invading intra-articular cartilage and other support structures of the joint [2]. These mesenchymal cells normally produce hyaluronic acid and other lubricants that facilitate joint movement and a low friction environment.

FLS display an aggressive phenotype in RA that persists in long-term culture [2,3]. These imprinted cells can migrate between joints and exhibit characteristics of locally invasive transformed cells [4]. The mechanism

This chapter was originally published under the Creative Commons Attribution License. Whitaker JW, Shoemaker R, Boyle DL, Hillman J, Anderson D, Wang W, and Firestein GS. An Imprinted Rheumatoid Arthritis Methylome Signature Reflects Pathogenic Phenotype. Genome Medicine 5,40 (2013). doi:10.1186/gm444

that contribute to functional alterations in RA FLS are only partially understood and include somatic mutations, alterations in cell survival and apoptosis genes, and persistent activation of signaling pathways [3]. Epigenetic changes, including aberrant miRNA expression [5], can also contribute to the aggressive RA FLS phenotype.

More recently, a characteristic DNA methylation signature that could affect cell function and distinguishes RA from osteoarthritis (OA) FLS was discovered [6]. Differentially methylated loci (DML) involve many key genes implicated in inflammation, immune responses, cell-cell interactions, and matrix regulation. The original study defining the RA methylation pattern was performed on a relatively limited number of cell lines and did not evaluate the stability of the signature over multiple passages. For the present analysis, we increased the number of OA and RA cell lines and included normal (NL) synoviocytes. The greater number of cells permitted a focused evaluation of promoter sequences and a more detailed pathway analysis. The results demonstrate a pattern of differentially methylated pathways in RA FLS that define pathogenic processes that could permit identification of novel therapeutic targets.

12.2 METHODS

12.2.1 FLS AND PATIENT PHENOTYPE

FLS were isolated from synovial tissues obtained from 11 RA and 11 OA patients at the time of joint replacement as described previously [7]. The diagnosis of RA conformed to the American College of Rheumatology 1987 revised criteria [8]. The protocol was approved by the UCSD Human Subjects Research Protection Program. Synoviocytes were used from passage 3 through 7, when FLS were a homogeneous population with < 1% CD11b, < 1% phagocytic, and < 1% FcR II positive cells. Normal human synoviocytes were provided by the San Diego Tissue Bank from autopsy specimens. Preparation of the genomic DNA from early, middle, and late passage cells (passages 3, 5, and 7, respectively) for the Infinium

HumanMethylation450 BeadChip (Illumina; San Diego, CA) and calculation of methylation frequencies (Beta values) was performed as previously reported [6]. The BeadChip data from the original 11 samples in reference 6 are available through the Gene Expression Omnibus (GEO) under the accession [GSE46364].

12.2.2 BEADCHIP PROCESSING AND VALIDATION

BeadChip data were processed in R 2.15 using the methylumi and minfi packages. Data were normalized via the minfi package (preprocessIllumina function). CpGs with detection P values > 0.001 were filtered out. For chip validation, biologic replicates within chips were performed and demonstrated a mean correlation coefficient $r^2 = 0.9338$. Replicates between chips demonstrated a mean correlation coefficient $r^2 = 0.9858$. Regarding potential performance differences between Infinium I and II probes on the BeadChip, we reasoned that since CpGs were tested independently, probe type-specific bias would be equally present in both phenotype populations. Therefore, the risk of false-positive detection due to probe-type differences is low.

12.2.3 METHYLATION HEAT MAPS AND HISTOGRAMS

Methylation frequencies of previously identified RA-OA differentially methylated CpGs [6] across FLS samples were multiplied by 100 to obtain values interpreted as methylation percentages. The Euclidian distances between FLS samples and CpGs were calculated and hierarchically clustered using complete linkage. The results were visualized in a heat map using the heatmap.2 function in the gplots R package as previously described [6]. Missing values were represented with a white color. For each FLS cell line, beta value differences of the previously identified 1,859 CpG signature between passages were calculated and plotted as histograms with bins for every 0.01 interval. The bar areas were normalized so that their total sum equaled unity.

12.2.4 CORRELATIONS BETWEEN FLS PASSAGE NUMBER

The FLS lines were experimentally processed the same day across three BeadChips. This approach minimized intra-dataset (that is, KEGG and passage FLS datasets) batch effects like BeadChip lot, reagent lot, lab processing, or temporal variability). The tight hierarchical clustering of P5 FLS samples across the KEGG and passage datasets demonstrates that inter-dataset batch effects are minor relative to the RA methylation signature (see Results). Furthermore, validation studies of duplicate samples on the same BeadChip, on different BeadChips, or performed on different runs showed very strong correlations (data not shown). For each cell line, the Spearman Rank correlation of beta values of the previously identified 1,859 CpG signatures was calculated across passages. For each pairwise correlation calculation, CpGs with missing data were omitted. For the correlation between replicates of passage 5 comparisons were made within the same cell line. To estimate passage correlation, the Spearman correlation coefficients between passage 5 and the other passages were calculated per cell line. An average was calculated based on these correlation coefficients.

12.2.5 IDENTIFYING DIFFERENTIALLY METHYLATED GENES (DMGS)

A Welch's t-test was used to calculate the significance of differential methylation. We chose to apply Welch's t-test as the samples may have unequal variance. All loci that are present on the array were tested and the resulting P values were converted into q values [9]. Additionally, the average difference in mean values at each position was calculated. Loci with q values < 0.05 and average mean differences > 0.1, or < -0.1, were labelled as differential methylated loci (DML). Missing values and values with detection P values > 0.01 were not included in this analysis. At a specific locus, if values were absent but at least three values present, for each of the two groups being considered, then comparison was made between only the existing values. If there were less than three values present in a single group, at a specific locus, then this locus was ignored from the analysis. The DMLs within the promoters of genes were identified and the DMLs were linked to the corresponding genes. The locations of refseq genes were obtained from the University of California, Santa Cruz. If a promoter contained one or more DMLs within a 3 kb window around a gene's transcription start site (TSS) (-2500 bps to +500 bps from the TSS) then the gene was labelled as a DMG.

The significance of DMG in 271 KEGG human pathways was assessed [10]. Enrichment factors (EF) were calculated as:

EF = (total DMGs in pathway / total genes in pathway)/(total DMGs/total genes in KEGG)

The "total genes in the pathway" and "total genes in KEGG" only considered genes that are present in a KEGG pathway and are covered by the BeadChip.

The hypergeometric distribution was used to calculate enrichment P values that were converted into q values. Resulting q values represented the fraction of randomly selected background gene sets that were at least as enriched in genes found in the tested pathway as the DMG set. A q value threshold of 0.05 determined significance. The significance of 34,449 GO categories was tested in the same way. The background for the GO analysis included all the genes whose promoters are covered by the methylation array and that are present in the GO database.

12.3 RESULTS

12.3.1 STABILITY OF THE METHYLOME SIGNATURE IN RA FLS

We previously identified a methylome signature in RA comprised of 1,859 DML and predicts the phenotype of passage 5 FLS (RA vs. OA). One critical question to answer before performing additional pathway analysis with more cell lines is whether this signature is stable. Therefore, we assayed

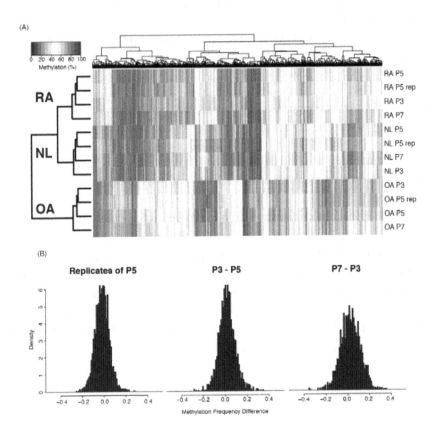

FIGURE 1: The RA methylome signature is stable over passages. (A) Hierarchical clustering RA, OA, and NL samples at P3, P5, and P7. Each column shows the methylation level at one of the 1,859 DML. Additionally, samples from P5 of Nakano et al. 2012 are shown as reference and are labeled as rep. (B) The distribution of the difference in beta values between passages for RA sample.

the methylomes of nine FLS cell lines (three RA, three OA, and three NL) at the 3rd, 5th, and 7th passage (P3, P5, and P7, respectively). Passage 3 cells were the earliest samples evaluated because passage 1 and 2 lines can include other cell types. By the 3rd passage, FLS are a homogeneous population of cells (< 1% CD11b positive, < 1% phagocytic, and < 1% FcR II and FcR III receptor positive) [2].

We first performed hierarchical clustering of RA, OA, and NL samples from the three passages. In addition, we included P5 samples from our previous study as an internal biological sample control. The RA, OA, and NL groups clustered separately at all passages, confirming that the RA methylome signature is stable over many passages (see Figure 1A for representative examples). Of note, the replicates of P5 clustered very closely and were also only slightly different from the other passages.

To further explore the stability of the RA methylome signature over time, we considered the difference in methylation percentages between different passages and the replicates of P5. Figure 1B shows that variation between replicates of P5 is comparable to the variation between P5-P3 and P5-P7. The correlation across the nine cell lines between P5 replicates is 0.950 while the correlation between P3-P5 is 0.943. These data show that P3 and P5 are as highly correlated as replicates of the same passage and that there is very little change in the methylation frequencies between P3 and P5. There is a slight decrease in correlation between P3 to P7 (0.883) as the cells approach senescence.

12.3.2 DETERMINATION OF DIFFERENTIALLY METHYLATED GENES IN RA FLS

Having confirmed that the RA methylome signature is stable we then investigated its relationship with clinical phenotype on a systems level. Previously, we had carried out KEGG and GO analysis on a limited set of samples (six RA and five OA FLS lines). We have advanced on this previous analysis by increasing the sample size to 11 RA and 11 OA and adding six NL lines. The increased number of samples from 11 to 28 allowed us to focus on the subset of DMLs within the gene promoters (-2500 to +500 bps from the TSS). DMLs were identified by calculating P values using

Welch's t test. Then the resulting P values were corrected for multiple testing to produce q values. Genes that contain DMLs within their promoters were labeled DMGs. An average mean difference of 0.1 or greater was required for a DML to be considered significant.

Identification of DMGs was carried out by comparing the RA samples to five combinations of OA and NL: "RA vs. OA," "RA vs. NL," "RA vs. OA+NL" (which combines the OA and NL databases), "RA vs. OA or NL" (which includes DMGs that are significant in either RA vs. OA or RA vs. NL) and "RA vs. (OA or NL) or (OA+NL)" (denoted as "combined"). We focused on comparisons that take account of both OA and NL as these are of greatest relevance to differentiating RA phenotype from non-RA. Furthermore, smaller NL sample size identified a reduced set of DMGs making this set of DMGs unsuitable for systems level analysis.

A summary of the number of genes identified in each of the comparisons is shown in Table 1 (for a full list of genes, see Supplemental Table 1). The majority (90%) of the 2,375 total genes identified (the combined) as DMGs were identified solely by comparison of RA and OA.

TABLE 1: A summary of the number of DMGs, pathways, and GO terms identified as significant

	Combined	OA+NL	OA or NL
DMGs	2,375	472	2,346
KEGG	20	19	25
GO	43	546	40

The sets were defined through the following comparisons: 'combined' combines the sets from the other two comparisons; "OA+NL" compares RA with a combined RA and NL database; "OA or NL" includes DMGs that are significant in either "RA vs. OA" or "RA vs. NL." A complete list of DMGs is provided in Additional file 1. DMGs: differentially methylated genes.

12.3.3 DETERMINATION OF DIFFERENTIALLY METHYLATED KEGG PATHWAYS IN RA FLS

Having established sets of DMGs, we identified the biological pathways and gene ontologies that were enriched within the sets. To identify enriched pathways, the DMGs where mapped to the KEGG pathways and GO databases. Enrichment P values were then calculated using the hypergeometric distribution. Then these P values were corrected for multiple testing to produce q values. A q values cut-off of < 0.05 was considered significant.

A summary of the total number of significant KEGG pathways and GO categories that were found significant is given in Table 2. The 221 additional DMGs that are included in the Combined set have a significant effect on KEGG pathway enrichment and result in 13 additional pathways identified as significantly enriched compared with the previous published analysis on a limited dataset.

TABLE 2: KEGG pathways that enriched with genes that contain DML within their promoters

Comparison name	Combined		OA+NL		OA or NL	
Comparison description	RA vs (OA or NL) or (OA+NL)		RA vs OA+NL		RA vs OA or NL	
Pathway name	EF (q-value)	# of DMGs (%)	EF (q-value)	# of DMGs (%)	EF (q-value)	# of DMGs (%)
Rheumatoid arthritis	2.5 (0.00266)	24 (27.0)	6.5 (1.91e-05)	12 (13.5)	2.3 (0.00467)	22 (24.7)
NOD-like receptor signaling pathway	2.5 (0.00741)	16 (27.6)	5.8 (0.0014)	7 (12.1)	2.3 (0.0374)	14 (24.1)
Cell adhesion molecules (CAMs)	1.8 (0.0294)	25 (19.4)	3.0 (0.0232)	8 (6.2)	1.8 (0.0343)	25 (19.4)
Focal adhesion	1.6 (0.0287)	35 (17.6)			1.6 (0.0321)	35 (17.6)
Cytosolic DNA-sensing pathway			4.6 (0.0202)	5 (9.6)		

TABLE 2: *Cont.*

Comparison name	Combined		OA+NL		OA or NL	
Comparison description	RA vs (OA or NL) or (OA+NL)		RA vs OA+NL		RA vs OA or NL	
Pathway name	EF (q-value)	# of DMGs (%)	EF (q-value)	# of DMGs (%)	EF (q-value)	# of DMGs (%)
Cytokine-cytokine receptor interaction			2.3 (0.0231)	12 (4.8)		
Toll-like receptor signaling pathway	1.9 (0.0377)	19 (20.7)				
Complement and coagulation cascades	2.0 (0.0494)	15 (21.7)				
Staphylococcus aureus infection	2.9 (0.00379)	16 (31.4)	4.7 (0.019)	5 (9.8)	2.9 (0.00457)	16 (31.4)
Graft-versus-host disease	2.7 (0.0211)	11 (29.7)	10.4 (2.66e-05)	8 (21.6)	2.5 (0.0468)	10 (27.0)
Allograft rejection	2.6 (0.031)	10 (28.6)	9.6 (0.000159)	7 (20.0)	2.7 (0.0389)	10 (28.6)
Leishmaniasis	2.0 (0.0451)	15 (22.1)	4.9 (0.00304)	7 (10.3)	2.1 (0.048)	15 (22.1)
Toxoplasmosis	1.7 (0.0435)	24 (18.8)	3.4 (0.00759)	9 (7.0)	1.7 (0.046)	24 (18.8)
Viral myocarditis	2.6 (0.00392)	19 (27.9)			2.6 (0.00457)	19 (27.9)
Dilated cardiomyopathy	2.3 (0.00489)	22 (24.7)			2.3 (0.00467)	22 (24.7)
Hypertrophic cardiomyopathy (HCM)	2.3 (0.00487)	21 (25.3)			2.2 (0.00904)	20 (24.1)
Aldosterone-regulated sodium reabsorption	2.8 (0.00761)	13 (31.0)			2.9 (0.00814)	13 (31.0)
Influenza A	1.7 (0.0308)	29 (18.4)	4.0 (0.000283)	13 (8.2)		
Type II diabetes mellitus	2.5 (0.0185)	13 (27.7)			2.6 (0.0203)	13 (27.7)

TABLE 2: *Cont.*

Comparison name	Combined		OA+NL		OA or NL	
Comparison description	RA vs (OA or NL) or (OA+NL)		RA vs OA+NL		RA vs OA or NL	
Pathway name	EF (q-value)	# of DMGs (%)	EF (q-value)	# of DMGs (%)	EF (q-value)	# of DMGs (%)
Carbohydrate digestion and absorption	2.6 (0.0225)	12 (27.9)			2.4 (0.0474)	11 (25.6)
Type I diabetes mellitus			8.2 (0.000269)	7 (17.1)		
Asthma			10.3 (0.000274)	6 (21.4)		
Tuberculosis			3.8 (0.000386)	13 (7.9)		
Antigen processing and presentation			5.7 (0.000668)	8 (11.9)		
Phagosome			3.7 (0.00131)	11 (7.7)		
Autoimmune thyroid disease			6.9 (0.00152)	6 (14.3)		
Intestinal immune network for IgA production			6.3 (0.00233)	6 (13.0)		
Chagas disease (American trypanosomiasis)	2.0 (0.0206)	22 (21.4)				
Prion diseases			5.5 (0.0246)	4 (11.4)		
African trypanosomiasis	2.6 (0.031)	10 (28.6)				

KEGG pathways that are found as significantly enriched (q < 0.05) in three comparisons are shown. Eight pathways especially relevant to RA are placed in the top part of the table. Within each section, the number of significant comparisons orders the pathways. If multiple pathways have the same number of comparison then an average q values is used for ordering. # denotes the number of DMGs in the selected pathway.

The enriched KEGG pathways out of a total of 271 pathways evaluated are summarized in Table 3 using the various groupings described above. The top ranked pathway is the KEGG "rheumatoid arthritis" pathway (see Figure 2) with 2.47-fold enrichment (P = 1.729e-05 and q = 0.0027) and 24 out of 89 genes identified as DMGs in the union set. This confirms that the observed alterations in DNA methylation are highly relevant to RA. Furthermore, eight additional immunological pathways relevant to RA were also identified as significantly enriched with DMGs in RA FLS. For example, KEGG "Complement and coagulation cascades" pathway (see Figure 3) is 1.99-fold enriched (P = 0.0064 and q = 0.0494) with 15 out of 69 genes labeled as DMGs in the union set. The KEGG "Focal Adhesion" pathway (see Figure 4) is 1.61-fold enriched (P = 0.0027 and q = 0.0420) with 35 out of 199 genes labeled as DMGs in the union set. The KEGG "Toll-like receptor signaling" pathway (see Figure 5) is 1.89-fold enriched (P = 0.0042 and q = 0.0377) with 19 out of 92 genes labeled as DMGs in the union set.

TABLE 3: Gene ontology terms that are enriched in two or more sets of genes

Comparison name		Combined		OA+NL		OA or NL	
Comparison description		RA vs OA or NL or OA+NL		RA vs OA+NL		RA vs OA or NL	
Pathway name	GO type	EF (q-value)	# of DMGs (%)	EF (q-value)	# of DMGs (%)	EF (q-value)	# of DMGs (%)
positive regulation of ERK1 and ERK2 cascade	BP	3.5 (0.000494)	18 (38.3)	9.0 (0.000111)	9 (19.1)	3.3 (0.00106)	17 (36.2)
proteinaceous extracellular matrix	CC	2.2 (7.07e-05)	48 (24.2)	3.3 (0.00287)	14 (7.1)	2.1 (0.000254)	46 (23.2)
signal transduction	BP	1.4 (0.000717)	174 (15.4)	1.5 (0.0263)	37 (3.3)	1.4 (0.000713)	172 (15.2)
extracellular matrix	CC	2.3 (0.00282)	30 (25.0)	2.3 (0.0441)	6 (5.0)	2.3 (0.00192)	30 (25.0)
inflammatory response	BP	1.8 (0.00821)	45 (20.1)	2.3 (0.0301)	11 (4.9)	1.8 (0.0106)	44 (19.6)

TABLE 3: *Cont.*

Comparison name		Combined		OA+NL		OA or NL	
Comparison description		RA vs OA or NL or OA+NL		RA vs OA+NL		RA vs OA or NL	
Pathway name	GO type	EF (q-value)	# of DMGs (%)	EF (q-value)	# of DMGs (%)	EF (q-value)	# of DMGs (%)
fibroblast growth factor receptor signaling'	BP	9.1 (0.02)	4 (100.0)	23.5 (0.0176)	2 (50.0)	9.2 (0.0177) 4 (100.0)	
MHC class II protein complex	CC	4.5 (0.0346)	7 (50.0)	20.1 (9.47e-05)	6 (42.9)	4.6 (0.0303)	7 (50.0)
focal adhesion	CC	2.1 (0.0176)	26 (23.6)	2.6 (0.0418)	6 (5.5)	2.2 (0.0136)	26 (23.6)
Rho guanyl-nucleotide exchange factor activity	MF	2.3 (0.0443)	18 (25.4)	3.3 (0.0375)	5 (7.0)	2.3 (0.0377)	18 (25.4)
regulation of Rho protein signal transduction	BP	2.3 (0.0481)	18 (25.0)	3.3 (0.038)	5 (6.9)	2.3 (0.0412)	18 (25.0)
positive regulation of inflammatory response	BP	3.3 (0.0173)	12 (36.4)			3.3 (0.0141)	12 (36.4)
cell adhesion	BP	1.4 (0.0425)	84 (15.7)			1.4 (0.0404)	83 (15.5)
extracellular region	CC	1.6 (2.4e-13)	306 (17.2)	1.8 (0.000356)	67 (3.8)	1.6 (4.11e-13)	302 (16.9)
extracellular space	CC	1.6 (2.91e-06)	133 (18.1)	2.2 (0.000971)	34 (4.6)	1.6 (7.7e-06)	130 (17.7)
immune response	BP	1.9 (0.000153)	64 (21.0)	3.1 (0.000722)	20 (6.6)	1.9 (0.000352)	62 (20.3)
plasma membrane	CC	1.3 (4.6e-08)	467 (14.3)	1.4 (0.00269)	99 (3.0)	1.3 (6.35e-08)	461 (14.1)
Z disc	CC	3.5 (0.00133)	16 (38.1)	5.6 (0.0161)	5 (11.9)	3.5 (0.00099)	16 (38.1)
scavenger receptor activity	MF	3.5 (0.00104)	16 (39.0)	4.6 (0.0327)	4 (9.8)	3.6 (0.000814)	16 (39.0)
odontogenesis	BP	4.2 (0.00175)	12 (46.2)	5.4 (0.0374)	3 (11.5)	4.2 (0.00132)	12 (46.2)
integral to plasma membrane	CC	1.4 (0.00501)	149 (15.2)	1.6 (0.0271)	33 (3.4)	1.4 (0.0102)	145 (14.8)

TABLE 3: *Cont.*

Comparison name		Combined		OA+NL		OA or NL	
Comparison description		RA vs OA or NL or OA+NL		RA vs OA+NL		RA vs OA or NL	
Pathway name	GO type	EF (q-value)	# of DMGs (%)	EF (q-value)	# of DMGs (%)	EF (q-value)	# of DMGs (%)
multicellular organismal development	BP	1.5 (0.000606)	143 (16.1)	1.4 (0.0435)	27 (3.0)	1.5 (0.000332)	143 (16.1)
structural molecule activity	MF	1.9 (0.00594)	42 (20.9)	2.1 (0.0414)	9 (4.5)	1.9 (0.0041)	42 (20.9)
positive regulation of cell proliferation	BP	1.6 (0.019)	58 (17.8)	2.9 (0.00105)	20 (6.2)	1.6 (0.0315)	56 (17.2)
positive regulation of interferon-gamma production	BP	3.2 (0.0439)	10 (35.7)	10.1 (0.00104)	6 (21.4)	3.3 (0.0383)	10 (35.7)
skeletal muscle contraction	BP	5.5 (0.0292)	6 (60.0)	9.4 (0.0378)	2 (20.0)	5.5 (0.0256)	6 (60.0)
sarcolemma	CC	2.5 (0.0352)	17 (27.0)	3.7 (0.0326)	5 (7.9)	2.5 (0.0296)	17 (27.0)
structural constituent of muscle	MF	2.7 (0.0487)	13 (29.5)	4.3 (0.0353)	4 (9.1)	2.7 (0.0423)	13 (29.5)
actin binding	MF	1.6 (0.0497)	49 (17.5)	2.0 (0.0373)	12 (4.3)	1.6 (0.0404)	49 (17.5)
myeloid cell differentiation	BP	4.2 (0.0456)	7 (46.7)	6.3 (0.0434)	2 (13.3)	4.3 (0.0403)	7 (46.7)
sarcomere	CC	3.3 (0.00145)	17 (36.2)			3.3 (0.00106)	17 (36.2)
skin morphogenesis	BP	9.1 (0.0036)	5 (100.0)			9.2 (0.00292)	5 (100.0)
potassium channel regulator activity	MF	3.8 (0.0172)	10 (41.7)			3.8 (0.0141)	10 (41.7)
response to organic cyclic compound	BP	2.2 (0.0177)	25 (24.0)	3.2 (0.0274)	7 (6.7)		

TABLE 3: *Cont.*

Comparison name		Combined		OA+NL		OA or NL	
Comparison description		RA vs OA or NL or OA+NL		RA vs OA+NL		RA vs OA or NL	
Pathway name	GO type	EF (q-value)	# of DMGs (%)	EF (q-value)	# of DMGs (%)	EF (q-value)	# of DMGs (%)
response to mechanical stimulus	BP	2.8 (0.0383)	13 (31.0)	5.6 (0.0161)	5 (11.9)		
response to glucocorticoid stimulus	BP	2.3 (0.0306)	20 (25.3)	3.6 (0.0273)	6 (7.6)		
response to prostaglandin E stimulus	BP	6.5 (0.0313)	5 (71.4)			6.6 (0.0277)	5 (71.4)
regulation of muscle contraction	BP	5.0 (0.0433)	6 (54.5)			5.0 (0.0383)	6 (54.5)
epidermis development	BP	2.2 (0.0448)	19 (24.7)	3.0 (0.0402)	5 (6.5)		
ion transport	BP	1.4 (0.0437)	84 (15.7)			1.4 (0.0415)	83 (15.5)
PR of GMSFP'	BP	7.3 (0.0493)	4 (80.0)			7.4 (0.0441)	4 (80.0)
troponin complex	CC	5.7 (0.0495)	5 (62.5)			5.7 (0.0442)	5 (62.5)
phosphatase binding	MF	5.7 (0.0495)	5 (62.5)			5.7 (0.0442)	5 (62.5)

GO categories that are significantly enriched (q < 0.05) during three comparisons are shown. Twelve pathways especially relevant to RA are placed in the top part of the table while other pathways are show at the bottom. Within each section, the number of significant comparisons orders the pathways. If multiple GO categories are significantly enriched in the same number of comparison then an average q values is used for ordering. Only GO categories found as significantly enriched in three or more comparisons are shown. # denotes the number of DMGs in the selected pathway. The GO category "positive regulation of granulocyte macrophage colony-stimulating factor production" is abbreviated to 'PR of GMSFP' and category 'regulation of fibroblast growth factor receptor signaling pathway' is abbreviated to "fibroblast growth factor receptor signaling." The GO types stand for: BP: biological process; CC: cellular component; MF: molecular function.

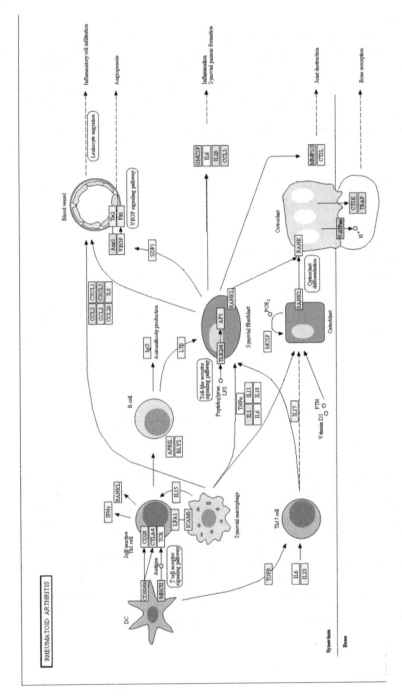

FIGURE 2: DMGs in the KEGG RA pathway. The methylation status at the promoters of genes within the pathway is shown.

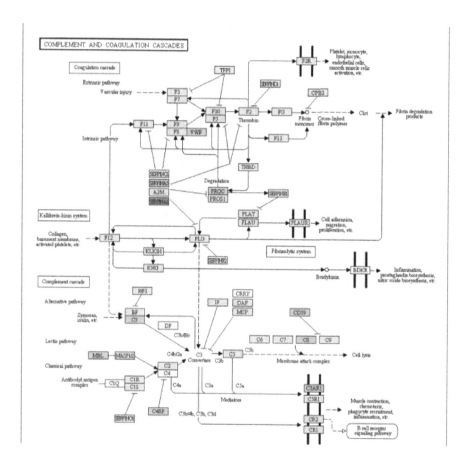

FIGURE 3: DMGs in the KEGG "Complement and coagulation cascades" pathway. The methylation status at the promoters of genes within the pathway is shown.

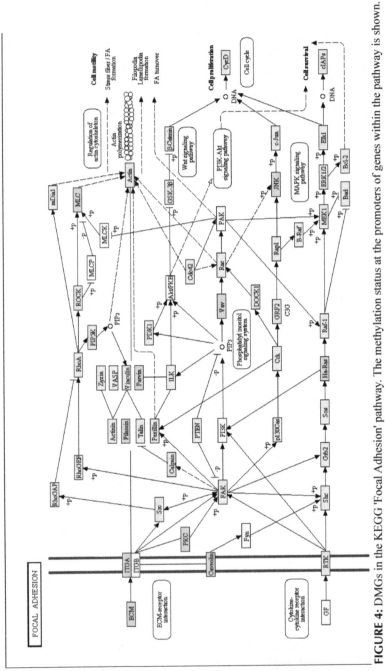

FIGURE 4: DMGs in the KEGG 'Focal Adhesion' pathway. The methylation status at the promoters of genes within the pathway is shown.

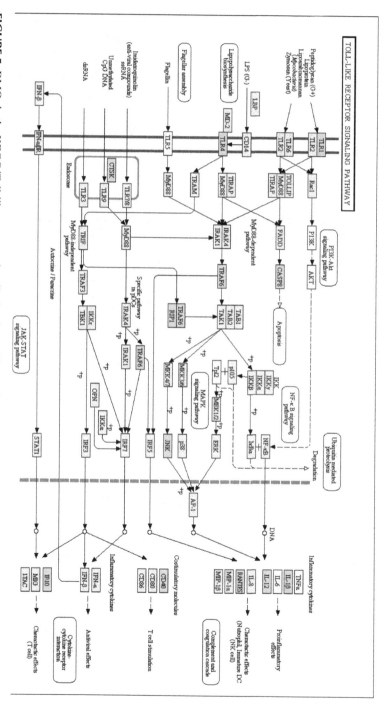

FIGURE 5: DMGs in the KEGG 'Toll-like receptor signaling' pathway. The methylation status at the promoters of genes within the pathway is shown.

Certain KEGG pathways and GO categories are significantly enriched in "OA+NL" or "OA or NL" but are not significantly enriched in "combined." This can occur because the increase in the total number of significant genes can affect the enrichment of a subset of genes within a particular pathway. For example, the KEGG pathway "cytosolic DNA sensing" is significantly enriched in "OA+NL" but not in combined despite the "OA+NL" containing five DMGs in the pathway whereas 'combined' contains eight. This occurs because the total number of DMGs increases from 472 in "OA+NL" to 2,375 in "combined."

12.3.4 DETERMINATION OF DIFFERENTIALLY METHYLATED GO PATHWAYS IN RA FLS

The enriched GO categories out of the full 34,449 category dataset are summarized in Table 4 where 10 categories especially relevant to RA are listed at the top of the table. Of particular interest is the overlap with KEGG because of the preponderance of matrix, adhesion, and signaling GO categories.

12.4 DISCUSSION

Fibroblast-like synoviocytes (FLS), which form the synovial intimal lining, play an integral role in the pathogenesis of RA by producing cytokines, small molecule mediators, and proteases [1]. The FLS are responsible for cartilage damage by virtue of their ability to adhere to and invade the cartilage extracellular matrix [11]. Rheumatoid FLS exhibit a unique aggressive phenotype that contributes to the cytokine milieu and joint destruction [12]. Functional studies suggest that RA cells are imprinted in situ and maintain these features after many passages in tissue culture. For example, RA FLS, unlike OA or NL synoviocytes, invade cartilage explants in SCID mice [13]. RA FLS can grow under anchorage-independent conditions, are less susceptible to contact inhibition, and resistant to apoptosis [14,15].

DNA methylation could play a critical role in joint damage by epigenetic imprinting FLS in RA. Evidence of abnormal methylation and a distinct methylation signature was recently described in RA synoviocytes [6]. Using a limited number of cell lines, hyper- and hypomethylated CpG sites were demonstrated in nearly 2,000 loci located in 1,200 genes. Methylation status determined by array analysis was confirmed by bisulfite sequencing and correlated with gene expression in that study. Additional analysis identified over 200 genes with multiple differentially methylated loci. Preliminary KEGG and GO analysis suggested that pathways involved with inflammation, matrix regulation, and immune responses are differentially methylated. The present study greatly expands upon the initial dataset by doubling the number of RA and OA FLS and adding normal FLS. The increased sample size also allowed us to focus our analysis on differentially methylated promoter sites. These data refined the KEGG and GO analysis and led to identification of additional key pathways implicated in disease.

Before extending our computational studies, we determined if the RA methylation signature is stable. Comparison of the methylation patterns between different passages of RA, OA, and NL FLS showed that the signature changes very little over time. These results correlate with previous studies demonstrating that the FLS transcriptome is also stable in culture [2,16]. By the 7th passage, a slight increase in methylation variability was detected, but the correlation was only slightly lower than between replicates of the same passage. Furthermore, the most significant methylation changes that may be associated with pathogenic processes appear to be very stable over time in FLS lines. These data suggest that the majority of the variation is a result of noise in the bead array assay.

Methylome stability has been observed with other long-term cultured cell lines. For instance, multiple passages of the cell lines IMR90 (human fetal lung fibroblast) and H1 (human embryonic stem cells) showed high concordance [17]. The methylome is not immutable, however, and can be modulated by the environment, different developmental stages [18], or prolonged tissue culture [19]. For example, dynamic changes in methylome occur in human embryonic stem cells, a fibroblastic differentiated derivative of the human embryonic stem cells, and neonatal fibroblasts.

Immortalized fibroblasts that evolve separately over 300 generations show stochastic methylation changes. Despite the random nature of changes, they resulted in a deterministic remodeling of the methylome that correlates with histone modification and CTCF binding.

The stability of the RA methylome signature from the earliest possible passage (P3) to cells approaching senescence (P7) suggests that it is imprinted in FLS rather than a transient phenomenon. However, it does not tell us the origin of the RA methylome signature. In particular, we are still unsure whether the imprinting predates disease, is brought about by interaction with the pre-RA synovium environment, or is modified by RA in a way that influences the behavior of FLS. Our recent study show that DNMT expression and function are suppressed in FLS when exposed to IL-1 [20]. However, this effect is transient and is reversed 2 weeks after the cytokine is removed from the cultures. Therefore, cytokines can potentially contribute to altered DNA methylation in FLS but probably do not account for the long-lasting effects. Evaluation of FLS from patients at high risk for RA but without clinical disease would be needed to resolve this issue with greater certainty. Also, specificity for RA, as opposed to other forms of inflammatory arthritis, will require evaluation of FLS from other forms of synovitis.

Systems level analysis of the RA methylome signature in our expanded dataset reveals that DMLs are highly enriched in the promoters of genes that belong to characteristic functional categories. Because we had three distinct cell populations, we used several different ways to evaluate how RA differed from OA and/or NL FLS. There were some differences in the genes and pathways that were differentially methylated depending on how the phenotypes were grouped. Relatively broad agreement among the various types of analyses was observed. The most gratifying was the RA pathway in the KEGG analysis, which was found in the three most robust comparisons and confirmed the relevance of our analysis to this disease.

We also found the enrichment of many pathways that are related to the RA phenotype and immune responses. The KEGG and GO analysis of differentially methylated pathways is, therefore, non-random and likely essential for establishment or maintenance of the RA FLS phenotype. Even many of the seemingly less relevant categories that were identified as enriched result from overlap in sets of genes that are shared with pathways that are more clearly relevant to RA. For example, the pathway 'Staphylococcus aureus infection' contains 16 DMGs; however, six of these are also present in the RA pathway.

The nature of the RA-associated pathways enriched in our KEGG and GO analysis provides clues regarding the pathogenesis of the disease. For example, the role of complement is well documented in animal studies [21]. This innate immune mechanism is also strongly implicated in the initiation and acute inflammatory reaction of RA [22]. Several complement components are produced by FLS in the intimal lining as well as cultured synoviocytes [23]. The pathway analysis indicates that regulation of complement is abnormal in addition to the fact that it is robustly consumed in the joints.

Altered methylation and, presumably, gene regulation in FLS is also observed for many other components of innate immunity. Notably, TLR, cytosolic DNA-sensing, and NOD-like receptor pathways are significantly enriched in the KEGG analysis for differentially methylated genes. Each pathway has been implicated as fundamental mechanisms that regulate the inflammatory response in RA [24-26]. Genes regulating innate immunity are emerging as potential therapeutic targets for RA, and the methylation data supports their participation in rheumatoid synovitis. Similarly, multiple cytokines are differentially methylated in the RA pathway and in the cytokine-cytokine receptor pathway, including TNF and other critical mediators of RA. Additional types of pathways involving inflammation, host defense, and immune responses are enriched in the GO analysis and are consistent with the insights gleaned from the KEGG pathways.

The data suggest that pathway analysis can provide other clues for disease pathogenesis and novel therapeutic interventions. For example, cell-cell and cell-matrix interactions are differentially methylated in the focal adhesion pathway and the cell adhesion molecule pathways. Several potential therapeutic targets are within these pathways and could be explored for diseases like RA. The specific genes that are differentially methylated are not necessarily the ones that should be the focus of drug development. Instead, more attractive proteins in the pathway that are more amenable to inhibition or modulation could be selected and achieve the same result.

12.5 CONCLUSIONS

An expanded dataset evaluating differentially methylated pathways confirmed the limited data and greatly extended the number of pathways that are enriched in RA. The relative stability of the signature was also demonstrated, supporting the notion that the cells are imprinted rather than merely reflecting transient cytokine effects. These data can provide insights into the pathogenesis of RA as well as identifying potential therapeutic targets.

REFERENCES

1. Firestein GS: Evolving concepts of rheumatoid arthritis. Nature 2003, 423:356-361.
2. Bartok B, Firestein GS: Fibroblast-like synoviocytes: key effector cells in rheumatoid arthritis. Immunol Rev 2010, 233:233-255.
3. Bottini N, Firestein GS: Duality of fibroblast-like synoviocytes in RA: passive responders and imprinted aggressors. Nat Rev Rheumatol 2013, 9:24-33.
4. Lefevre S, Knedla A, Tennie C, Kampmann A, Wunrau C, Dinser R, Korb A, Schnaker EM, Tarner IH, Robbins PD, Evans CH, Sturz H, Steinmeyer J, Gay S, Scholmerich J, Pap T, Muller-Ladner U, Neumann E: Synovial fibroblasts spread rheumatoid arthritis to unaffected joints. Nat Med 2009, 15:1414-1420.
5. Filkova M, Jungel A, Gay RE, Gay S: MicroRNAs in rheumatoid arthritis: potential role in diagnosis and therapy. BioDrugs 2012, 26:131-141.
6. Nakano K, Whitaker JW, Boyle DL, Wang W, Firestein GS: DNA methylome signature in rheumatoid arthritis. Ann Rheum Dis 2013, 72:110-117.
7. Rosengren S, Firestein GS, Boyle DL: Measurement of inflammatory biomarkers in synovial tissue extracts by enzyme-linked immunosorbent assay. Clin Diagn Lab Immunol 2003, 10:1002-1010.
8. Arnett FC, Edworthy SM, Bloch DA, McShane DJ, Fries JF, Cooper NS, Healey LA, Kaplan SR, Liang MH, Luthra HS, Medsger TA, Mitchell DM, Neustadt DH, Pinals RS, Schaller JG, Sharp JT, Wilder RL, Hunder GG: The American Rheumatism Association 1987 revised criteria for the classification of rheumatoid arthritis. Arthritis Rheum 1988, 31:315-324.
9. Storey JD, Tibshirani R: Statistical significance for genomewide studies. Proc Natl Acad Sci USA 2003, 100:9440-9445.
10. Kanehisa M, Goto S, Sato Y, Furumichi M, Tanabe M: KEGG for integration and interpretation of large-scale molecular data sets. Nucleic Acids Res 2012, 40:D109-114.

11. Lee DM, Kiener HP, Agarwal SK, Noss EH, Watts GF, Chisaka O, Takeichi M, Brenner MB: Cadherin-11 in synovial lining formation and pathology in arthritis. Science 2007, 315:1006-1010.

12. Firestein GS: Invasive fibroblast-like synoviocytes in rheumatoid arthritis. Passive responders or transformed aggressors?. Arthritis Rheum 1996, 39:1781-1790.

13. Muller-Ladner U, Kriegsmann J, Franklin BN, Matsumoto S, Geiler T, Gay RE, Gay S: Synovial fibroblasts of patients with rheumatoid arthritis attach to and invade normal human cartilage when engrafted into SCID mice. Am J Pathol 1996, 149:1607-1615.

14. Lafyatis R, Remmers EF, Roberts AB, Yocum DE, Sporn MB, Wilder RL: Anchorage-independent growth of synoviocytes from arthritic and normal joints. Stimulation by exogenous platelet-derived growth factor and inhibition by transforming growth factor-beta and retinoids. J Clin Invest 1989, 83:1267-1276.

15. Baier A, Meineckel I, Gay S, Pap T: Apoptosis in rheumatoid arthritis. Curr Opin Rheumatol 2003, 15:274-279.

16. Hirth A, Skapenko A, Kinne RW, Emmrich F, Schulze-Koops H, Sack U: Cytokine mRNA and protein expression in primary-culture and repeated-passage synovial fibroblasts from patients with rheumatoid arthritis. Arthritis Res 2002, 4:117-125.

17. Lister R, Pelizzola M, Dowen RH, Hawkins RD, Hon G, Tonti-Filippini J, Nery JR, Lee L, Ye Z, Ngo QM, Edsall L, Antosiewicz-Bourget J, Stewart R, Ruotti V, Millar AH, Thomson JA, Ren B, Ecker JR: Human DNA methylomes at base resolution show widespread epigenomic differences. Nature 2009, 462:315-322.

18. Laurent L, Wong E, Li G, Huynh T, Tsirigos A, Ong CT, Low HM, Kin Sung KW, Rigoutsos I, Loring J, Wei CL: Dynamic changes in the human methylome during differentiation. Genome Res 2010, 20:320-331.

19. Landan G, Cohen NM, Mukamel Z, Bar A, Molchadsky A, Brosh R, Horn-Saban S, Zalcenstein DA, Goldfinger N, Zundelevich A, Gal-Yam EN, Rotter V, Tanay A: Epigenetic polymorphism and the stochastic formation of differentially methylated regions in normal and cancerous tissues. Nat Genet 2012, 44:1207-1214.

20. Nakano K, Boyle DL, Firestein GS: Regulation of DNA methyltransferases and DNA methylation in rheumatoid arthritis synoviocytes. J Immunol 2012, 190:1297-1303.

21. Kyburz D, Corr M: The KRN mouse model of inflammatory arthritis. Springer Semin Immunopathol 2003, 25:79-90.

22. Maciejewska Rodrigues H, Jungel A, Gay RE, Gay S: Innate immunity, epigenetics and autoimmunity in rheumatoid arthritis. Mol Immunol 2009, 47:12-18.

23. Firestein GS, Paine MM, Littman BH: Gene expression (collagenase, tissue inhibitor of metalloproteinases, complement, and HLA-DR) in rheumatoid arthritis and osteoarthritis synovium. Quantitative analysis and effect of intraarticular corticosteroids. Arthritis Rheum 1991, 34:1094-1105.

24. Brentano F, Kyburz D, Schorr O, Gay R, Gay S: The role of Toll-like receptor signalling in the pathogenesis of arthritis. Cell Immunol 2005, 233:90-96.

25. Carrion M, Juarranz Y, Perez-Garcia S, Jimeno R, Pablos JL, Gomariz RP, Gutier-rez-Canas I: RNA sensors in human osteoarthritis and rheumatoid arthritis synovial fibroblasts: immune regulation by vasoactive intestinal peptide. Arthritis Rheum 2011, 63:1626-1636.

26. Ospelt C, Brentano F, Jungel A, Rengel Y, Kolling C, Michel BA, Gay RE, Gay S: Expression, regulation, and signaling of the pattern-recognition receptor nucleotide-binding oligomerization domain 2 in rheumatoid arthritis synovial fibroblasts. Arthritis Rheum 2009, 60:355-363.

AUTHOR NOTES

CHAPTER 1

Competing Interests
The authors declare that they have no competing interests.

Author Contributions
SWK carried out the molecular genetic studies, analyzed all data and drafted the manuscript. PBS performed the statistical analysis. ROM was in charge of the patient database and the design of the study. MM, SK and NB carried out the biochemical assays. FR was in charge of the healthy control database. LY performed the methylation analysis. JB, RM, and AT were in charge of the ICU patient database. RLM and DTOC were involved in the design of the study, analyzed all data and responsible for the project. All authors read and approved the final manuscript.

Acknowledgments
The work was supported by the National Institutes of Health: HL58120; RR00827 (UCSD General Clinical Research Center); MD000220 (UCSD Comprehensive Research Center in Health Disparities (CRCHD); and DK079337 (UAB/UCSD O'Brien Kidney Disease Research Center). SWK was supported by the Inje Research and Scholarship Foundation. SWK, PBS, and ROM were supported by post-doctoral research fellowships from the National Kidney Foundation.

CHAPTER 2

Competing Interests
The authors declare that they have no competing interests.

Author Contributions

AG carried out the study design, gene expression studies, DNA methylation and drafted the manuscript. HC participated in DNA methylation analysis. MA participated in extraction of RNA/DNA and carried out gene expression experiment. CL participated in study design and gene expression analysis. KKL participated in gene expression analysis. KL conceived of the study and participated in study design and helped drafted the manuscript. All authors have read and approved the manuscript.

Acknowledgments

Supported in parts by grants from the Swedish Cancer Society (2014), the Swedish Research Council (08712), Assar Gabrielsson Foundation (AB Volvo), Jubileumskliniken Foundation, IngaBritt & Arne Lundberg Research Foundation, Swedish and Gothenburg Medical Societies, the Medical Faculty, University of Gothenburg and Sahlgrenska University Hospital Foundation. We would like to thank the Swegene Gothenburg Genomics resource unit for providing access to the ABI 3730 Sequencer.

CHAPTER 3

Competing Interests

The authors declare that they have no competing interests.

Author Contributions

JL performed the experiments and prepare the manuscript. YY and FT performed the experiments. HMZ and SC designed and performed the viral challenge experiment. JZS designed and wrote the paper.

Acknowledgments

The study was grant-supported by NIFA 2008-35204-04660
This article has been published as part of BMC Proceedings Volume 5 Supplement 4, 2011: Proceedings of the International Symposium on Animal Genomics for Animal Health (AGAH 2010). The full contents of the supplement are available online at http://www.biomedcentral.com/1753-6561/5?issue=S4.

CHAPTER 4

Competing Interests

The authors declare that they have no competing interests.

Author Contributions

KR and SB carried out the sample collection. KR drafted the manuscript. KR and GB performed the PCR and pyrosequencing experiments. MB and MW and SP carried out the microarrays and their analyses. MW, SP, KH and KS helped with the experiments. BS performed the statistical analysis. SB and MB participated in the study design and coordination and MB, OR and DW helped to draft the manuscript. All authors read and approved the final manuscript.

Ethics Approval

This study was conducted with the approval of the Ethics Review Board of Eberhard-Karls-University, Tuebingen, Germany.

Acknowledgments

The authors thank all patients who participated in this study.
KR was the recipient of a temporary research fellowship within the PATE/fortüne program of the Eberhard-Karls-University of Tuebingen, number: 1835-0-0.

CHAPTER 5

Acknowledgments

Work on epigenetics in our lab is supported by a grant from Instituto de Salud Carlos III-Fondo de Investigaciones Sanitarias (09/539). JDC is recipient of a contract from IFIMAV.

CHAPTER 6

Competing Interests

The authors declare that they have no competing interests.

Author Contributions

MT, MM, DF, RB, and PY designed the study. MT and RB drafted the manuscript. MT, MM, DF, and BR analyzed the data. RB, PY, and BR critically reviewed the manuscript. PY, BR, and JC generated the data. GM procured samples. RB, PY, and GM oversaw the project.

Acknowledgments

This work was supported by NCI Comprehensive Cancer Center Support Grant P30 CA016058 (P.Y. and G.M.) and CA102031 (G.M.), 5 P50 CA140158-03 (G.M. and R.B.), National Center For Advancing Translational Sciences Grant 8TL1TR000091-05 (M.T.), and in part by an allocation of computing time from the Ohio Supercomputer Center. We would also like to acknowledge Yi-Wen Huang and Tim H-M. Huang for generating and sharing the endometrial dataset, and Rita Huang and Hung-Cheng Lai for generating and sharing the ovarian dataset.

This article has been published as part of BMC Genomics Volume 13 Supplement 8, 2012: Proceedings of The International Conference on Intelligent Biology and Medicine (ICIBM): Genomics. The full contents of the supplement are available online athttp://www.biomedcentral.com/bmcgenomics/supplements/13/S8.

CHAPTER 7

Competing Interests

The authors declare that they have no competing interests.

Author Contributions

SG participated in developing the graphical and statistical aspects of the approach and methods proposed in the paper. VG participated in developing the approach and method proposed in the paper and applying it to the case of Parkinson's. MK participated in the development of the approach and method proposed in this paper and advised on its relevance to gene-environment interactions and epidemiology. MP participated in the development of the approach and methods proposed in this paper and advised on its relevance to molecular genetics and epidemiology. VP participated in the development of the approach and method proposed in the paper with particular focus on how to combine the graphical and causal Bradford-Hill criteria in the context of genetic causation.

Acknowledgments

This work has been made possible by a grant to ECNIS (Environmental Cancer Risk, Nutrition and Individual Susceptibility), a network of excellence operating within the European Union 6th Framework Program, Priority 5: "Food Quality and Safety" (Contract No 513943). Paolo Vineis would like to acknowledge the European Union grant HEALTH-2007-201550 HyperGenes. Sara Geneletti would like to acknowledge the support of the Economic and Social Research Council (award number RES-576-25-5003). This work does not necessarily represent the official position of the Centers for Disease Control and Prevention.

CHAPTER 8

Competing Interests

The authors declare that they have no competing interests.

Author Contributions

MX carried out the experimental design, data analysis, interpretation and drafted the manuscript. KG directed the experimental design, data analysis, interpretation and participated in manuscript editing. AW and AL provided the phenotype information. JC participated in the experimental design. BEH imputed the missing values and participated in manuscript editing. AM provided the genotype files and participated in manuscript editing. STW had overall oversight of the study and helped prepare the manuscript. All authors read and approved the final manuscript.

Acknowledgments

This work was supported by NIH U01 HL65899, P01 HL083069, and K23 HG3983. We thank all CAMP subjects for their ongoing participation in this study. We acknowledge the CAMP investigators and research team, supported by NHLBI, for collection of CAMP Genetic Ancillary Study data. All work on data collected from the CAMP Genetic Ancillary Study was conducted at the Channing Laboratory of the Brigham and Women's Hospital under appropriate CAMP policies and human subject's protections. The CAMP Genetics Ancillary Study is supported by U01 HL075419, U01 HL65899, P01 HL083069, R01 HL086601, and T32 HL07427 from the National Heart, Lung and Blood Institute, National Institutes of Health.

CHAPTER 9

Competing Interests
The authors declare that they have no competing interests.

Author Contributions
SIK, JZ, IAK, LAW and AKD are contributed in literature review, graphics work and writing the manuscript. All authors read and approved the final manuscript.

Author Information
Shabana I. Khan is the Senior Scientist at the National Center for Natural Products Research and Associate Professor of the Department of Pharmacognosy at the University of Mississippi, University, MS 38677, USA. Jianping Zhao is the Associate Research Scientist at the National Center for Natural Products Research at the University of Mississippi, University, MS 38677, USA. Ikhlas A. Khan is the Assistant Director of the National Center for Natural Products Research and Professor of Pharmacognosy, School of Pharmacy of the University of Mississippi, University, MS 38677, USA. Larry A. Walker is the Director of the National Center for Natural Products Research at the University of Mississippi, and Associate Director for Basic Research Oxford, University of Mississippi Cancer Institute and the Professor of Pharmacology, School of Pharmacy of the University of Mississippi, University, MS 38677, USA, Asok K. Dasmahapatra is the Research Scientist at the National Center for Natural Products Research and Assistant Professor of the Department of Pharmacology, School of Pharmacy of the University of Mississippi, University, MS 38677, USA.

Acknowledgments

United States Department of Agriculture (USDA), Agriculture Research Service Specific Cooperative Agreement No 58-6408-2-0009 is acknowledged for partial support of this work.

CHAPTER 10

Competing Interests

The authors declare that they have no competing interests.

Author Contributions

The authors' contributions to this research work are reflected in the order shown, with the exception of BL who supervised the research and finalized the report. JM, SW, and MZ carried out all of the experiments. JM and BL drafted the manuscript. XSD, CKL, XDY, and BL conceived of the study, and participated in its design and coordination. All authors read and approved the final manuscript.

CHAPTER 11

Competing Interests

None of the authors has any competing interests associated with the studies described in this review article.

Author Contributions

TK drafted the manuscript. KM participated in writing the section entitled 'MeCP2: a molecule that bridges epigenetics and neuroscience'. TH participated in making the figures and helped to draft the manuscript. All authors read and approved the final manuscript.

Acknowledgments

The research described in this article was partially supported by the Ministry of Education, Science, Sports and Culture (MEXT), grants-in-aid (KAKENHI) for Scientific Research (A) and (B) (23390272) (to TK), for Exploratory Research (23659519) (to TK), for Young Scientists (B) (23791156) (to KM), and a for Scientific Research (C) (23591491) (to TH).

CHAPTER 12

Competing Interests

Dr. Firestein and Dr. Wang serve on the Scientific Advisory Board of Ignyta, Inc. and have equity positions. Dr. Anderson and Dr. Shoemaker are employees of Ignyta, Inc. The remaining authors declare that they have no competing interests.

Author Contributions

Conception and design: JWW, RS, DLB, DA, WW, and GSF. Acquisition of data: JWW, RS, and JH. Analysis and interpretation of data: JWW, RS, DA, WW, and GSF. Writing manuscript: JWW, WW, and GSF. All authors read and approved the final manuscript.

Acknowledgments

This project was supported by grants from the Research Foundation (GSF) and NIH National Center for Advancing Translational Science (UL1TR000100) (GSF) and funding from Ignyta, Inc. (DLB).

INDEX

Printed in the United States
by Baker & Taylor Publisher Services